PERSONAL GROWTH AND BEHAVIOR 97/98

Seventeenth Edition

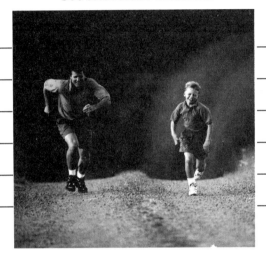

Editor

Karen G. Duffy
SUNY College, Geneseo

Karen G. Duffy holds a doctorate in psychology from Michigan State University and is currently a professor of psychology at SUNY at Geneseo. She sits on the executive board of the New York State Employees Assistance Program and is a certified community and family mediator. She is a member of the American Psychological Society and the Eastern Psychological Association.

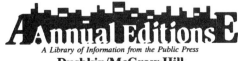

A Library of Information from the Public Press
Dushkin/McGraw·Hill
Sluice Dock, Guilford, Connecticut 06437

Visit us on the Internet—http://www.dushkin.com

The Annual Editions Series

ANNUAL EDITIONS is a series of over 65 volumes designed to provide the reader with convenient, low-cost access to a wide range of current, carefully selected articles from some of the most important magazines, newspapers, and journals published today. ANNUAL EDITIONS are updated on an annual basis through a continuous monitoring of over 300 periodical sources. All ANNUAL EDITIONS have a number of features that are designed to make them particularly useful, including topic guides, annotated tables of contents, unit overviews, and indexes. For the teacher using ANNUAL EDITIONS in the classroom, an Instructor's Resource Guide with test questions is available for each volume.

VOLUMES AVAILABLE

Abnormal Psychology
Adolescent Psychology
Africa
Aging
American Foreign Policy
American Government
American History, Pre-Civil War
American History, Post-Civil War
American Public Policy
Anthropology
Archaeology
Biopsychology
Business Ethics
Child Growth and Development
China
Comparative Politics
Computers in Education
Computers in Society
Criminal Justice
Criminology
Developing World
Deviant Behavior
Drugs, Society, and Behavior
Dying, Death, and Bereavement

Early Childhood Education
Economics
Educating Exceptional Children
Education
Educational Psychology
Environment
Geography
Global Issues
Health
Human Development
Human Resources
Human Sexuality
India and South Asia
International Business
Japan and the Pacific Rim
Latin America
Life Management
Macroeconomics
Management
Marketing
Marriage and Family
Mass Media
Microeconomics

Middle East and the
    Islamic World
Multicultural Education
Nutrition
Personal Growth and Behavior
Physical Anthropology
Psychology
Public Administration
Race and Ethnic Relations
Russia, the Eurasian Republics,
    and Central/Eastern Europe
Social Problems
Social Psychology
Sociology
State and Local Government
Urban Society
Western Civilization,
    Pre-Reformation
Western Civilization,
    Post-Reformation
Western Europe
World History, Pre-Modern
World History, Modern
World Politics

Cataloging in Publication Data
Main entry under title: Annual Editions: Personal growth and behavior. 1997/98.
    1. Personality—Periodicals. 2. Adjustment (Psychology)—Periodicals. I.
Duffy, Karen G., *comp.* II. Title: Personal growth and behavior.
ISBN 0-697-37336-3
155'.2'05   75-20757   ISSN. 0732-0779

© 1997 by Dushkin/McGraw·Hill, Guilford, CT 06437, A Division of The McGraw·Hill Companies, Inc.

Copyright law prohibits the reproduction, storage, or transmission in any form by any means of any portion of this publication without the express written permission of Dushkin/McGraw·Hill, and of the copyright holder (if different) of the part of the publication to be reproduced. The Guidelines for Classroom Copying endorsed by Congress explicitly state that unauthorized copying may not be used to create, to replace, or to substitute for anthologies, compilations, or collective works.

Annual Editions® is a Registered Trademark of Dushkin/McGraw·Hill,
A Division of The McGraw·Hill Companies, Inc.

Seventeenth Edition

Cover image © 1996 PhotoDisc, Inc.

Printed in the United States of America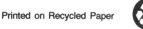

Editors/Advisory Board

Members of the Advisory Board are instrumental in the final selection of articles for each edition of ANNUAL EDITIONS. Their review of articles for content, level, currentness, and appropriateness provides critical direction to the editor and staff. We think that you will find their careful consideration well reflected in this volume.

EDITOR

Karen G. Duffy
SUNY College, Geneseo

ADVISORY BOARD

Sonia L. Blackman
California State Polytechnic University

Stephen S. Coccia
Orange County Community College

Linda Corrente
Community College of Rhode Island

Robert DaPrato
Solano Community College

Jack S. Ellison
University of Tennessee

Mark J. Friedman
Montclair State University

Roger Gaddis
Gardner-Webb University

Don Hamachek
Michigan State University

Richard A. Kolotkin
Moorhead State University

Angela J. C. LaSala
Community College of
Southern Nevada

David M. Malone
Duke University

Donald McGuire
Dalhousie University

Karla K. Miley
Black Hawk College

Terry F. Pettijohn
Ohio State University
Marion

Alex J. Rakowski
Chicago State University

Victor L. Ryan
University of Colorado
Boulder

Pamela E. Stewart
Northern Virginia Community College

Leora C. Swartzman
University of Western Ontario

Kenneth L. Thompson
Central Missouri State University

Robert S. Tomlinson
University of Wisconsin, Eau Claire

Charmaine Wesley
Modesto Junior College

Lois J. Willoughby
Miami Dade Community College

Staff

Ian A. Nielsen, Publisher

EDITORIAL STAFF

Roberta Monaco, Developmental Editor
Addie Raucci, Administrative Editor
Cheryl Greenleaf, Permissions Editor
Deanna Herrschaft, Permissions Assistant
Diane Barker, Proofreader
Lisa Holmes-Doebrick, Program Coordinator
Joseph Offredi, Photo Coordinator

PRODUCTION STAFF

Brenda S. Filley, Production Manager
Charles Vitelli, Designer
Shawn Callahan, Graphics
Lara M. Johnson, Graphics
Laura Levine, Graphics
Mike Campbell, Graphics
Juliana Arbo, Typesetting Supervisor
Jane Jaegersen, Typesetter
Marie Lazauskas, Word Processor
Larry Killian, Copier Coordinator

To the Reader

In publishing ANNUAL EDITIONS we recognize the enormous role played by the magazines, newspapers, and journals of the *public press* in providing current, first-rate educational information in a broad spectrum of interest areas. Many of these articles are appropriate for students, researchers, and professionals seeking accurate, current material to help bridge the gap between principles and theories and the real world. These articles, however, become more useful for study when those of lasting value are carefully *collected, organized, indexed,* and *reproduced* in a *low-cost format,* which provides easy and permanent access when the material is needed. That is the role played by ANNUAL EDITIONS. Under the direction of each volume's *academic editor,* who is an expert in the subject area, and with the guidance of an *Advisory Board,* each year we seek to provide in each ANNUAL EDITION a current, well-balanced, carefully selected collection of the best of the public press for your study and enjoyment. We think that you will find this volume useful, and we hope that you will take a moment to let us know what you think.

Have you ever watched children on a playground? Some children are reticent; watching the other children play, they sit demurely and shun becoming involved in the fun. Some children readily and happily interact with their playmates. They take turns, share their toys, and follow the rules of the playground. Other children are bullies who brazenly taunt the playing children and aggressively take others' possessions. What makes each child so different? Do childhood behaviors forecast adult behaviors? Can children's (or adults') antisocial behaviors be changed?

These questions are not new. Lay persons and social scientists alike have always been curious about human nature. The answers to our questions, though, are incomplete, because attempts to address these issues are relatively new or just developing. Psychology, the science that can and should answer questions about individual differences and that is the primary focus of this book, has existed for just over one hundred years. That may seem old to you, but it is young when other disciplines are considered. Mathematics, medicine, and philosophy are thousands of years old.

By means of psychology and related sciences, this anthology will help you explore the issues of individual differences and their origins, methods of coping, personality change, and other matters of human adjustment. The purpose of this anthology is to compile the newest, most complete and readable articles that examine individual behavior and adjustment as well as the dynamics of personal growth and interpersonal relationships. The readings in this book offer interesting insights into both the everyday and scientific worlds, a blend welcomed by most of today's specialists in human adjustment.

This anthology is revised each year to reflect both traditional viewpoints and emerging perspectives about people's behavior. Thanks to the editorial board's valuable advice, the present edition has been completely revised and includes a large number of new articles representing the latest thinking in the field.

Annual Editions: Personal Growth and Behavior 97/98 is comprised of six units, each of which serves a distinct purpose. The first unit is concerned with issues related to self-identity. For example, one theory addressed in this anthology, humanism, hypothesizes that self-concept, our feelings about who we are and how worthy we are, is the most valuable component of personality. This unit includes articles that supplement the theoretical articles by providing applications of, or alternate perspectives on, popular theories about individual differences and human adjustment. These include all of the classic and major theories of personality: humanistic, behavioral, psychoanalytic, and trait theories.

The second unit provides information on *how* and *why* a person develops in a particular way—in other words, what factors determine or direct individual growth: physiology, heredity, experience, or some combination. The third unit pertains to problems commonly encountered in the different stages of development: infancy, childhood, adolescence, and adulthood.

The fourth and fifth units are similar in that they address problems of adjustment—problems that occur in interpersonal relationships and problems that are created for individuals by the prevailing social environment or our culture. Unit 4 concerns topics such as competition, love, and friendship, while unit 5 discusses racism, trends in violent crime, and the rapid increase in use of technology in America. The final unit focuses on adjustment, or how most people cope with some of these and other issues.

This anthology will challenge you and interest you in a variety of topics. It will provide you with many answers but will also stimulate many questions. Perhaps it will inspire you to continue your study of the burgeoning field of psychology, which is responsible for exploring personal growth and behavior. As has been true in the past, your feedback on this edition would be valuable for future revisions. Please take a moment to fill out and return the postage-paid *article rating form* on the last page. Thank you.

Karen Groves Duffy

Karen G. Duffy
Editor

Contents

To the Reader   iv
Topic Guide   2

Overview   4

UNIT 1

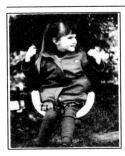

Becoming a Person: Seeking Self-Identity

Seven selections discuss the psychosocial development of an individual's personality. Attention is given to values, emotions, lifestyles, and self-concept.

1. **The 'Soul': Modern Psychological Interpretations,** Morton Hunt, *Free Inquiry,* Fall 1994.   6
   Morton Hunt traces the concept of *soul,* or more loosely, mind, from early philosophers through to the contemporary concept of *consciousness* provided by today's psychologists. As he develops history, Hunt reveals important points, for example, that humans are the only creatures that think about thinking.

2. **The Last Interview of Abraham Maslow,** Edward Hoffman, *Psychology Today,* January/February 1992.   11
   Although initially "sold on behaviorism," Abraham Maslow became one of the founders of a comprehensive human psychology or *humanistic psychology.* In an important last interview, Maslow shares his philosophy on the nature of human beings and of the potential for world peace and understanding.

3. **Should Schools Try to Boost Self-Esteem?** Roy F. Baumeister, *American Educator,* Summer 1996.   15
   Noted psychologist Roy Baumeister defines what *self-esteem* is. He then explores its upside and downside, with an eye toward examining whether or not *boosting self-esteem* is as beneficial as parents and teachers believe.

4. **The Shrink Is In,** Jonathan Lear, *The New Republic,* December 25, 1995.   22
   Psychoanalysis or Freudian theory is quite old; however, attacks on the theory continue today. Jonathan Lear takes a look at psychoanalytic concepts such as the *Oedipal complex, fantasy, and the unconscious.* He examines why the attacks occur and whether, in fact, Sigmund Freud has made significant contributions to our understanding of human nature. Lear also contrasts Freud with other philosophers who addressed human nature.

5. **How Useful Is Fantasy?** Paul M. Insel, *Healthline,* March 1995.   29
   Daydreams can be adaptive. They can prepare us for future events, substitute for impulsive behavior, and get us past anger. Paul Insel explores these and other aspects of *fantasy* life.

6. **The Rewards of Learning,** Paul Chance, *Phi Delta Kappan,* November 1992.   31
   The author reviews important principles of *behaviorism* such as *positive reinforcement* and *punishment.* He argues that there is an appropriate place in teaching for both *intrinsic* and *extrinsic rewards.*

7. **The Stability of Personality: Observations and Evaluations,** Robert R. McCrae and Paul T. Costa Jr., *Current Directions in Psychological Science,* December 1994.   36
   There is substantial evidence for the *stability of personality* as well as for *individual differences* in personality traits. The authors review research on personality that supports their view, and they critique research that does not.

The concepts in bold italics are developed in the article. For further expansion please refer to the Topic Guide, the Glossary, and the Index.

UNIT 2

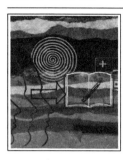

Determinants of Behavior: Motivation, Environment, and Physiology

Eight articles examine the effects of culture, genes, and emotions on an individual's behavior.

Overview   40

8. **Nature, Nurture, Brains, and Behavior,** Kenneth J. Mack, *The World & I,* July 1996.   42
   Genes and the environment interact to affect *development*. Some researchers maintain that a complex environment that promotes learning excites nerve cells and can therefore alter genetic expression. Behavioral research, for example, with children in Head Start programs, is helping psychologists better understand the complex interplay between genes, environments, the *nervous system, and learning.*

9. **Unraveling the Mystery of Life,** Mariette DiChristina, *Bostonia,* Fall 1995.   48
   Genome research that attempts to determine which *genes* are responsible for which human traits is enabling scientists to predict which individuals might suffer from a particular disease as well as indicating how to treat or prevent certain *disorders.*

10. **The New Social Darwinists,** John Horgan, *Scientific American,* October 1995.   51
    A second Darwinian revolution may be occurring. *Evolutionary psychologists* view *natural selection* as responsible for sexuality, male dominance, language, stepparent murders of stepchildren, and other behaviors. This position contrasts sharply with cultural explanations and is, of course, not without criticisms.

11. **Revealing the Brain's Secrets,** Kathleen Cahill Allison, *Harvard Health Letter,* January 1996.   57
    Discoveries in molecular biology and *genetics* are unlocking the mysteries of Alzheimer's disease, depression, and other *brain disorders.* From these discoveries, scientists hope to find new forms of *treatment* for such disabling neuronal problems.

12. **Man's World, Woman's World? Brain Studies Point to Differences,** Gina Kolata, *New York Times,* February 28, 1995.   61
    The use of functional *Magnetic Resonance Imaging* provides scientists with a noninvasive technique to study the *brain.* Using resting and active images, scientists are uncovering some interesting cognitive, behavioral, and emotional differences in the brain functioning of *men* and *women.*

13. **Kernel of Fear,** Mark Caldwell, *Discover,* June 1995.   64
    Researchers now know that the *amygdala* of the brain monitors fear responses. Finding a chemical or drug to overcome the effects of this chickpea-size part of the brain may help individuals with *posttraumatic stress disorder.*

14. **The Brain Manages Happiness and Sadness in Different Centers,** Daniel Goleman, *New York Times,* March 28, 1995.   68
    Scientists are remapping the human *brain,* with a surprising result for emotions. Opposite emotions such as *happiness* and *sadness* are not registered in one place in the brain. Rather, each emotion entails quite independent brain activity.

15. **Faith & Healing,** Claudia Wallis, *Time,* June 24, 1996.   71
    Faith healers have frequented various cultures at various points in history. Some medical studies demonstrate that faith indeed leads to better *health* and faster recovery; however, more evidence exists of a *mind-body connection.*

The concepts in bold italics are developed in the article. For further expansion please refer to the Topic Guide, the Glossary, and the Index.

UNIT 3

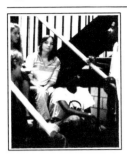

Problems Influencing Personal Growth

Ten articles consider aging, development, self-image, depression, and social interaction and their influences on personal growth.

Overview 74

16. **Clipped Wings,** Lucile F. Newman and Stephen L. Buka, *American Educator,* Spring 1991. 76
A recent report for the Education Commission of the States is excerpted here. Details of research compilations demonstrate that *prenatal exposure* to drugs, alcohol, and nicotine hampers *children's development,* especially their *learning.*

17. **How Kids Benefit from Child Care,** Vivian Cadden, *Working Mother,* April 1993. 82
When surveyed, *working mothers* nearly unanimously agree that children benefit from *early child care.* The mothers report enhanced *educational* and *social development.*

18. **Fathers' Time,** Paul Roberts, *Psychology Today,* May/June 1996. 86
Fathers and mothers parent their children differently. The influence of the father on the child is now considered important and complex. Fathers, for example, are more physical, joking, and playful with their children than are mothers, who are more comforting and protective. The *father's style* may be what promotes *autonomy in adolescence.*

19. **Lies of the Mind,** Leon Jaroff, *Time,* November 29, 1993. 93
Many adults are discovering memories of *childhood abuse.* Real or imagined, these memories are wreaking psychological havoc on individuals and families. New support groups and therapies are available, but some of the *therapy* may be prompting memories that are not accurate.

20. **Why Schools Must Tell Girls: 'You're Smart, You Can Do It,'** Myra Sadker and David Sadker, *USA Weekend,* February 4–6, 1994. 97
No matter what *school* grade they are in, *boys* tend to capture teachers' attention. To their detriment, education has become a spectator sport for many girls.

21. **It Takes a School,** Margot Hornblower, *Time,* June 3, 1996. 100
Schools need to become learning, caring, *holistic communities.* Such holistic schools offer preschool, parent education, surrogate parents, and other features that increase attendance, enhance standardized test scores, and hopefully reduce delinquency.

22. **Helping Teenagers Avoid Negative Consequences of Sexual Activity,** Jeannie I. Rosoff, *USA Today Magazine (Society for the Advancement of Education),* May 1996. 102
Most *adolescents* have normal *sexual urges,* so how can they be taught to resist these urges, particularly with all the sex portrayed in the American media? Jeannie Rosoff explores data on *teen sexuality* and offers practical advice on how to reduce it.

23. **New Passages,** Gail Sheehy, *U.S. News & World Report,* June 12, 1995. 105
Renowned author Gail Sheehy examines what she calls a revolution in the *adult life cycle.* She says we pass through three distinct adulthoods, rather than one. Sheehy places particular emphasis on *midlife* in this essay.

The concepts in bold italics are developed in the article. For further expansion please refer to the Topic Guide, the Glossary, and the Index.

24. **Is It Normal Aging—Or Alzheimer's?** *Consumer Reports on Health,* October 1995. 110
This concise selection describes the causes and consequences of *Alzheimer's disease.* More importantly, a home test enables the reader to differentiate *normal memory failure* due to aging or depression from the more disabling memory failure of Alzheimer's disease.

25. **The Mystery of Suicide,** David Gelman, *Newsweek,* April 18, 1994. 113
Through analysis of the suicide of rock singer Kurt Cobain, David Gelman helps the reader understand the *frequency* and *causes* of *suicide* and the *interventions* used with those individuals who attempt suicide.

UNIT 4

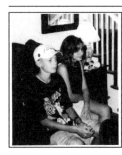

Relating to Others

Ten articles examine some of the dynamics involved in relating to others. Topics discussed include friendship, love, the importance of family ties, and self-esteem.

Overview 116

26. **The EQ Factor,** Nancy Gibbs, *Time,* October 2, 1995. 118
Emotional intelligence, our ability to understand our own and others' *emotions,* may be more important to success than cognitive intelligence. But emotional intelligence (EQ) may be as useless as IQ is without a *moral* compass. This article explores psychological research that investigates how these concepts relate to one another and how emotional intelligence develops.

27. **The Enduring Power of Friendship,** Susan Davis, *American Health,* July/August 1996. 123
Adult friendships are not studied as often as adult romances or childhood friendships. Research indicates that most adult friendships end due to *life transitions* and that they dissolve with a whimper, unlike some of our romantic relationships.

28. **Are You Shy?** Bernardo J. Carducci with Philip G. Zimbardo, *Psychology Today,* November/December 1995. 126
Shy people suffer not just from *shyness* but also from inability to think clearly in the presence of others, from the perception by others that they are snobby, and from an overall lack of success. The *social, cultural, and physiological causes* of shyness are elaborated here.

29. **Hotheads and Heart Attacks,** Edward Dolnick, *Health,* July/August 1995. 133
The Type H (for hostility) theory is replacing the concept of the Type A personality. Type A's are competitive, hostile, and deadline oriented. It is *hostility,* especially when acted on, that may be the real culprit in *heart attack proneness.*

30. **Go Ahead, Say You're Sorry,** Aaron Lazare, *Psychology Today,* January/February 1995. 138
Apologies are important for restoring self-esteem and *interpersonal relationships.* Apologies, however, are antithetical to our values of winning, success, and perfection. Aaron Lazare describes the content of a successful apology.

31. **The Heart and the Helix,** Jeffrey Kluger, *Discover,* February 1995. 141
Jeffrey Kluger takes a tongue-in-cheek look at six types of *love styles.* Referring to research, he reports that *identical twins* rarely have the same styles as each other but frequently match the styles of their spouses.

The concepts in bold italics are developed in the article. For further expansion please refer to the Topic Guide, the Glossary, and the Index.

32. **Back Off!** Geraldine K. Piorkowski, *Psychology Today*, January/February 1995. — 144
    As a culture, we seem too preoccupied with *intimacy*. Perhaps we need to back off from our close relationships and not demand so much of them.

33. **Preventing Failure in Intimate Relationships,** J. Earl Thompson Jr., *USA Today Magazine (Society for the Advancement of Education)*, March 1996. — 147
    Several myths regarding *likelihood of divorce* are countered here. Data are used to show why couples' relationships disintegrate. Advice is also given about what strategies work for *keeping relationships healthy*.

34. **Patterns of Abuse,** *Newsweek*, July 4, 1994. — 150
    Two million women are beaten every year; they are *victims of domestic violence*. This article focuses on who they are, who the *abusers* are, why the women stay or leave, and where they can get help.

35. **The Secret World of Siblings,** *U.S. News & World Report*, January 10, 1994. — 155
    The importance of *siblings* is being recognized by scientists because siblings are taking over parental roles. Why siblings are similar yet different and how and why siblings develop *relationships in childhood* and adulthood are being scrutinized.

UNIT 5

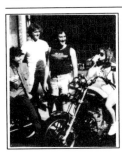

Dynamics of Personal Adjustment: The Individual and Society

Five selections discuss some of the problems experienced by individuals as they attempt to adjust to society.

Overview — 160

36. **Disintegration of the Family Is the Real Root Cause of Violent Crime,** Patrick F. Fagan, *USA Today Magazine (Society for the Advancement of Education)*, May 1996. — 162
    The popular assumption that there is an *association between race and crime* is false. When other factors are controlled, there is at least one variable that seems to account for our crime wave—*lack of a nuclear family*—which generally means that one of the child's parents is missing. Patrick Fagan traces the development of violence from childhood through adulthood in a person from a single-parent home, whether white or black.

37. **Mixed Blood,** Jefferson M. Fish, *Psychology Today*, November/December 1995. — 165
    The American concept of *race* is quite different from the concept of race in other cultures; thus, the American concept is just one of many "folk taxonomies." Because race as construed by Americans does not exist, discussions of *racial differences in IQ* are moot, according to Jefferson Fish.

38. **Media, Violence, Youth, and Society,** Ray Surette, *The World & I*, July 1994. — 170
    Violence is a cultural product. Years of research have linked violence on our streets to *mass media*. Other reasons for our epidemic of violence, as well as solutions for decreasing violence, are suggested.

The concepts in bold italics are developed in the article. For further expansion please refer to the Topic Guide, the Glossary, and the Index.

39. **The Evolution of Despair,** Robert Wright, *Time,* August 28, 1995.   177

Evolutionary psychologists suggest that our modern lives are at odds with our ancestral past. Specifically, *modern technology* isolates us, when in order to spread our genes through the *gene pool* we need to be more, not less, *social.*

40. **Psychotrends: Taking Stock of Tomorrow's Family and Sexuality,** Shervert H. Frazier, *Psychology Today,* January/February 1994.   181

The AIDS epidemic has expanded rather than dimmed our interest in *sex.* The sexual revolution is not over. Demographers are continuing to track changes in sexual behavior, attitudes, families, gender roles, and other important trends.

UNIT 6

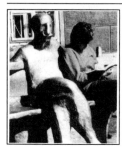

Enhancing Human Adjustment: Learning to Cope Effectively

Nine selections examine some of the ways an individual learns to cope successfully within today's society. Topics discussed include therapy, depression, stress, and interpersonal relations.

Overview   186

41. **What You Can Change and What You Cannot Change,** Martin E. P. Seligman, *Psychology Today,* May/June 1994.   188

Americans seem to be on constant *self-improvement* kicks, many of which fail. Martin Seligman explains which attempts to change are a waste of time and which are worthwhile. He discusses *diets* and *psychological disorders* in particular.

42. **Frontiers of Psychotherapy,** Saúl Fuks, *The UNESCO Courier,* February 1996.   196

In the past, *psychotherapists* were construed as powerful healers. However, the trend today is to *empower clients* to assume responsibility for their own lives. Thus, the roles, practices, contexts, and forms of therapy are changing.

43. **Prescriptions for Happiness?** Seymour Fisher and Roger P. Greenberg, *Psychology Today,* September/October 1995.   198

Antidepressant drugs, which are medications used to treat and manage *psychological disorders,* are discussed here. The *studies* verifying these drugs' utility are highly questionable in terms of design and interpretation. Seymour Fisher and Roger Greenberg question whether such medications should indeed be prescribed.

44. **Upset? Try Cybertherapy,** Kerry Hannon, *U.S. News & World Report,* May 13, 1996.   203

More psychologists are offering *computerized or electronic consultation* for fees. *Ethical standards* lag the growth of Web sites. This article lists several legitimate sites for finding psychological information, including therapy.

45. **Defeating Depression,** Nancy Wartik, *American Health,* December 1993.   205

Millions are afflicted with *depression.* Scientists believe that a combination of *genetics, personality structure,* and *life events* triggers major depression. A self-assessment quiz is included as well as a discussion of a variety of all-important interventions.

The concepts in bold italics are developed in the article. For further expansion please refer to the Topic Guide, the Glossary, and the Index.

46. **Addiction: A Whole New View,** Joann Ellison Rodgers, *Psychology Today,* September/October 1994. 211
   Is *addiction* a lifelong disease or a behavior similar in several respects to other behaviors? The latter view is adopted in this reading, which examines successful versus unsuccessful *treatment* methods.

47. **Stress: It's Worse than You Think,** John Carpi, *Psychology Today,* January/February 1996. 217
   Stress, at epidemic proportions in today's society, affects both our physical and psychological well-being. *Managing stress* is important, and John Carpi shares a multitude of techniques for coping with it.

48. **The New Frontiers of Happiness . . . Happily Ever Laughter,** Peter Doskoch, *Psychology Today,* July/August 1996. 225
   Humor is a full-cortex experience that leaves us less depressed, less anxious, and more creative. However, new research discloses that the use of humor as a *coping mechanism* has its limits.

49. **On the Power of Positive Thinking: The Benefits of Being Optimistic,** Michael F. Scheier and Charles S. Carver, *Current Directions in Psychological Science,* February 1993. 228
   Two psychologists discuss *optimism* and its relationship to *psychological and physical well-being* and to other psychological constructs such as *self-efficacy.*

Glossary 233
Index 241
Article Review Form 244
Article Rating Form 245

The concepts in bold italics are developed in the article. For further expansion please refer to the Topic Guide, the Glossary, and the Index.

Topic Guide

This topic guide suggests how the selections in this book relate to topics of traditional concern to students and professionals involved with the study of personal growth and behavior. It is useful for locating articles that relate to each other for reading and research. The guide is arranged alphabetically according to topic. Articles may, of course, treat topics that do not appear in the topic guide. In turn, entries in the topic guide do not necessarily constitute a comprehensive listing of all the contents of each selection.

TOPIC AREA	TREATED IN	TOPIC AREA	TREATED IN
Addiction	46. Addiction: A Whole New View	Drugs/Medication	43. Prescriptions for Happiness?
Adolescence	22. Helping Teenagers Avoid Negative Consequences of Sexual Activity		46. Addiction: A Whole New View
		Emotions/ Emotional Intelligence	26. EQ Factor
Adulthood	19. Lies of the Mind 23. New Passages		
		Evolutionary Psychology	10. New Social Darwinists 39. Evolution of Despair
Aging	24. Is it Normal Aging?—Or Alzheimers		
AIDS	40. Psychotrends	Faith Healers	15. Faith and Healing
Apologies	30. Go Ahead, Say You're Sorry	Families	36. Disintegration of the Family Is the Real Root Cause of Violent Crime
Brain	11. Revealing the Brain's Secrets 12. Man's World, Woman's World? 13. Kernel of Fear 14. Brain Manages Happiness and Sadness in Different Centers	Fantasy	5. How Useful Is Fantasy?
		Fear	13. Kernel of Fear
		Freud, Sigmund	4. The Shrink Is In
Child Abuse	19. Lies of the Mind	Friendship	27. Enduring Power of Friendship
Children	17. How Kids Benefit from Child Care 18. Fathers' Time 19. Lies of the Mind 20. Why Schools Must Tell Girls: 'You're Smart, You Can Do It'	Gender	12. Man's World, Woman's World? 20. Why Schools Must Tell Girls: 'You're Smart, You Can Do It'
		Genes	8. Nature, Nurture, Brains, and Behavior 9. Unraveling the Mystery of Life 11. Revealing the Brain's Secrets 39. Evolution of Despair
Computers/ Technology	39. Evolution of Despair 44. Upset? Try Cybertherapy		
Consciousness	1. 'Soul': Modern Psychological Interpretations		
		Happiness	14. Brain Manages Happiness and Sadness in Different Centers 48. New Frontiers of Happiness
Day Care	17. How Kids Benefit from Child Care		
Daydreams	5. How Useful Is Fantasy?	Health	15. Faith and Healing
Depression	45. Defeating Depression	Hostility	29. Hotheads and Heart Attacks
Development	16. Clipped Wings	Humanistic Psychology	2. Last Interview of Abraham Maslow 4. The Shrink Is In
Divorce	33. Preventing Failure in Intimate Relationships	Humor	48. New Frontiers of Happiness
Domestic Violence	34. Patterns of Abuse	Interpersonal Relations	27. Enduring Power of Friendship 30. Go Ahead, Say You're Sorry

TOPIC AREA	TREATED IN	TOPIC AREA	TREATED IN
IQ	37. Mixed Blood	Reinforcement	6. Rewards of Learning
Love	31. Heart and the Helix 32. Back Off! 33. Preventing Failure in Intimate Relationships	Schools	3. Should Schools Try to Boost Self-Esteem? 20. Why Schools Must Tell Girls: 'You're Smart, You Can Do It' 21. It Takes a School
Marriage	33. Preventing Failure in Intimate Relationships	Self-Efficacy	49. On the Power of Positive Thinking
Mind-Body Connection	15. Faith and Healing	Self-Esteem	3. Should Schools Try to Boost Self-Esteem?
Natural Selection	10. New Social Darwinists	Sex/Sexuality	22. Helping Teenagers Avoid Negative Consequences of Sexual Activity
Nature/Nuture	8. Nature, Nurture, Brains, and Behavior	Shyness	28. Are You Shy?
Nervous System	8. Nature, Nurture, Brains, and Behavior	Soul	1. 'Soul': Modern Psychological Interpretations
Oedipal Complex	4. The Shrink Is In	Stress	47. Stress: It's Worse than You Think
Optimism	49. On the Power of Positive Thinking	Suicide	25. Mystery of Suicide
Personality	7. Stability of Personality	Television	38. Media, Violence, Youth, and Society
Prenatal Stage	16. Clipped Wings	Thinking	1. 'Soul': Modern Psychological Interpretations
Psychoanalysis	4. The Shrink Is In	Traits	7. Stability of Personality
Psychotherapy	41. What You Can Change and What You Cannot Change 42. Frontiers of Psychotherapy 44. Upset? Try Cybertherapy	Type A Behavior	29. Hotheads and Heart Attacks
		Unconscious	4. The Shrink Is In
Punishment	6. Rewards of Learning	Violence	36. Disintegration of the Family Is the Real Root Cause of Violent Crimes 38. Media, Violence, Youth, and Society
Race	37. Mixed Blood		

Becoming a Person: Seeking Self-Identity

A baby sits in front of a mirror and looks at herself. A chimpanzee sorts through photographs while its trainer carefully watches its reactions. A college student answers a survey on how she feels about herself. What do each of these events share in common? All are examples of techniques used to investigate self-concept.

That baby in front of the mirror has a red dot on her nose. Researchers watch to see if the baby reaches for the dot in the mirror or touches her own nose. Recognizing the fact that the image she sees in the mirror is her own, the baby touches her real nose, not the nose in the mirror.

The chimpanzee has been trained to sort photographs into two piles—human pictures or animal pictures. If the chimp has been raised with humans, the researcher wants to know into which pile (animal or human) the chimp will place its own picture. Is the chimp's concept of itself animal or human? Or does the chimp have no concept of self at all?

The college student taking the self-survey answers questions about her body image, whether or not she thinks she is fun to be with, whether or not she spends large amounts of time in fantasy, and her feelings about her personality and intelligence.

These research projects are designed to investigate how self-concept develops and steers our behaviors and thoughts. Most psychologists believe that people develop a personal identity or a sense of self, which is a sense of who we are, our likes and dislikes, our characteristic feelings and thoughts, and an understanding of why we behave as we do. *Self-concept* is our knowledge of our gender, race, and age, as well as our sense of self-worth and more. Strong positive or negative feelings are usually attached to this identity. Psychologists are studying how and when this sense of self develops. Most psychologists do not believe that infants are born with a sense of self but rather that children slowly develop self-concept as a consequence of their experiences.

This unit delineates some of the popular viewpoints regarding how sense of self and personality develop and how, or if, they guide behavior. This knowledge of how self develops provides an important foundation for the rest of the units in this book. This unit explores three major theories or forces in psychology: self or humanistic, psychoanalytic, and trait theories. For each theory, related research, applications, or concepts are examined in companion articles.

First, "The 'Soul': Modern Psychological Interpretations" introduces the concept of mind, or soul, the mechanism by which self-concept perhaps develops. Morton Hunt reviews the concept of consciousness from its treatment by the earliest philosophers through to today's psychologists.

With this general introduction in mind, the next two selections are devoted to humanistic psychology, the school of psychology with a strong interest in self-concept. In fact, many of the humanistic theorists also are called self-theorists. In "The Last Interview of Abraham Maslow," this founder of humanistic psychology discusses the evolution of his theory. In the interview, Maslow talks about his philosophy of human nature and its potential for peaceful living and other positive outcomes for humans. In a companion article, "Should Schools Try to Boost Self-Esteem?" the issue of whether we should indeed try to raise self-esteem, particularly in our schools, is addressed. The author, Roy Baumeister, a noted psychologist, reveals that while attempts to manipulate self-esteem are noble, they do have their pitfalls.

The next two essays relate to psychoanalysis, a theory and form of therapy to which humanism was a reaction. The main proponent of psychoanalysis was Sigmund Freud, who believed that individuals possess a dark, lurking unconscious that often motivates negative behaviors. These essays explore Freudian concepts. "The Shrink Is In" is a fairly balanced review of Freud's theory. It examines both the attacks on Freud's concepts, such as the Oedipal conflict and the unconscious, and his contributions to our understanding of personality. In the second companion article, "How Useful Is Fantasy?" fantasies are examined. Freud claimed that the unconscious expresses itself in our fantasies. Thus, to know more about the unconscious, all we need to do is understand or interpret our fantasies. This piece will help you to understand what fantasies mean and what their value is in everyday life.

One other formal and important theory of human nature is behaviorism, the theory of B. F. Skinner. Two main principles of behavioral theory are reinforcement and punishment. In fact, Skinner posited that these principles shape and guide most of our behaviors. In "The Rewards of Learning," Paul Chance reviews these principles and concludes, as do most psychologists, that rewarding prosocial behavior is a better strategy than punishing antisocial or negative behaviors.

UNIT 1

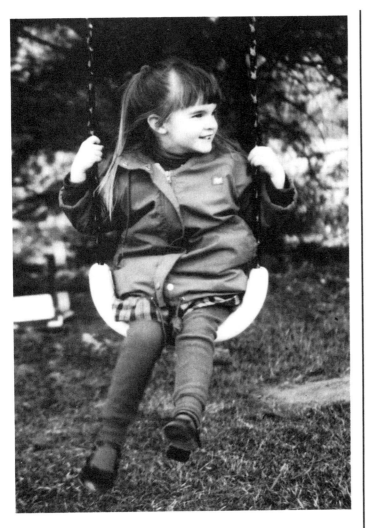

The last article in the unit offers a contrasting viewpoint of human nature, known as the trait or dispositional approach. Trait theories in general hold that our personalities are comprised of various traits possibly tied together by our self-concept. This review of relevant research, claims that most personality traits remain constant over time, in sharp contrast especially with the growth theory of Maslow and the psychoanalytic stage theory of Freud.

Looking Ahead: Challenge Questions

What is consciousness? How have conceptions of consciousness or mind changed over the centuries? Do you think one theory about the mind is better than the others? Why or why not?

Does the sense of self develop the same way in each individual? What, if any, aspects of self, such as gender, develop faster than other aspects? Can one type of experience influence identity more than another experience? How and when does self-concept influence us?

What does Abraham Maslow propose about self in his theory? How can his humanistic theory help us produce a more peaceful world and strengthen positive human attributes?

How can we study self-perception? Person perception? What has research revealed about these processes? Why is information about these processes valuable?

Is self-concept stable, or does it seem to change regularly? What events create change? How could an individual change his or her self-concept? Is psychotherapy the best or only way to create change? Can people change spontaneously or as a result of a growth experience?

How can we raise children with high self-esteem? What happens to children and adults with low self-esteem? Should schools try to enhance or raise self-esteem, one important aspect of self-concept? What are the advantages of such programs? What are the drawbacks?

How and when do you think children develop a sense of self? How do people show others that they have a sense of self? Do children understand their own behavior first or others' behavior first? Which word, "yes" or "no," is usually added first to the child's vocabulary? What impact does this have on the child's development of self-concept?

Is self-concept the only guide for our behaviors? Do individuals have a number of selves and show different ones to different people? If so, is this normal, or does it signal some kind of maladjustment?

Suppose someone developed on a desert island with no human contact. What might this individual be like? How might she or he appear to others who have been raised in civilization?

Do you believe in the unconscious? Why or why not? Give examples from your own life of its influence. What scientific evidence exists that demonstrates the potential of the unconscious? What other concepts are important to Freud's concept of humans? Define and give examples of each. Discuss whether or not dreams reveal unconscious wishes. What do various fantasies mean to you? To Freudians? Why do people fantasize?

What are the important principles of behavioral theory? Define reinforcement and punishment. Under what circumstances should each be used, if at all? Should parents and teachers use both reward and punishment? Why or why not?

Do you think personality traits remain stable over a lifetime? Do traits remain stable across situations; are they carried from church to school, for example? Do traits collectively comprise self-concept or is self comprised of more than traits? Explain.

Which theory of human personality (humanistic, psychoanalytic, behavioral, or trait) do you think is best and why?

The 'Soul': Modern Psychological Interpretations

Morton Hunt

Morton Hunt is the author of several books on human nature and the mind, including The Compassionate Beast *(1990) and* The Story of Psychology *(Doubleday, 1993), from which this article is adapted.*

A few years ago I drove past the scene of an accident, where police and an ambulance crew were clustered near two smashed cars. In one, a middle-aged man was resting, it seemed, with his head halfway out the open window. But then I had the sickening realization that he was dead. Moments ago this had been a person on his way to some appointment, his mind busy with plans and filled with the knowledge gathered over a lifetime—and then suddenly only an inert body in which the brain was cooling down, its neuronal currents shut off, everything stored in it erased and lost.

It was a reality difficult to grasp. At my sister's funeral nine years ago, I looked at her in her casket and found it hard to believe that the person I had known and loved all my life would never again kiss me, sing Schubert's "Lieder," offer me more of her pot roast, ask how my work was going—hard to believe that this body resembled her but that *she herself* was . . . nowhere.

No wonder the belief in a soul that inhabits the body but endures elsewhere after death is, as anthropologist Weston La Barre wrote some years ago, "the most ancient and pervasive of beliefs. . . . No other single belief has so profoundly influenced so many human beings for so unimaginably long a time."

Of course, that doesn't mean that such a thing as a soul exists. As human beings have increasingly understood the world, they have discarded many age-old erroneous beliefs about it. We know that the sun, moon, and stars do not revolve around the Earth, though they seem to; we know that the universe is between ten and twenty billion years old and was not made in six days, 5,998 years ago.

Yet today, when the evidence of psychology and biology indicates that soul is an erroneous explanation of what we see, many or most Americans still believe in it. Even among non-churchgoing Protestants, according to a recent national poll, nearly three quarters believe the soul lives on after death.

Here are three examples of how entrenched the concept of soul is in our culture:

• Not long ago I saw a full-hour documentary on prime-time TV about a haunted house. Its occupants, several experts in haunted houses, and a priest who does exorcisms all explained the creaks, bumps in the night, and knocked-over lamps as the work of spirits unable to go to their final rest.

• In New York, the American Society for Psychical Research holds yearly seminars and conferences in which people, some of them holding Ph.D.'s in learned fields, earnestly discuss out-of-body experiences and back-from-death experiences, both of which they consider realities, not illusions.

• Many millions of Americans have bought and take seriously books by that noted expert on spiritual matters, Shirley MacLaine, that tell how to retrieve memories of your past lives when your soul inhabited other bodies. (Odd, isn't it, that people never find they used to be louse-infested, stinking, illiterate medieval peasants but always Roman senators, seventeenth-century ladies-in-waiting to the queen, or something of the sort.)

But it isn't good enough to scoff at the belief in the soul; as secular humanists, we need to understand the grounds for that belief and to find a modern interpretation of soul that harmonizes human experience with reason and scientific knowledge.

Why have all sorts of human beings, from primitives who could not count or write to such great thinkers as Socrates and St. Thomas Aquinas, believed in the soul?

Anthropologists say that animism—the belief, virtually universal among preliterate peoples, that there are spirits in all living things—is an attempt to account for the central mystery of life and death: namely, why is a tree, an animal, or a person alive and then dead? What *disappears* from the living thing?

The answer of primitive peoples was

1. 'Soul'

that there is a spirit or ghost-soul in each living thing that escapes from the body at the moment of death. Most often, they identified this spirit with air or breath. In the *Iliad* a dying warrior is said to breathe out his *psyche* (soul) in his last gasp, and the ancient Hebrews believed it was when God breathed into a lifeless piece of clay that it became the living Adam.

Other great mysteries that early peoples explained in terms of the soul included dreaming (in which, they thought, the soul leaves the body and travels), the hallucinations of fever, the reliving of past experiences, and birth itself. Such beliefs about soul were, said Professor La Barre, "plausible conclusions, deriving from genuine and identifiable experiences . . . [a kind of] crude folk science."

Upon this foundation, the Greeks and later the Christians built complex mythologies about what happens to the soul after it leaves the body—in the Greek version, crossing the river Styx to Hades and there being judged and sent on either to Tartarus (hell) or the Elysian Fields (heaven); in the Christian version, going to heaven, or to purgatory for a period of suffering before rising to heaven, or to everlasting torment in hell.

But there is a serious problem with this concept, as Greek philosophers recognized as early as the fifth century B.C.E. It was clear to them that the mind develops from infancy to adulthood; how, then, is the soul related to the mind—is it identical, or something else? If identical, then after death the ghost of a child would be forever a child, the ghost of a senile person forever senile. Maybe the soul is not identical with the mind, but then, what is it after death—an empty nothing?

Socrates had an answer. His way of teaching—the Socratic method—consisted of slyly asking a friend or a student questions as if he, Socrates, knew nothing, but the answers to which led the friend or student step by step to conclusions it seemed he must have known without realizing that he did—until the questioning caused him to "remember" them. In the *Meno* dialogue, by means of leading questions he gets a young slave boy to seemingly recall geometrical theorems he hadn't known he knew. This was Socrates' chief ground for asserting that we possess an immortal soul that exists before we are born and comes to us equipped with innate knowledge; experience and learning only cause us to remember what we already know. The soul is mind, but it can exist independently of the body.

Other philosophers then asked how other forms of conscious experience—perceptions, and the emotions that so often overpower our thinking minds—were related to the soul. Socrates' great pupil, Plato, had an answer: The soul has three parts—appetites, will, and reason, which tries to govern the first two. In this view, which came to dominate not only Greek philosophy but Christian theology, the soul experiences feelings and desires, and is often misled by them, especially by lustful desires.

> The body fills us full of loves and lusts and fears and fancies of all kinds. . . . We are slaves to [the body's] service. If we would have true knowledge of anything we must be quit of the body—the soul in herself must behold things in themselves; then we shall attain the wisdom we desire, be pure and have converse with the pure. . . . And what is purification but the separation of the soul from the body?

Does that sound like one of the church fathers, or perhaps Saint Augustine or the angelic doctor, Aquinas himself? I'd say so—but in fact it's from the *Phaedo* dialogue of Plato.

For indeed Plato saw the soul as trapped in the body and subject to its desires, and as liberated by death to live in the realm of purity and truth. That theme is repeated endlessly over the centuries by pagan philosophers and Christian theologians alike.

But the Christians could not accept Plato's view that the soul exists before birth and is equipped with innate knowledge. For one thing, Genesis says that Adam came to life only when God breathed life into him, so the soul, in the Christian view, is newly created at birth—although today some Right-to-Lifers say it is created at the moment of conception.

For another thing—even more troublesome—Plato maintained that the mind was the only immortal part of the soul; although the soul experienced perceptions, desires, and feelings while it inhabited the body, it was freed from them when it departed. But according to Christian doctrine, after death the soul goes either to heaven and there lives in joy, or to hell and there suffers eternal agony—and unless it could perceive and feel when detached from the body, how could it either sense delight or suffer torment?

Accordingly, most of the fathers of the church concluded that the soul, even when separated from the body's sense organs, could feel both pleasure or pain. How it could do so they never explained, but they and their successors throughout the centuries described in wonderful detail the agonies of souls in hell. About the pleasures of the souls in heaven, they were less specific, though they felt sure those pleasures were not fleshly. Tertullian, a father of the church, advised his wife that when they met again after death, they would no longer be enslaved by the disgusting habits their bodily desires had led to:

> Translated as [we] will be into the condition and sanctity of angels . . . there will be . . . no resumption of voluptuous disgrace between us. No such frivolities, no such impurities, does God promise to His servants.

I'm sorry to say that history does not record what Tertullian's wife thought of this description of their married lovemaking.

While philosophers and theologians struggled with the problems inherent in the concept of the soul, uneducated people believed simply in all those traditional notions we know so well: that the soul escapes from the body at death in the form of a vapor, sometimes faintly visible; that when seen in séances or in graveyards on dark and stormy nights, the soul looks and talks like the person whose body it used to inhabit and retains all that person's knowledge; and that in heaven it lives in everlasting bliss (doing what, no one knows) and in hell under-

1. BECOMING A PERSON: SEEKING SELF-IDENTITY

goes the torture of sulfurous flames for all eternity.

But with the advent of the scientific era, it became more difficult, at least for the educated, to maintain that the soul was wholly incorporeal. René Descartes, one of the greatest minds of Western history, knew that feelings, impulses, and ideas were due to specific currents of some kind in the nervous system. He thought that "animal spirits," a rarefied kind of fluid, flowed through the nerves like the water that flowed through the pipes of the lifelike automatons in the Royal Gardens and caused them to move. But being a Roman Catholic, he had to find a way to reconcile this physical account with the existence of a soul. He conjectured that the pineal gland, a tiny body in the middle of the brain whose function no physiologist knew, was a junction point where the nervous system's currents were somehow transformed into disembodied messages that could reach the soul—and where, in reverse, the soul's commands were turned into a flow of animal spirits in the nerves, activating the body. There is no evidence whatever that this is anything but the philosopher's wishful thinking.

Meanwhile, in England, where the physical sciences and biology, unhampered by the restructuring of Catholic doctrine, were making great strides, a very different school of philosopher-psychologists regarded such speculations as mystical nonsense. These down-to-earth thinkers—they're known as the empiricists—felt that since the soul has no traits that we can perceive, there is no point in even talking about it.

John Locke, the great seventeenth-century philosopher-psychologist, and David Hume, prominent a century later, both maintained that the mind of the infant is a blank slate on which experience writes what the individual comes to know; they both, therefore, totally rejected the concept of innate ideas. While neither of them dared say outright that the soul did not exist, they both said it was unknowable, and that nothing could be said about it.

In the late eighteenth and the nineteenth centuries, physiologists in England and on the Continent made a series of historic discoveries linking nerve transmissions to specific bodily processes, making it ever clearer that what happens in the mind is built up of physical events.

- The Italian Luigi Galvani found that nerve impulses involve measurable amounts of electric current.
- Various other physiologists found that nerve impulses also rely on specific chemical reactions. For instance, in the cells of the retina three different kinds of chemicals react to different colors of light; the cells richest in each chemical notify the brain when that color activates them.
- Still others found that special areas of the brain perform specific functions. On the left side, two small areas processed language; if either is damaged by an accident, the person still knows who he is and what he wants to say but cannot express his thoughts in intelligible words and sentences.

For such reasons, by the middle of the nineteenth century some avant-garde psychologists and physiologists were beginning to think that:

- Experiences, feelings, perceptions, and thoughts were the result of biological events in specific networks of brain cells.
- There was no need or reason to suppose we have an incorporeal soul.
- Everything formerly attributed to the workings of an incorporeal mind or soul could be, or some day would be, explained in physiological terms. As

> "There *is* something like a soul in us; something over and above the bodily stuff of which we are made. That something is the set of functions, resulting from an organization of the materials, that each of us calls 'I.' The existence of that 'I' is a marvel, a wonder—but not a supernatural mystery."

Emil DuBois-Reymond, a young German physiologist and the leader of the Berlin Physical Society, a little group of anti-mentalist, anti-supernaturalist physiologists, boldly proclaimed in 1842:

No forces other than the common physical-chemical ones are active within the organism. In those cases which cannot at this time be explained by these forces, one must . . . [search for] new forces, [comparable] to the chemical-physical forces inherent in matter and reducible to the force of attraction and repulsion.

As a colleague of his said, this was a "psychology without a soul."

In the 150 years since then, psychology has become a science. It has been dominated first by one, then another, school of thought—functionalism, behaviorism, cognitivism, information processing, and others—each adding something to our understanding of the causes of perceptions, emotions, and thoughts. Some examples:

- Ivan Pavlov, John Watson, and other behaviorists found that much of what the individual animal or person becomes, in the course of development, is due to "conditioning"—the linking or association of certain stimuli to certain responses. Pat a puppy every time he comes when you call him and soon he will come at your call. Scold him every time he pees on the rug and soon he will whine or bark to be let out when he needs to pee.
- Developmental psychologists like Jean Piaget found that as the mind develops from its experiences of the world, the child becomes capable of increasingly complex thinking. Show a three-year-old a row of eight closely spaced buttons and another row of eight widely spaced buttons, ask her which row has more buttons, and she'll say the longer row. Ask her again when she's six or seven and she'll know they have the same number. But at six or seven she can't reason about abstract ideas such as justice—although by fourteen she can.
- Cognitive psychologists studied reasoning by a method they called "protocol analysis." They'd give a volunteer a chess problem or cryptogram to solve and have him talk out loud as he worked on it; from what he said they'd plot out how his mind drew on memory for clues, thought up possibilities, tested what each would lead to, backed up and

tried again when a line of thought led to a dead end, and so step by step arrived at a solution.

• Neuropsychologists studied the structure and electrochemical workings of the brain during perception, emotion, and thinking. One finding: the brain of an animal or person living in an interesting environment develops a richer network of neuron (brain cell) connections than the animal or person living in a boring and impoverished environment. Another finding: neurotransmitters are chemicals emitted by a neuron when it fires that cross a microscopic gap to an adjourning neuron and cause *it* to fire, sending a message further; when any of those chemicals is in short supply due to disease or aging, thinking is altered in specific ways.

What is the relation between these minuscule electrical and chemical events and the mind's perceptions, feelings, and, most important, thoughts? One current theory is that the firing of neurons is like the switching on and off of semiconductors in a computer. As everyone knows, in a computer those patterns of ons and offs can represent numbers, letters, words, thoughts of all sorts. And in fact, the thoughts of a person solving a cryptogram can be translated into steps of a computer program—which can solve a cryptogram just as a person would.

Multiply these examples ten thousandfold and you get some idea of the extent to which modern psychology explains what takes place in the mind.

There is no room in this explanation for the soul; there is nothing for it to do. Moreover, if all mental processes are built up of cellular chemistry, synaptic connections, conditioned responses, and programs, how can the soul—which has no such machinery—possibly see, feel, or think?

And yet, when we put together all that we know about nerve transmission, specialized brain structures, and the computerlike programs by means of which we think, we still haven't explained the most important of all mental phenomena—human consciousness.

I am always aware that I am I—but no computer knows who it is. All of you are aware that it is *you* who are experiencing this day, the light—*you* and not just a stupendously intricate assembly of brain cells. What is this sense of self that no computer program has ever simulated, no brain-wave tracing has shown, no microscopic analysis of neuron networks can pinpoint? Could it be . . . the soul?

Today several leading research psychologists have tentative explanations of the phenomenon of consciousness. Francis Crick, Nobel Laureate (for his co-discovery of the structure DNA), talks about the "self-activating" nature of the brain's neural activity; activity in the brain generates other activity—which reactivates the source of that activity. (In simpler terms, we can think about our own thoughts—something no other animal and no computer does.)

Gerald Edelman, another Nobel Laureate, believes that consciousness arises from the interaction between the linguistic and the concept-forming parts of the brain; our ability to label things, by means of words, and fit them into categories frees the mind from subservience to events in real time and enables us to be aware of our own thoughts and our own self.

The explanation of consciousness and other high-level mental processes that I like best, and that is favored by many contemporary psychologists, has to do with the level of organization of a phenomenon, and of the functions that that form of organization serves. An organized group of molecules, cells, or persons has a reality over and above that of the sum of its molecules, cells, or persons. A candle flame isn't an object but trillions of molecular events occurring in an organized way. A wave, breaking at the beach, isn't an object but trillions of molecules of water acting in an organized fashion. The action of each molecule is a primary reality; the form of organization of all those molecules that we call a flame or a wave is itself a reality on another level, a reality due to organization. So, too, the cells of your stomach function together to perform functions that are possible only because they are organized into layers with special purposes and capacities—some to secrete digestive fluids, others to secrete mucous that protects the cells from digesting themselves.

Let me offer a metaphor that may be helpful. Consider a building. It may be made of beams, timber, nails, glass, wiring, pipes. If all these materials were neatly stacked on the ground, would they be, say, the Institute for Rational-Emotive Therapy? Of course not. But assembled as they are, they *are* the Institute—although nothing has been added.

No, something *has* been added: a meaningful, useful organization of those materials. Organization isn't a thing; you can't hold it, weigh it, or move it to some other place while leaving the materials here. But it, too, is a reality.

So with the human mind, or self, or, if you wish, the soul. You can't find it under the microscope, and when a person dies, there is no immediate loss of body weight due to the departure of the soul, because the soul isn't a thing, it's a set of functions or processes arising from organization. The brain has about 100 billion cells, none of which is capable of a thought, but which function as a thinking mechanism by virtue of the trillions of connections established among them, partly by the chemical tropisms of development during the child's first years, when neurons group and seek to connect with others according to genetic planning. But by far the largest part of the organization of the neurons is due to experiences and learning, which strengthens some connections and prunes away unnecessary others until the result is the individual's own mind, consciousness, Self.

But that organization exists among the cells of the living brain. Out-of-body experiences are no more possible than for the Institute for Rational-Emotive

1. BECOMING A PERSON: SEEKING SELF-IDENTITY

Therapy building to exist on West End Avenue while all the beams, wood, nails, windows, and so on remain here. After death, when the currents are turned off, no messages flow, no memories and ideas can be summoned up from the bank of connections, the organization has ceased to exist. The person who used to inhabit that brain and body has ceased to be in exactly the same way that this building would cease to be if it were completely disassembled.

That is what contemporary psychologist tells us about the soul. There *is* something like a soul in us; something over and above the bodily stuff of which we are made. That something is the set of functions, resulting from an organization of the materials, that each of us calls "I." The existence of that "I" is a marvel, a wonder—but not a supernatural mystery.

This interpretation of soul is a long way from the distant past. Yet there *is* comfort in it; one who believes in this concept of soul fears neither eternal torment in hell nor the prospect of an eternity of nothing to do in heaven. I'll settle for that, and I'd guess that you will, too.

The Last Interview of
ABRAHAM MASLOW

Edward Hoffman, Ph.D.

About the author: Edward Hoffman received his doctorate from the University of Michigan. A clinical psychologist on New York's Long Island, he is the author of several books, including The Right to be Human: A Biography of Abraham Maslow *(Tarcher).*

When Abraham Maslow first shared his pioneering vision of a "comprehensive human psychology" in this magazine in early 1968, he stood at the pinnacle of his international acclaim and influence.

HIS ELECTION AS PRESIDENT OF THE American Psychological Association some months before capped an illustrious academic career spanning more than 35 productive years, during which Maslow had steadily gained the high regard—even adulation—of countless numbers of colleagues and former students. His best-known books, *Motivation and Personality* and *Toward a Psychology of Being*, were not only being discussed avidly by psychologists, but also by professionals in fields ranging from management and marketing to education and counseling. Perhaps even more significantly, Maslow's iconoclastic concepts like peak experience, self-actualization, and synergy had even begun penetrating popular language.

Nevertheless, it was a very unsettling time for him: Recovering from a major heart attack, the temperamentally restless and ceaselessly active Maslow was finding forced convalescence at home to be almost painfully unbearable. Suddenly, his extensive plans for future research, travel, and lecturing had to be postponed. Although Maslow hoped for a speedy recovery, frequent chest pains induced a keen sense of his own mortality. As perhaps never before, he began to ponder his career's accomplishments and his unrealized goals.

In 1968 PSYCHOLOGY TODAY was a precocious one-year-old upstart, but such was its prestige that it was able to attract perhaps the country's most famous psychologist for an interview.

Maslow likely regarded the PT interview as a major opportunity to outline his "comprehensive human psychology" and the best way to actualize it. At 60, he knew that time permitted him only to plant seeds (in his own metaphor) of research and theory—and hope that later generations would live to see the flowering of human betterment. Perhaps most prescient at a time of global unrest is Maslow's stirring vision of "building a psychology for the peace table." It was his hope that through psychological research, we might learn how to unify peoples of differing racial and ethnic origins, and thereby create a world of peace.

Although the complete audiotapes of the sessions, conducted over three days, disappeared long ago under mysterious circumstances, the written condensation that remains provides a fascinating and still-relevant portrait of a key thinker at the height of his prowess. Intellectually, Maslow was decades ahead of his time; today the wide-ranging ideas he offers here are far from outdated. Indeed, after some twenty-odd years, they're still on the cutting edge of American psychology and social science. Emotionally, this interview is significant for the rare—essentially unprecedented—glimpse it affords into Maslow's personal history and concerns: his ancestry and upbringing; his mentors and ambitions; his courtship, marriage, and fatherhood; and even a few of his peak experiences.

Maslow continued to be puzzled and intrigued by the more positive human phenomenon of self-actualization. He was well aware that his theory about the "best of humanity" suffered from methodological flaws. Yet he had become ever more convinced of its intuitive validity, that self-actualizers provide us with clues to our highest innate traits: love and compassion, creativity and aesthetics, ethics and spirituality. Maslow longed to empirically verify this lifelong hunch.

1. BECOMING A PERSON: SEEKING SELF-IDENTITY

In the two years of his life that remained, this gifted psychologist never wrote an autobiography, nor did he ever again bare his soul in such a public and wide-ranging way. It may have been that Maslow regarded this unusually personal interview as a true legacy. More than 20 years later, it remains a fresh and important document for the field of psychology.

Mary Harrington Hall, for PSYCHOLOGY TODAY: A couple of William B. Yeats's lines keep running through my head: "And in my heart, the daemons and the gods wage an eternal battle and I feel the pain of wounds, the labor of the spear." How thin is the veneer of civilization, and how can we understand and deal with evil?

Abraham H. Maslow: It's a psychological puzzle I've been trying to solve for years. Why are people cruel and why are they nice? Evil people are rare, but you find evil behavior in the majority of people. The next thing I want to do with my life is to study evil and understand it.

PT: By evil here, I think we both mean destructive action without remorse. Racial prejudice is an evil in our society which we must deal with. And soon. Or we will go down as a racist society.

Maslow: You know, when I became A.P.A. president, the first thing I wanted to do was work for greater recognition for the Negro psychologists. Then I found that there were no Negroes in psychology, at least not many. They don't major in psychology.

PT: Why should they? Why would I think that psychology would solve social problems if I were a Negro living in the ghetto, surrounded by despair?

Maslow: Negroes have really had to take it. We've given them every possible blow. If I were a Negro, I'd be fighting, as Martin Luther King fought, for human recognition and justice. I'd rather go down with my flag flying. If you're weak or crippled, or you can't speak out or fight back in some way, then people don't hesitate to treat you badly.

PT: Could you look at evil behavior in two ways: evil from below and evil from above? Evil as a sickness and evil as understood compassionately?

Maslow: If you look at evil from above, you can be realistic. Evil exists. You don't give it quarter, and you're a better fighter if you can understand it. You're in the position of a psychotherapist. In the the same way, you can look at neurosis. You can see neurosis from below—as a sickness—as most psychiatrists see it. Or you can understand it as a compassionate man might: respecting the neurosis as a fumbling and inefficient effort toward good ends.

PT: You can understand race riots in the same way, can't you?

Maslow: If you can only be detached enough, you can feel that it's better to riot than to be hopeless, degraded, and defeated. Rioting is a childish way of trying to be a man, but it takes time to rise out of the hell of hatred and frustration and accept that to be a man you don't have to riot.

PT: In our society, we see all behavior as a demon we can vanquish and banish, don't we? And yet good people do evil things.

Maslow: Most people are nice people. Evil is caused by ignorance, thoughtlessness, fear, or even the desire for popularity with one's gang. We can cure many such causes of evil. Science is progressing, and I feel hope that psychology can solve many of these problems. I think that a good part of evil behavior bears on the behavior of the normal.

PT: How will you approach the study of evil?

Maslow: If you think only of evil, then you become pessimistic and hopeless like Freud. But if you think there is no evil, then you're just one more deluded Pollyanna. The thing is to try to understand and realize how it's possible for people who are capable of being angels, heroes, or saints to be bastards and killers. Sometimes, poor and miserable people are hopeless. Many revenge themselves upon life for what society has done to them. They enjoy hurting.

PT: Your study of evil will have to be subjective, won't it? How can we measure evil in the laboratory?

Maslow: All the goals of objectivity, repeatability, and preplanned experimentation are things we have to move toward. The more reliable you make knowledge, the better it is. If the salvation of man comes out of the advancement of knowledge—taken in the best sense—then these goals are part of the strategy of knowledge.

PT: What did you tell your own daughters, Ann and Ellen, when they were growing up?

Maslow: Learn to hate meanness. Watch out for anybody who is mean or cruel. Watch out for people who delight in destruction.

PT: How would you describe yourself? Not in personality, because you're one of the warmest and sweetest men I've ever met. But who are you?

Maslow: I'm someone who likes plowing new ground, then walking away from it. I get bored easily. For me, the big thrill comes with the discovering.

PT: Psychologists all love Abe Maslow. How did you escape the crossfire?

Maslow: I just avoid most academic warfare. Besides, I had my first heart attack many years ago, and perhaps I've been unconsciously favoring my body. So I may have avoided real struggle. Besides, I only like fights I know I can win, and I'm not personally mean.

PT: Maybe you're just one of the lucky few who grew up through a happy childhood without malice.

Maslow: With my childhood, it's a wonder I'm not psychotic. I was the little Jewish boy in the non-Jewish neighborhood. It was a little like being the first Negro enrolled in the all-white school. I grew up in libraries and among books, without friends.

Both my mother and father were uneducated. My father wanted me to be a lawyer. He thumbed his way across the whole continent of Europe from Russia and got here at the age of 15. He wanted success for me. I tried law school for two weeks. Then I came home to my poor father one night after a class discussing "spite fences" and told him I couldn't be a lawyer. "Well, son," he said, "what do you want to study?" I answered: "Everything." He was uneducated and couldn't understand my passion for learning, but he was a nice man. He didn't understand either that at 16, I was in love.

PT: All 16-year-olds are in love.

Maslow: Mine was different. We're talking about my wife. I loved Bertha. You know her. Wasn't I right? I was extremely shy, and I tagged around after her. We were too young to get married. I tried to run away with her.

PT: Where did you run?

Maslow: I ran to Cornell for my sophomore year in college, then to Wisconsin. We were married there when I was 20 and Bertha was 19. Life didn't really start for me until I got married.

I went to Wisconsin because I had just discovered John B. Watson's work, and I was sold on behaviorism. It was an explosion of excitement for me. Bertha came to pick me up at New York's 42nd Street library, and I was dancing down Fifth Avenue with exuberance. I embarrassed her, but I was so excited about

Watson's behaviorist program. It was beautiful. I was confident that here was a real road to travel: solving one problem after another and changing the world.

PT: A clear lifetime with built-in progress guaranteed.

Maslow: That was it. I was off to Wisconsin to change the world. I went there to study with psychologist Kurt Koffka, biologist Hans Dreisch, and philosopher Alexander Meiklejohn. But when I showed up on the campus, they weren't there. They had just been visiting professors, but the lying catalog had included them anyway.

Oh, but I was so lucky, though. I was young Harry Harlow's first doctoral graduate. And they were angels, my professors. I've always had angels around. They helped me when I needed it, even fed me. Bill Sheldon taught me how to buy a suit. I didn't know anything of amenities. Clark Hull was an angel to me, and later, Edward L. Thorndike.

PT: You're an angelic man. I've heard too many stories to let you deny it. What kind of research were you doing at Wisconsin?

Maslow: I was a monkey man. By studying monkeys for my doctoral dissertation, I found that dominance was related to sex, and to maleness. It was a great discovery, but somebody had discovered it two months before me.

PT: Great ideas always go in different places and minds at the same time.

Maslow: Yes, I worked on it until the start of World War II. I thought that working on sex was the easiest way to help mankind. I felt if I could discover a way to improve the sexual life by even one percent, then I could improve the whole species.

One day, it suddenly dawned on me that I knew as much about sex as any man living—in the intellectual sense. I knew everything that had been written; I had made discoveries with which I was pleased; I had done therapeutic work. This was about 10 years before the Kinsey report came out. Then I suddenly burst into laughter. Here was I, the great sexologist, and I had never seen an erect penis except one, and that was from my own bird's-eye view. That humbled me considerably.

PT: I suppose you interviewed people the way Kinsey did?

Maslow: No, something was wrong with Kinsey. I really don't think he liked women, or men. In my research, I interviewed 120 women with a new form of interview. No notes. We just talked until I got some feeling for the individual's personality, then put sex against that background. Sex has to be considered in regard to love, otherwise it's useless. This is because behavior can be a defense—a way of hiding what you feel—particularly regarding sex.

I was fascinated with my research. But I gave up interviewing men. They were useless because they boasted and lied about sex. I also planned a big research project involving prostitutes. I thought we could learn a lot about men from them, but the research never came off.

PT: You gave up all your experimental research in these fields.

Maslow: Yes, around 1941 I felt I must try to save the world, and to prevent the horrible wars and the awful hatred and prejudice. It happened very suddenly. One day just after Pearl Harbor, I was driving home and my car was stopped by a poor, pathetic parade. Boy Scouts and old uniforms and a flag and someone playing a flute off-key.

As I watched, the tears began to run down my face. I felt we didn't understand—not Hitler, nor the Germans, nor Stalin, nor the Communists. We didn't understand any of them. I felt that if we could understand, then we could make progress. I had a vision of a peace table, with people sitting around it, talking about human nature and hatred, war and peace, and brotherhood.

I was too old to go into the army. It was at that moment I realized that the rest of my life must be devoted to discovering a psychology for the peace table. That moment changed my whole life. Since then, I've devoted myself to developing a theory of human nature that could be tested by experiment and research. I wanted to prove that humans are capable of something grander than war, prejudice, and hatred. I wanted to make science consider all the people: the best specimen of mankind I could find. I found that many of them reported having something like mystical experiences.

PT: Your work with "self-actualizing" people is famous. You have described some of these mystical experiences.

Maslow: Peak experiences come from love and sex, from aesthetic moments, from bursts of creativity, from moments of insight and discovery, or from fusion with nature.

I had one such experience in a faculty procession here at Brandeis University. I saw the line stretching off into a dim future. At its head was Socrates. And in the line were the ones I love most. Thomas Jefferson was there. And Spinoza. And Alfred North Whitehead. I was in the same line. Behind me, that infinite line melted into the dimness. And there were all the people not yet born who were going to be in the same line.

I believe these experiences can be studied scientifically, and they will be.

PT: This is all part of your theory of metamotivation, isn't it?

Maslow: But not all people who are metamotivated report peak experiences. The "nonpeakers" are healthy, but they lack poetry and soaring flights of the imagination. Both peakers and nonpeakers can be self-actualized in that they're not motivated by basic needs, but by something higher.

PT: Real self-actualization must be rare. What percentage of us achieve it?

Maslow: I'd say only a fraction of one percent.

PT: People whose basic needs have been met, then, will pursue life's ultimate values?

Maslow: Yes, the ultimate happiness for man is the realization of pure beauty and truth, which are the ultimate values. What we need is a system of thought—you might even call it a religion—that can bind humans together. A system that would fit the Republic of Chad as well as the United States: a system that would supply our idealistic young people with something to believe in. They're searching for something they can pour all that emotion into, and the churches are not much help.

PT: This system must come.

Maslow: I'm not alone in trying to make it. There are plenty of others working toward the same end. Perhaps their efforts, aided by the hundreds of youngsters who are devoting their lives to this, will develop a new image of man that rejects the chemical and technological views. We've technologized everything.

PT: The technologist is the person who has fallen in love with a machine. I suppose that has also happened to those in psychology?

Maslow: They become fascinated with the machine. It's almost a neurotic love. They're like the man who spends Sundays polishing his car instead of stroking his wife.

PT: In several of your papers, you've said that you stopped being a behaviorist when your first child was born.

Maslow: My whole training at Wiscon-

1. BECOMING A PERSON: SEEKING SELF-IDENTITY

sin was behaviorist. I didn't question it until I began reading some other sources. Later, I began studying the Rorschach test.

At the same time, I stumbled into embryology and read Ludwig von Bertalanffy's *Modern Theories of Development*. I had already become disillusioned with Bertrand Russell and with English philosophy generally. Then, I fell in love with Alfred North Whitehead and Henri Bergson. Their writings destroyed behaviorism for me without my recognizing it.

When my first baby was born, that was the thunderclap that settled things. I looked at this tiny, mysterious thing and felt so stupid. I felt small, weak, and feeble. I'd say that anyone who's had a baby couldn't be a behaviorist.

PT: As you propose new ideas, and blaze new ground, you're bound to be criticized, aren't you?

Maslow: I have worked out a lot of good tricks for fending off professional attacks. We all have to do that. A good, controlled experiment is possible only when you already know a hell of a lot. If I'm a pioneer by choice and I go into the wilderness, how am I going to make careful experiments? If I tried to, I'd be a fool. I'm not against careful experiments. But rather, I've been working with what I call "growing tip" statistics.

With a tree, all the growth takes place at the growing tips. Humanity is exactly the same. All the growth takes place in the growing tip: among that one percent of the population. It's made up of pioneers, the beginners. That's where the action is.

PT: You were the one who helped publish Ruth Benedict's work on synergy. What's it about?

Maslow: That it's possible to set up social institutions that merge selfishness and unselfishness, so that you can't benefit yourself without benefiting others. And the reverse.

PT: How can psychology become a stronger force in our society?

Maslow: We all should look at the similarities within the various disciplines and think of enlarging psychology. To throw anything away is crazy. Good psychology should include all the methodological techniques, without having loyalty to one method, one idea, or one person.

PT: I see you as a catalyst and as a bridge between many disciplines, theories, and philosophies.

Maslow: My job is to put them all together. We shouldn't have "humanistic psychology." The adjective should be unnecessary. I'm not antibehaviorist. I'm antidoctrinaire.

PT: Abe, when you look back on your own education, what kind would you recommend for others?

Maslow: The great educational experiences of my life were those that taught me most. They taught me what kind of a person I was. These were experiences that drew me out and strengthened me. Psychoanalysis was a big thing for me. And getting married. Marriage is a school itself. Also, having children. Becoming a father changed my whole life. It taught me as if by revelation. And reading particular books. William Graham Sumner's *Folkways* was a Mount Everest in my life: It changed me.

My teachers were the best in the world. I sought them out: Erich Fromm, Karen Horney, Ruth Benedict, Max Wertheimer, Alfred Adler, David Levy, and Harry Harlow. I was there in New York City during the 1930s when the wave of distinguished émigrés arrived from Europe.

PT: Not everyone can have such an illustrious faculty.

Maslow: It's the teacher who's important. And if this is so, then what we are doing with our whole educational structure—with credits and the idea that one teacher is as good as another? You look at the college catalog and it says English 342. It doesn't even bother to tell you the instructor's name, and that's insane. The purpose of education—and of all social institutions—is the development of full humaneness. If you keep that in mind, all else follows. We've got to concentrate on goals.

PT: It's like the story about the test pilot who radioed back home: "I'm lost, but I'm making record time."

Maslow: If you forget the goal of education, then the whole thing is lost.

PT: If a rare, self-actualizing young psychologist came to you today and said, "What's the most important thing I can do in this time of crisis?", what advice would you give?

Maslow: I'd say: Get to work on aggression and hostility. We need the definitive book on aggression. And we need it now. Only the pieces exist: the animal stuff, the psychoanalytic stuff, the endocrine stuff. Time is running out. A key to understanding the evil which can destroy our society lies in this understanding.

There's another study that could be done. I'd like to test the whole, incoming freshman class at Brandeis University in various ways: psychiatric interviews, personality tests, everything. I want to follow them for four years of college. For a beginning, I want to test my theory that emotionally healthy people perceive better.

PT: You could make the college study only a preliminary, and follow them through their whole life span, the way Lewis Terman did with his gifted kids.

Maslow: Oh yes! I'd like to know: How good a father or mother does this student become? And what happens to his/her children? This kind of long-term study would take more time than I have left. But that ultimately doesn't make any difference. I like to be the first runner in the relay race. I like to pass on the baton to the next person.

SHOULD SCHOOLS TRY TO BOOST SELF-ESTEEM?

Beware the dark side

ROY F. BAUMEISTER

Roy F. Baumeister is the Elsie Smith professor of psychology at Case Western Reserve University in Cleveland, Ohio. For a fuller discussion of the relationship between self-esteem and violence, see "Relation of Threatened Egotism to Violence and Aggression: The Dark Side of High Self-Esteem," by Roy F. Baumeister, Laura Smart, and Joseph M. Boden (Psychological Review, 1996, Vol. 103, No. 1).

"WE MUST raise children's self-esteem!" How often has this sentiment been expressed in recent years in schools, homes, and meeting rooms around the United States? The sentiment reflects the widespread, well-intentioned, earnest, and yet rather pathetic hope that if we can only persuade our kids to love themselves more, they will stop dropping out, getting pregnant, carrying weapons, taking drugs, and getting into trouble, and instead will start achieving great things in school and out.

Unfortunately, the large mass of knowledge that research psychologists have built up around self-esteem does not justify that hope. At best, high self-esteem is a mixed blessing whose total effects are likely to be small and minor. At worst, the pursuit of high self-esteem is a foolish, wasteful, and self-destructive enterprise that may end up doing more harm than good.

Writers on controversial topics should acknowledge their biases, and so let me confess mine: I have a strong bias in favor of self-esteem. I have been excited about self-esteem ever since my student days at Princeton, when I first heard that it was a topic of study. Over the past two decades I have probably published more studies on self-esteem than anybody else in the United States (or elsewhere). It would be great for my career if self-esteem could do everything its boosters hope: I'd be dining frequently at the White House and advising policymakers on how to fix the country's problems.

It is therefore with considerable personal disappointment that I must report that the enthusiastic claims of the self-esteem movement mostly range from fantasy to hogwash. The effects of self-esteem are small, limited, and not all good. Yes, a few people here and there end up worse off because their self-esteem was too low. Then again, other people end up worse off because their self-esteem was too high. And most of the time self-esteem makes surprisingly little difference.

Self-esteem is, literally, how favorably a person regards himself or herself. It is perception (and evaluation), not reality. For example, I think the world would be a better place if we could all manage to be a little nicer to each other. But that's hard: We'd all have to discipline ourselves to change. The self-esteem approach, in contrast, is to skip over the hard work of changing our actions and instead just let us all *think* we're nicer. That won't make the world any better. People with high self-esteem are not in fact any nicer than people with low self-esteem—in fact, the opposite is closer to the truth.

High self-esteem means thinking well of oneself, re-

1. BECOMING A PERSON: SEEKING SELF-IDENTITY

gardless of whether that perception is based on substantive achievement or mere wishful thinking and self-deception. High self-esteem can mean *confident* and *secure*—but it can also mean *conceited, arrogant, narcissistic,* and *egotistical.*

A recent, widely publicized study dramatized the fact that self-esteem consists of perception and is not necessarily based on reality. In an international scholastic competition, American students achieved the lowest average scores among all participating nationalities. But the American kids rated themselves and their performance the highest. This is precisely what comes of focusing on self-esteem: poor performance accompanied by plenty of empty self-congratulation. Put another way, we get high self-esteem as inflated perceptions covering over a rather dismal reality.

Looking ahead, it is alarming to think what will happen when this generation of schoolchildren grows up into adults who may continue thinking they are smarter than the rest of the world—while actually being dumber. America will be a land of conceited fools.

All of this might fairly be discounted if America were really suffering from an epidemic of low self-esteem, such as if most American schoolchildren generally had such negative views of themselves that they were unable to tackle their homework. But that's not the case. On the contrary, as I'll explain shortly, self-esteem is already inflated throughout the United States. The average American already regards himself or herself as above average. At this point, any further boosting of self-esteem is likely to approach the level of grandiose, egotistical delusions.

Benefits of Self-Esteem

Let us begin with the positive consequences of high self-esteem. Much has been claimed, but very little has been proven. Some years ago California formed a task force to promote self-esteem, and its manifesto was filled with optimistic assertions about how raising self-esteem would help solve most of the personal and social problems in the state. Here is a sample of its rhetoric: "the lack of self-esteem is central to most personal and social ills plaguing our state and nation," and indeed self-esteem was touted as a social vaccine that might inoculate people "against the lures of crime, violence, substance abuse, teen pregnancy, child abuse, chronic welfare dependency, and educational failure."[1]

Such rhetoric is especially remarkable in light of another fact. That same task force commissioned a group of researchers to assemble the relevant facts and findings about self-esteem. Here is what the experts in charge of the project concluded from all the information they gathered: "The news most consistently reported, however, is that the associations between self-esteem and its expected consequences are mixed, insignificant, or absent."[2] In short, self-esteem doesn't have much impact.

Even when the occasional study does link low self-esteem to some problem pattern, there is often a serious chicken-and-egg ambiguity about which comes first. For example, if someone showed that drug-addicted pregnant unmarried school-dropout teenagers with criminal records have low self-esteem, this might mean only that people stop bragging after they mess up their lives. It would not prove that low self-esteem caused the problems. The few researchers who have tried to establish causality have usually concluded that self-esteem is mainly an outcome, not a cause. At best there is a mutual influence of spiraling effects.

To be sure, there are some benefits of high self-esteem. It helps people bounce back after failure and try again. It helps them recover from trauma and misfortune. In general, high self-esteem makes people feel good. Low self-esteem accompanies various emotional vulnerabilities, including depression and anxiety. (Again, though, there is no proof that low self-esteem causes these problems, or that raising self-esteem will prevent them.)

Children who do well in school have slightly higher self-esteem than those who do poorly. Unfortunately the effect is small, and in fact anyone who believes in the value of education should wish for a stronger effect simply on the basis that successful students *deserve* higher self-esteem. Across multiple studies, the average correlation between grades and self-esteem is .24, which means about 6 percent of the variance.[3] In other words, moving from the very highest self-esteem scores to the very lowest would yield about a 6 percent difference in school performance. A small increase in self-esteem, such as might be produced by a school program aimed at boosting self-esteem, would probably make only a 1 percent difference or less. And even that assumes that self-esteem is the cause, not the effect, contrary to many indications. To the extent that it is school success or failure that alters self-esteem, and not the other way around, any independent effort to raise self-esteem would have no effect at all on school performance.

Once again I must say how disappointing I've found these facts to be. Self-esteem is not altogether useless, but its benefits are isolated and minor, except for the fact that it feels good. When I embarked on a career of research on self-esteem, I had hoped for a great deal more.

The Dark Side of High Self-Esteem

The very idea that high self-esteem could have bad consequences strikes some people as startling. The self-esteem movement wants to present self-esteem as having many good and no bad effects. But very few psychological traits are one-sidedly good, and those few are mostly abilities (like intelligence or self-control). High self-esteem can certainly cause its share of problems. If you pause to recall that the category of high self-esteem includes people who think they are great without necessarily *being* great, this conclusion may seem less startling.

A large, important study recently adopted a novel approach to separating self-esteem from all its causes and correlates.[4] The researchers measured how each individual rated himself or herself compared to how that person was rated by others who knew him or her. They were particularly interested in the category of

> *The very idea that high self-esteem could have bad consequences strikes some people as startling.*

people with inflated self-esteem—the ones who rated themselves higher than their friends rated them. This, after all, is where the self-esteem movement leads: Concentrate on getting kids to think well of themselves, regardless of actual accomplishments. The researchers had no difficulty finding plenty of students who fit that category. They are, in a sense, the star products and poster children of the self-esteem movement.

And what were they like? The researchers' conclusions did not paint an encouraging picture of health, adjustment, or success. On the contrary, the long-term outcomes of these people's lives found above average rates of interpersonal and psychological problems. A second study, with laboratory observations of live interactions, showed these people to be rather obnoxious. They were more likely than others to interrupt when someone else was speaking. They were more prone to disrupt the conversation with angry and hostile remarks. They tended to talk *at* people instead of talking *to* or *with* them. In general, they irritated the other people present. Does any of this sound familiar? This is what comes of inflated self-esteem.

The picture is one of a self-centered, conceited person who is quick to assert his or her own wants but lacks genuine regard for others. That may not be what the self-esteem movement has in mind, but it is what it is likely to produce. In practice, high self-esteem usually amounts to a person thinking that he or she is better than other people. If you think you're better than others, why should you listen to them, be considerate, or keep still when you want to do or say something?

Over the past several years, I have been writing a book on evil and violence (*Evil: Inside Human Violence and Cruelty*, to be published by Freeman this fall). Given my longstanding interest in self-esteem, I naturally wanted to acknowledge any part that it plays. Various pundits and so-called experts have long asserted that low self-esteem causes violence, but I've had enough experience with self-esteem to know that I'd better check the data rather than relying on vague generalizations and ostensibly "common" knowledge.

Two graduate students and I reviewed literally hundreds of studies on the topic. What we found was so surprising that, in addition to my book, we recently published a lengthy article in psychology's most eminent journal, the *Psychological Review*.[5] We combined evidence from all spheres of violence we could find: murder, assault, rape, terrorism, bullies, youth gangs, repressive governments, tyranny, family violence, warfare, oppression, genocide, and more.

We concluded that the idea that low self-esteem causes violence is simply and thoroughly wrong. It is contradicted by a huge mass of information and evidence. People with low self-esteem are generally shy, humble, modest, self-effacing individuals. Violent perpetrators—from Hitler, Hussein, and Amin, down to the common wife-beater or playground bully—are decidedly not like that.

If anything, high self-esteem is closer to the violent personality. Most perpetrators of violence are acting out of some sense of personal superiority, especially one that has been threatened or questioned in some way. I am not saying that high self-esteem, per se, directly causes violence. Not all people with high self-esteem become violent. But violent people are a subset of people with high self-esteem. The main recipe for violence is *threatened egotism*—that is, a belief in personal superiority that is challenged, questioned, or "dissed" by somebody else. Inflated self-esteem often leads to that pattern.

Consider some of the evidence. In the first place, whenever there are two groups with different levels of self-esteem, the more egotistical group is nearly always the more violent one. The most familiar example is gender: Men have higher self-esteem and higher rates of violence. When self-esteem fluctuates, the risk of violence rises with the favorable views of self, such as in manic-depressive illness. Indeed, people who are intoxicated with alcohol show increases in self-esteem and increases in violent tendencies.

A recent study[6] found that nowadays many homicides occur in connection with other crimes such as robbery, but in the remaining cases the homicide is often the result of an altercation that begins with challenges and insults, in which someone's favorable self-opinion is disputed by the other person. The person who feels he (or less often she) is losing face in the argument may resort to violence and murder.

Even within samples of offenders, it appears that indicators of egotism can discriminate violent and troublesome tendencies, and it is the favorable views of self that are linked to the worse actions. A group of researchers administered the California Psychological Inventory to young men (in their late teens) on parole.[7] The researchers were able to predict future parole violations (recidivism) better than previous attempts. Among the traits that predicted high recidivism were being egotistical and outspoken (as well as "touchy," which suggests being easily offended). Meanwhile, being modest and unassuming (associated with low self-esteem) were among the traits linked to being least likely to violate parole. These results all seem to fit the view linking favorable views of self to violent tendencies.

Aggression starts in childhood, and bullies are the most notable examples. They are of particular importance because childhood bullies have been found to be four times more likely than other children to engage in

1. BECOMING A PERSON: SEEKING SELF-IDENTITY

serious criminal behavior during their subsequent adult life. Dan Olweus is an expert who has studied bullies for years, and he recently summarized the conclusions that his program of research has yielded. Unlike victims of bullying (who show multiple indications of low self-esteem), the bullies themselves seemed relatively secure and free from anxiety. "In contrast to a fairly common assumption among psychologists and psychiatrists, we have found no indicators that the aggressive bullies (boys) are anxious and insecure under a tough surface," said Olweus, adding that multiple samples and methods had confirmed this conclusion, and concluding that bullies "do not suffer from poor self-esteem."[8]

One of the most earnest and empathic efforts to understand the subjective experience of committing crimes was that of sociologist Jack Katz.[9] Homicide as well as assault emerged in his study as typically caused by threats to the offender's public image. In Katz's view, the offender privately holds a positive view of self, but the eventual victim impugns that view and implicitly humiliates the offender, often in front of an audience. The response is unplanned violence resulting in injury or death. Katz insisted that feelings of being humiliated are quickly transformed into rage. He argued that many men feel that almost anyone can judge them and impugn their esteem, whereas for women self-esteem is most heavily invested in their intimate relationships—with the result that men will attack strangers while women mainly just murder their intimate partners, because only the partners can threaten their self-esteem to a sufficient degree to provoke such a violent response.

Another example of the relationship between inflated self-esteem and violence focuses on juvenile delinquency. The classic study by Glueck and Glueck compared juvenile delinquents against a matched sample of nondelinquent boys.[10] Although the study was an early one and has been criticized on methodological grounds, it benefited from a large sample and extensive work, and nearly all of their findings have been replicated by subsequent studies. The Glueck and Glueck study did not measure self-esteem directly (indeed it antedated most modern self-esteem scales), but there were plenty of related variables. The pattern of findings offers little to support the hypothesis that low self-esteem causes delinquency. Delinquent boys were more likely than controls to be characterized as self-assertive, socially assertive, defiant, and narcissistic, none of which seems compatible with low self-esteem. Meanwhile, the delinquents were less likely than the comparison group to be marked by the factors that do indicate low self-esteem, including severe insecurity, feelings of helplessness, feelings of being unloved, general anxiety (a frequent correlate of low self-esteem), submissiveness, and fear of failure. Thus, the thoughts and actions of juvenile delinquents suggested that they held quite favorable opinions of themselves.

It is useful to look for convergences between the Gluecks' study and more recent studies of youthful violence, not only because of the seminal nature of the Gluecks' work, but also because their data were col-

> *Far, far more Americans of all ages have accurate or inflated views of themselves than underestimate themselves. They don't need boosting.*

lected several decades ago and on an almost entirely white sample, unlike more recent studies. Converging findings thus confer especially high confidence in conclusions that can be supported across time and ethnicity.

One of the most thorough research projects on youth gangs was that of Martin Sanchez Jankowski, whose work involved 10 years, several cities, and 37 gangs.[11] Although as a sociologist he was disinclined to use self-esteem or personality factors as explanatory constructs, his study did furnish several important observations. Jankowski specifically rejected the notion that acting tough is a result of low self-esteem or feelings of inadequacy. In his words, "There have been some studies of gangs that suggest that many gang members have tough exteriors but are insecure on the inside. This is a mistaken observation" (p. 27). He said that for many members, the appeal of the gang is the positive respect it enjoys in the community as well as the respectful treatment from other gang members, which he found to be an important norm in nearly all gangs he studied. He said most gang members "expressed a strong sense of self-competence and a drive to compete with others" (p. 102). When they failed, they always blamed something external rather than personal inadequacy or error. This last observation is especially relevant because several controlled studies have shown that it is characteristic of high self-esteem and contrary to the typical responses of people with low self-esteem.

Recently I appeared on a radio talk show. The hostess seemed to have difficulty accepting the conclusion that low self-esteem is not a cause of violence, possibly because she had swallowed the propaganda line that all good things come from high self-esteem. To explain our findings, I offered the example of the Ku Klux Klan. The KKK has long advocated beliefs in white superiority and has turned violent in response to efforts to extend full equality to black citizens (thereby eroding the superior status of whites). I thought KKK violence was a good, clear example of threatened egotism.

For a moment the hostess seemed to see the point, but then she jumped back on the self-esteem bandwagon. "What about deep down inside?" she asked. I inquired whether she thought that Klansmen believed that they, as whites were inferior to blacks, which would fit the low self-esteem view. She balked at the word "inferior" but offered that the violent Klansmen believe deep down inside that they are "not superior"—in other words, equal—to blacks.

I didn't know what to say to this basically loony argument. Her theory that Klan violence could be traced to a "deep down" inner belief that blacks are equal to whites has two parts, both of which are bizarre: first, that members of the KKK truly believe in racial equality, and second, that belief in racial equality causes violence. It struck me that attempts to defend the self-esteem movement against the facts end up having to make such preposterous assertions.

Although this particular hostess's idea was absurd, she was invoking a point that the proponents of self-esteem have on occasion raised as a possibly valid defense. When obnoxious or socially undesirable acts are performed by egotistical people, thus contradicting the belief that high self-esteem is generally good, some propose that these obnoxious individuals must secretly have low self-esteem. Indeed, the editorial reviewers who evaluated our article on violence for the *Psychological Review* insisted that we tackle this theoretical question head-on in the final published version of the paper.

There are two main reasons to reject the "hidden low self-esteem" view. The first is that plenty of researchers have tried and failed to find any indications of this allegedly hidden low self-esteem. It's not for lack of trying, and indeed it would be quite a feather in any researcher's cap to show that actions are caused by low self-esteem hidden under a veneer of high self-esteem. Studies of childhood bullies, teen gang members, adult criminals, and various obnoxious narcissists keep coming to the same conclusion: "We've heard the theory that these people have low self-esteem or a negative self-image underneath, but we sure can't find any sign of it."

The other reason is even more compelling. Suppose it were true (which it does not seem to be) that some violent people have high self-esteem on the surface but low self-esteem inside. Which view of self (the surface veneer or the hidden one) would be the one responsible for violence? We already know that genuine low self-esteem, when *not* hidden, does not cause violence. Hence one would have to say that low self-esteem is only linked to violence when it is hidden. That means that the crucial cause of violence is what is *hiding* the secret insecurity—which means that the "veneer" of high self-esteem is the cause, and so we are back anyway to the position that egotism is the cause.

There isn't space here to exhaust the dark side of high self-esteem, but let me touch on a few other features. People with high self-esteem are less willing than others to heed advice, for obvious reasons—they usually think they know better. (Whether children with inflated self-esteem are less willing to listen to teachers is one possible implication of this, but to my knowledge this has not yet been studied.) They respond to failure by blaming everyone and everything but themselves, such as a flawed test, a biased or unfair teacher, or an incompetent partner. They sometimes extend their favorable self-opinion to encompass people close to or similar to themselves, but unfortunately this often translates into prejudice and condescension toward people who differ from them. (High self-esteem is in fact linked to prejudice against outgroups.) Finally, when their egotism is threatened, they tend to react irrationally in ways that have been shown to be risky, self-defeating, and even self-destructive.

Boosting Self-Esteem: The Problem of Inflation

Most (though not all) of the problems linked to high self-esteem involve inflated self-esteem, in the sense of overestimating oneself. Based on the research findings produced in laboratories all over North America, I have no objection to people forming a sober, accurate recognition of their actual talents and accomplishments. The violence, the self-defeating behaviors, and the other problems tend to be most acute under conditions of threatened egotism, and inflated self-esteem increases that risk. After all, if you really are smart, your experiences will tend to confirm that fact, and so there's not much danger in high self-esteem that is based on accurate recognition of your intelligence. On the other hand, if you overestimate your abilities, reality will be constantly showing you up and bursting your bubble, and so your (inflated) self-opinion will be bumping up against threats—and those encounters lead to destructive responses.

Unfortunately, a school system that seeks to boost self-esteem in general is likely to produce the more dangerous (inflated) form of self-esteem. It would be fine, for example, to give a hard test and then announce the top few scores for general applause. Such a system recognizes the successful ones, and it shows the rest what the important criteria are (and how much they may need to improve). What is dangerous and worrisome is any procedure that would allow the other students to think that they are just as accomplished as the top scorers even though they did not perform as well. Unfortunately, the self-esteem movement often works in precisely this wrong-headed fashion.

Some students will inevitably be smarter, work harder, learn more, and perform better than others. There is no harm (and in fact probably some positive value) in helping these individuals recognize their superior accomplishments and talents. Such self-esteem is linked to reality and hence less prone to causing dangers and problems.

On the other hand, there is considerable danger and harm in falsely boosting the self-esteem of the other students. It is fine to encourage them to work harder and try to gain an accurate appraisal of their strengths and weaknesses, and it is also fine to recognize their talents and accomplishments in other (including nonacademic) spheres, but don't give them positive feedback that they have not earned. (Also, don't downplay the importance of academic achievement as the central goal of school, such as by suggesting that success at sports or crafts is just as good.) To encourage the lower-performing students to regard their performance just as favorably as the top learners—a strategy all too popular with the self-esteem movement—is a tragic mistake. If successful, it results only in inflated self-esteem, which is the recipe for a host of problems and destructive patterns.

The logical implications of this argument show exactly when self-esteem should be boosted. When people seriously underestimate their abilities and accomplishments, they need boosting. For example, a student who falsely believes she can't succeed at math may end up short-changing herself and failing to fulfill her potential unless she can be helped to realize that yes, she does have the ability to master math.

In contrast, self-esteem should not be boosted when it is already in the accurate range (or higher). A student who correctly believes that math is not his strong point should not be given exaggerated notions of what he can accomplish. Otherwise, the eventual result will be failure and heartbreak. Along the way he's likely to be angry, troublesome, and prone to blame everybody else when something goes wrong.

In my years as an educator I have seen both patterns. But which is more common? Whether boosting self-esteem in general will be helpful or harmful depends on the answer. And the answer is overwhelmingly clear. Far, far more Americans of all ages have accurate or inflated views of themselves than underestimate themselves. They don't need boosting.

Dozens of studies have documented how inflated self-esteem is.[12] Research interest was sparked some years ago by a survey in which 90 percent of adults rated themselves "above average" in driving ability. After all, only half can really be above average. Similar patterns are found with almost all good qualities. A survey about leadership ability found that only 2 percent of high school students rated themselves as below average. Meanwhile, a whopping 25 percent claimed to be in the top 1 percent! Similarly, when asked about ability to get along with others, no students at all said they were below average.[13]

Responses to scales designed to measure self-esteem show the same pattern. There are always plenty of scores at the high end and plenty in the middle, but only a few straggle down toward the low end. This seems to be true no matter which of the many self-esteem scales is used. Moreover, the few individuals who do show the truly low self-esteem scores probably suffer from multiple problems that need professional therapy. Self-esteem boosting from schools would not cure them.

Obviously there's precious little evidence of low self-esteem in such numbers. By definition, plenty of people are in reality below average, but most of them refuse to acknowledge it. Meanwhile large numbers of people clearly overestimate themselves. The top 1 percent can really only contain 1 percent, not the 25 percent who claim to belong there. Meanwhile, the problem that would justify programs aimed at boosting self-esteem—people who significantly underestimate themselves—is extremely rare.

Conclusion

What is to be done? In response to the question about whether schools should boost self-esteem, my answer is: Don't bother. Efforts at boosting self-esteem probably feel good both for students and for teachers, but the real benefits and positive consequences are likely to be minor. Meanwhile, inflated self-esteem carries an assortment of risks and dangers, and so efforts to boost self-esteem may do as much harm as good, or possibly even more. The time, effort, and resources that schools put into self-esteem will not be justified by any palpable improvements in school performance, citizenship, or other outcomes.

There is one psychological trait that schools could help instill and that is likely to pay off much better than self-esteem. That trait is self-control (including self-discipline). Unlike self-esteem, self-control (or lack thereof) is directly and causally involved in a large set of social and personal problems.[14] Addiction, crime, violence, unwanted pregnancy, venereal disease, poor school performance, and many other problems have self-control failure as a core cause. Also unlike self-esteem, self-control brings benefits to both the individual and society. People with better self-control are more successful (socially and academically), happier, and better adjusted, than others. They also make better parents, spouses, colleagues, and employees. In other words, their self-control benefits the people close to them.

Indeed, I am convinced that weak self-control is a crucial link between family breakdown and many social problems. Study after study has shown that children of single parents show up worse than average on almost every measure, ranging from math achievement tests to criminal convictions. Most single parents I know are loving, dedicated, hard-working individuals, but all their energy goes toward providing food and shelter and their children's other basic needs. It seems to take a second parent to provide the supervision and consistent rule enforcement that foster self-control in the child.

How much the schools can do to build self-control is unclear. Still, just recognizing the priority and value of self-control will help. Obviously, self-control is not something that is instilled directly (as in a "self-control class") but rather should be cultivated like a cluster of good habits in connection with regular academic work, especially in the context of clear, consistent enforcement of academic and behavioral standards. The disciplinary and academic culture of a school should be aimed at recognizing and encouraging the self-control of individual students, including rewarding good self-control and punishing its failures or absences. With each new plan, policy, or procedure, school officials might pause to ask "Will this help strengthen self-control?" instead of "Might this hurt anybody's self-esteem?"

In the long run, self-control will do far more for the individuals and for society as a whole than will self-esteem. Moreover, self-control gives people the ability to change and improve themselves, and so it can bring about changes in substantive reality, not just in perception. And if one can make oneself into a better person, self-esteem is likely to increase too. Raising self-control may thus end up boosting self-esteem—but not in the dangerous or superficial ways that flourish now.

My final message to all the people working in today's schools and seeking to help the next generation get a good start is, therefore, as follows: Forget about self-esteem, and concentrate on self-control.

REFERENCES

[1] California Task Force (1990), *Toward a State of Self-Esteem*, p. 4.

[2] Mecca, Smelser, & Vasconcellos, 1989, *The Social Importance of Self-Esteem*, p. 15.

[3] Hattie & Hansford (1982), in the *Australian Journal of Education*. Note that percent of variance is calculated by squaring the correlation coefficient.

[4] Colvin, Block, & Funder (1995), in the *Journal of Personality and Social Psychology*.

[5] Baumeister, Smart, & Boden, 1996, in *Psychological Review*, Vol. 103, No. 1. Interested readers may wish to consult that article for the full details and findings.

[6] Polk, 1993, in *Journal of Criminal Justice*.

[7] Gough, Wenk, and Rozynko (1965), in *Journal of Abnormal Psychology*.

[8] Olweus, 1994, p. 100. In R. Huesmann (Ed.), *Aggressive Behavior*.

[9] Katz, 1988, *Seductions of crime*.

[10] Glueck & Glueck, 1950, *Unraveling Juvenile Delinquency*.

[11] Jankowski, 1991, *Islands in the Street*.

[12] For reviews, see Taylor & Brown, 1988, in *Psychological Bulletin*; Taylor, 1989, *Positive Illusions*.

[13] These findings are covered in Gilovich's book. A rare exception to this general inflation is that American females are dissatisfied with their bodies and in particular think they are overweight.

[14] For review, see Baumeister, Heatherton, & Tice (1994), *Losing Control*.

A counterblast in the war on Freud.

THE SHRINK IS IN

Jonathan Lear

JONATHAN LEAR is currently Visiting Professor at the Committee on Social Thought at the University of Chicago.

In an extraordinary decision, the Library of Congress this week bowed to pressure from angry anti-Freudians and postponed for as long as a year a major exhibition called "Sigmund Freud: Conflict and Culture." According to a front-page story in *The Washington Post*, some library officials blamed the delay on budget problems; but others contended that the real reason was heated criticism of a show that might take a neutral or even favorable view of the father of psychoanalysis. Some fifty psychologists and others, including Gloria Steinem and Oliver Sacks, signed a petition denouncing the proposed exhibit; as Steinem complained to the *Post*, it seemed to "have the attitude of 'He was a genius, *but...*' instead of 'He's a very troubled man, *and....*'" Though the library assured them that the exhibit "is not about whether Freudians or Freud critics, of whatever camp, are right or wrong," the critics refused an offer to contribute to the catalog or advise on the show.

Though this was perhaps the most blatant recent episode in the campaign against Freud, it is far from the only one. From *Time* to *The New York Times*, Freud-bashing has gone from an argument to a movement. In just the past few weeks Basic Books has brought out a long-winded tirade with what it no doubt hopes will be the sensational title *Why Freud Was Wrong*; and *The New York Review of Books* has collected some of its already-published broadsides against Freud into a new book.

In many cases, even the images accompanying these indictments seem to convey an extra dimension of hostility. "Is Freud dead?" *Time* magazine asked on its cover, Thanksgiving week, 1993. Whether or not this was really a question, it was certainly a repetition; for in the spring of 1966, *Time* had asked, "Is God Dead?" From a psychoanalytic point of view, repetitions are as interesting for their differences as for their similarities. With God, *Time* avoided any graven images and simply printed the question in red type against a black background, perhaps out of respect for the recently deceased. For Freud, by contrast, the magazine offered what was ostensibly a photograph of his face, but with his head blown open. One can tell it is *blown* open because what is left of the skull is shaped like a jigsaw puzzle, with several of the missing pieces flying off into space. The viewer can peer inside Freud's head and see: *there is nothing there.*

How can we explain the vehemence of these attacks on a long-dead thinker? There are, I think, three currents running through the culture that contribute to the fashion for Freud-bashing. First, the truly remarkable advances in the development of mind-altering drugs, most notably Prozac, alongside an ever-increasing understanding of the structure of the brain, have fueled speculation that one day soon all forms of talking therapy will be obsolete. Second, consumers increasingly rely on insurance companies and health maintenance organizations that prefer cheap pharmacology to expensive psychotherapy.

Finally, there is the inevitable backlash against the inflated claims that the psychoanalytic profession made for itself in the 1950s and '60s, and against its hagiography of Freud. Many reputable scholars now believe (and I agree) that Freud botched some of his most important cases. Certainly a number of his hypotheses are false; his analytic technique can seem flat-footed and intrusive; and in his speculations he was a bit of a cowboy.

It is also true that the American Psychoanalytic Association is a victim of self-inflicted wounds. In the original effort to establish psychoanalysis as a profession in this country, culminating in the 1920s, American analysts insisted that psychoanalytic training be restricted to medical doctors. The major opponent of such a restriction was Freud himself, who argued that this was "virtually equivalent to an attempt at repression." There was nothing about medical training, Freud thought, which peculiarly equipped one to become an analyst; and he suspected the Americans were motivated by the exclusionary interests of a guild. Freud lost: it was the one matter on which the American analysts openly defied the master. In the short run, this allowed the psychoanalytic profession to take advantage of the powerful positive transference that the American public extended to doctors through most of this century. Every profession in its heyday—and psychoanalysis was no exception—tends to be seduced by its own wishful self-image and to make claims for itself that it cannot ultimately sustain. In the longer run, though, psychoanalysis set itself up for revisionist criticism.

Yet, for all that, it also seems to me clear that, at his best, Freud is a deep explorer of the human condition, working in a tradition which goes back to Sophocles and which extends through Plato, Saint Augustine and Shakespeare to Proust and Nietzsche. What holds this tradition together is its insistence that there are significant meanings for human well-being which are obscured from immediate awareness. Sophoclean tragedy locates another realm of meaning in a divine world that humans can at most glimpse through oracles. In misunderstanding these strange meanings, humans usher in catastrophe.

Freud's achievement, from this perspective, is to locate these meanings fully inside the human world. Humans *make* meaning, for themselves and for others, of which they have no direct or immediate awareness. People make more meaning than they know what to do with. This is what Freud meant by the unconscious. And whatever valid criticisms can be aimed at him or at the psychoanalytic profession, it is nevertheless true that psychoanalysis is the most sustained and successful attempt to make these obscure meanings intelligible. Since I believe that this other source of meaning is of great importance for human development, I think that psychoanalytic therapy is invaluable for those who can make use of it; but, crazy as this may seem, I also believe that psychoanalysis is crucial for a truly democratic culture to thrive.

Take a closer look at the culture of criticism that has come to envelop psychoanalysis. You do not need to be an analyst to notice that more is going on here than a search for truth. Consider, for example, the emotionally charged debate over alleged memories of child abuse. No matter what side an author is on, Freud is blamed for being on the other. Jeffrey Masson, the renegade Freud scholar who believes that child abuse is more widespread than commonly acknowledged, made a name for himself by accusing Freud of suppressing the evidence in order to gain respectability. On the lecture circuit and in books like *The Assault on Truth* and *Against Therapy*, Masson has emerged as the most charismatic of the Freud-bashers, a self-styled defender of women and children against Freud's betrayals of them. Yet his critique of Freud is dependent on a willful misreading.

It is certainly true that at the beginning of his career, Freud hypothesized that hysteria and obsessional neurosis in adulthood were caused by memories of actual seductions in childhood. Because these memories were so upsetting, they were repressed, or kept out of conscious memory, but they still operated in the mind to cause psychological disease. By the fall of 1897, Freud had abandoned this view, which came to be known as the seduction theory. His explanation was that he had become increasingly skeptical that all the reports of childhood seduction—"not excluding my own"—could be straightforward memories. Masson, however, argues that this was merely Freud's attempt to fall into line with the prejudices of his German colleagues and thus to advance his career.

I find it impossible to read through Freud's writings without coming to the conclusion that it is Masson who is suppressing the evidence in order to advance his career. In fact, Freud never abandoned the idea that abuse of children caused them serious psychological harm, and throughout his career he maintained that it occurred more often than generally acknowledged. In 1917, for instance, twenty years after the abandonment of the seduction theory, Freud writes, "Phantasies of being seduced are of particular interest, because so often they are not [merely] phantasies but real memories." Even at the very end of his career, in 1938, Freud writes that while "the sexual abuse of children by adults" or "their seduction by other children (brothers or sisters) slightly their seniors" "do not apply to all children, … they are common enough." It is, therefore, misleading to say that Freud ever abandoned belief in the sexual abuse of children. What he abandoned was blind faith in the idea that alleged memories of abuse are always and everywhere what they purport to be.

Besides, to focus on child abuse is to miss the point. What is really at stake in the abandonment of the seduction theory is not the prevalence of abuse, but the nature of the mind's own activity. In assuming, as he first did, that all purported memories of child abuse were true, Freud was treating the mind as though it were merely a recipient of experience, recording reality in the same passive way a camera does light. Though the mind might be active in keeping certain memories out of conscious awareness, it was otherwise passive. In realizing that one could not take all memory-claims at face value, Freud effectively discovered that the *mind* is active and imaginative in the organization of its own experience. This is one of the crucial moments in the founding of psychoanalysis.

Of course, there is a tremendous difference—both clinical and moral—between actual and merely imagined child abuse. But from the point of view of the significance of Freud's discovery the whole issue of abuse or its absence, of seduction or its absence, is irrelevant. Once we realize that the human mind is *everywhere* active and imaginative, then we need to understand the routes of this activity if we are to grasp how the mind works. This is true whether the mind is trying to come to grips with painful reality, reacting to trauma, coping with the everyday or "just making things up."

Freud called this imaginative activity fantasy, and he argued both that it functions unconsciously and that it plays a powerful role in the organization of a person's experience. This, surely, contains the seeds of a profound insight into the human condition; it is the central insight of psychoanalysis, yet in the heated debate over child abuse, it is largely ignored. In fact, the discovery of unconscious fantasy does not itself tilt

1. BECOMING A PERSON: SEEKING SELF-IDENTITY

one way or the other in this debate. Freud himself became skeptical about whether all the purported memories of childhood seduction were actual memories—but that is because he took himself to have been overly credulous. One can equally well argue in the opposite direction: precisely because fantasy is a pervasive aspect of mental life, one needs a much more nuanced view of what constitutes real-life seduction. Because fantasy is active in parents as well as children, parents do not need to be crudely molesting their children to be seducing them. Ironically, *Freud*'s so called "abandonment of the seduction theory" can be used to widen the scope of what might be considered real seductions.

The irony is that while those who believe in the prevalence of childhood seductions attack Freud for abandoning the cause, those who believe that repressed memories of child abuse are overblown blame him for fomenting this excess. Its real origins, though, are in "recovered-memory therapy," an often quackish practice in which so-called therapists actively encourage their clients to "remember" incidents of abuse from childhood. After some initial puzzlement as to what was being asked of them, clients have been only too willing to oblige: inventing the wildest stories of satanic rituals, cannibalism and other misdemeanors of suburban life.

The consequences of believing these stories have in some cases been devastating. "As I write," Frederick Crews observes in *The New York Review of Books*, "a number of parents and child-care providers are serving long prison terms, and others are awaiting trial, on the basis of therapeutically induced 'memories' of child sexual abuse that never in fact occurred." But instead of giving Freud credit for being the first person to warn us against taking purportedly repressed memories of abuse at face value, Crews continues:

> Although the therapists in question are hardly Park Avenue psychoanalysts, the tradition of Freudian theory and practice unmistakably lies behind their tragic deception of both patients and jurors.

Crews, who is a professor of English at Berkeley and the éminence grise of Freud-bashers, acknowledges that his claim will "strike most readers as a slur." "Didn't psychoanalysis arise," he asks rhetorically, "precisely from a *denial* that certain alleged molestations were veridical?" Yes, it did. "It may seem calumnious," he writes later, "to associate the skeptical, thoroughly secular founder of psychoanalysis with the practices of Bible-thumping incest counselors who typically get their patient-victims to produce images of revolting satanic rituals." Yes, it does. But Crews is undeterred. He feels entitled to make this accusation, first, because Freud spent the earliest years of his career searching for repressed memories and, second, because Freud *did* suggest certain conclusions to his patients. That is, on occasion he took advantage of the charismatic position which people regularly assign to their doctors, teachers and political leaders and told patients how to think about themselves or what to do—sometimes to their profound detriment. Like most successful slurs, there is truth in each claim.

What is missing is the massive evidence on the other side. No one in the history of psychiatry has more openly questioned the veracity of purported childhood memories than Freud did. No one did more to devise a form of treatment which avoids suggestion. Looking back, I regularly find Freud's clinical interventions too didactic and suggestive. But the very possibility of "looking back" is due to Freud. It was Freud who first set the avoidance of suggestion as a therapeutic ideal—and it is Freud who devised the first therapeutic technique aimed at achieving it. Psychoanalysis distinguishes itself from other forms of talking cure by its rigorous attempt to work out a procedure which genuinely avoids suggestion.

This is of immense importance, for psychoanalysis thus becomes the first therapy which sets *freedom* rather than some specific image of human *happiness* as its goal. Other kinds of therapy posit particular outcomes—increased self-esteem, overcoming depression—and, implicitly or explicitly, give advice about how to get there. Psychoanalysis is the one form of therapy which leaves it to analysands to determine for themselves what their specific goals will be. Indeed, it leaves it to them to determine whether they will have specific goals. Of course, as soon as freedom becomes an ideal, enormous practical problems arise as to how one avoids compromising an analysand's freedom by unwittingly suggesting certain goals or outlooks. But if we can now criticize Freud's actual practice, it is largely due to technical advances which Freud himself inspired.

One might wonder: Why isn't Freud the hero of both these narratives, rather than the villain? Why doesn't Masson portray Freud as the pioneer who linked memories of child abuse with later psychological harm; why doesn't Crews lionize Freud as the first person to call the veracity of such memories into question? There are rational answers to these questions—in one case that he reversed his position, in the other that even though he reversed himself, he is responsible for a tradition—but neither of them are very satisfying. Rather, an emotional tide has turned, and reasons are used to cover over irrational currents. Part of this may be a healthy reversal, a reaction against previous idealizations. But it is also true that Freud is being made a scapegoat, and in the scapegoating process, nuance is abandoned.

To see nuance disappear, one has only to look at the supposed debate over the scientific standing of psychoanalysis. In a series of books and articles, Professor Adolf Grunbaum of the University of Pittsburgh has argued that psychoanalysis cannot *prove* the cause-and-effect connections it claims between unconscious motivation and its visible manifestations in ordinary life and in a clinical setting. Grunbaum argues correctly that Freud made genuine causal claims for psychoanalysis; notably, that it cures neurosis. But Grunbaum goes on to argue, much less plausibly, that in a clinical setting psychoanalysis cannot substantiate its claims. It is remarkable how many mainstream publications—*Time*, *The New York Times*, *The Economist* to name a few—have fallen all over themselves to give respectful mention to such abstruse work as Grunbaum's. Mere mention of the work lends a cloak of scientific legitimacy to the attack on Freud, while the excellent critiques of Grunbaum's work are ignored.

There is no doubt that the causal claims of psychoanalysis cannot be established in the same way as a causal claim in a hard-core empirical science like experimental physics. But neither can any causal claim of any form of psychology which interprets people's actions on the basis of their motives—including the ordinary psychology of everyday life. We watch a friend get up from her chair and head to the refrigerator: we assume she is hungry and is getting something to eat. We can, if we like, try to confirm this interpretation, but in nothing like the way we confirm something in physics. Of course, we can "test" our hypothesis by asking her what she is doing, and she may correct us, telling us that she is thirsty and getting something to drink. But it's possible that she's not telling us the truth. Indeed, it's possible, though unlikely, that she believes that the refrigerator is capable of sending messages to outer space, which will save the world from catastrophe. We cannot *prove* that our ordinary interpretation is correct. At best, we can gather more interpretive evidence of the same type to support or revise our hypothesis.

What are we to do, abandon our ordinary practice of interpreting people? If we want to know what caused the outbreak of the Peloponnesian War, why there is a crisis in the Balkans, what were the origins of the Renaissance, how slavery became institutionalized, we turn to history, economics and other social sciences for answers. No historical account is immune to skeptical challenge; no historical-causal claims can be verified in the same way as a causal claim in physics. But no one suggests giving up on history or the other interpretive sciences.

Meaning is like that. Humans are inherently makers and interpreters of meaning. It is meaning—ideas, desires, beliefs—which causes humans to do the interesting things they do. Yet as soon as one enters the realm of meaningful explanation one has to employ different methods of validating causal claims than one finds in experimental physics. And it is simply a mistake to think that therefore the methods of validation in ordinary psychology or in psychoanalysis must be less precise or fall short of the methods in experimental physics. To see this for yourself, take the following multiple-choice test:

> Question: Which is more precise, Henry James, in his ability to describe how a person's action flows from his or her motivations; or a particle accelerator, in its ability to depict the causal interactions of subatomic particles?
> Answers: *(a)* Henry James
> *(b)* the accelerator
> *(c)* none of the above

You do not have to flip to the end of the article or turn the page upside-down to learn that the answer is *(c)*. Actually, a better answer is to reject the question as ridiculous. There is no single scale on which one can place both Henry James and a particle accelerator to determine which is more precise. Within the realm of human motivation and its effects, *Portrait of a Lady* is more precise than a Peanuts cartoon; within the realm of measuring atomic movements, some instruments are more precise than others.

If psychoanalysis *were* to imitate the methods of physical science, it would be useless for interpreting people. Psychoanalysis is an extension of our ordinary psychological ways of interpreting people in terms of their beliefs, desires, hopes and fears. The extension is important because psychoanalysis attributes to people other forms of motivation—in particular wish and fantasy—which attempt to account for outbreaks of irrationality and other puzzling human behavior. In fact, it is a sign of psychoanalysis's *success* as an interpretive science that its causal claims cannot be validated in the same way as those of the physical sciences.

How, then, might we set appropriate standards of confirmation for causal claims in psychoanalysis? This genuine and important question tends to be brushed aside by the cliché of the analyst telling a patient who disagrees with an interpretation that she is just resisting. The apotheosis of this cliché can be found in Sir Karl Popper's *The Open Society and Its Enemies*, in which Popper argues that psychoanalysis is a pseudo-science because its discoveries cannot be falsified: what counts as evidence is too large and elusive for the total claim of the discipline to be either checked or challenged. Of course, in this broad sense nothing could "falsify" history or economics or our ordinary psychological interpretation of persons, but no one would think of calling these forms of explanation pseudo. And there *is* something that would count as a global refutation of psychoanalysis: if people always and everywhere acted in rational and transparently explicable ways, one could easily dismiss psychoanalysis as unnecessary rubbish. It is because people often behave in bizarre ways, ways which cause pain to themselves and to others, ways which puzzle even the actors themselves, that psychoanalysis commands our attention.

Unfortunately, there is some truth to the cliché of the analyst unfairly pulling rank on the analysand. Would that there were no such thing as a defensive analyst! Yet I believe that when psychoanalysis is done properly there is no form of clinical intervention—in psychology, psychiatry or general medicine—that pays greater respect to the individual client or patient. The proper attitude for an analyst is one of profound humility in the face of the infinite complexity of another human being. Because humans are self-interpreting animals, one must always be ready to defer to their explanations of what they mean. And yet, suppose just for the sake of argument that it is true that humans actively keep certain unpleasant meanings away from conscious awareness. Then one might expect that any process which brings those meanings closer to consciousness will be accompanied by a certain resistance. It then becomes an important technical and theoretical problem how to elicit those meanings without

1. BECOMING A PERSON: SEEKING SELF-IDENTITY

falling into the cliché, without provoking a massive outbreak of resistance, and all the while working closely with and maintaining deep respect for the analysand. We need to know in specific detail when and how it is appropriate to cite resistance in a clinical setting, and when it is not. Some of the best recent work in psychoanalytic theory addresses just this issue.

Consider this elementary example: an analysand may come precisely five minutes late every day for his session. For a while, there may be no point in inviting him to speculate about why. Any such question, no matter how gently or tentatively put, might only provoke a storm of protest: "you don't know how busy I am, how many sacrifices I make to get here," and so on. Even if the habitual lateness and the protests *are* examples of what analysts call resistance, there is one excellent reason not to say anything about it yet: the analysis is for the analysand. Any interpretation that he cannot make use of in his journey of self-understanding is inappropriate, even if the interpretation is accurate. *If* coming late is a resistance, and if the analyst is sufficiently patient, there will come a time when he will relax enough to become puzzled by his own behavior. He might say, "it's funny, I always seem to come exactly five minutes late," or "I've thought about asking you to start our sessions five minutes late, but I realized I'd only come five minutes later than that." At this point it would be a mistake not to pursue the issue, for a wealth of material may spontaneously emerge: for example, that he wanted to feel that he was in control, that he wanted the analyst to acknowledge him as a serious professional in his own right, etc. Once these desires are recognized, they can be explored—and sometimes that exploration can make a big difference in how the analysand sees himself and how he goes on to live the rest of his life. Should all of this be avoided because of some flat-footed assumption that the analyst is always pulling rank when she talks about resistance? The problem with the cliché is that it ignores all specifics. It uses the very possibility of invoking resistance to impugn psychoanalysis generally.

What is at stake in all of these attacks? If this were merely the attack on one historical figure, Freud, or on one professional group, psychoanalysts, the hubbub would have died down long ago. After all, psychoanalysis nowadays plays a minor role in the mental health professions; Freud is less and less often taught or studied. There is, of course, a certain pleasure to be had in pretending one is bravely attacking a powerful authority when one is in fact participating in a gang-up. But even these charms fade after a while. The real object of attack—for which Freud is only a stalking horse—is the very idea of humans having unconscious motivation. A battle may be fought over Freud, but the war is over our culture's image of the human soul. Are we to see humans as having depth—as complex psychological organisms who generate layers of meaning which lie beneath the surface of their own understanding? Or are we to take ourselves as transparent to ourselves?

Certainly, the predominant trend in the culture is to treat human existence as straightforward. In the plethora of self-help books, of alternative therapies, diets and exercise programs, it is assumed that we already know what human happiness is. These programs promise us a shortcut for getting there. And yet we can all imagine someone whose muscle tone is great, who is successful at his job, who "feels good about himself," yet remains a shell of a human being. Breathless articles in the science section of *The New York Times* suggest that the main obstacle to human flourishing is technological. And even this obstacle—in the recent discovery of a gene, or the location of a neuron in the brain, or in the synthesis of a new psychopharmacological agent—may soon be put out of the way. Candide is the ideal reader of the "Science Times." Of course, the *Times* did not invent this image of the best of all possible worlds: it is merely the bellwether for a culture that wishes to ignore the complexity, depth and darkness of human life.

It is difficult to make this point without sounding like a Luddite; so let me say explicitly that psychopharmacology and neuro-psychiatry have made, and will continue to make, valuable contributions in reducing human suffering. But it is a fantasy to suppose that a chemical or neurological intervention can solve the problems posed in and by human life. That is why it is a mistake to think of psychoanalysis and Prozac as two different means to the same end. The point of psychoanalysis is to help us develop a clearer, yet more flexible and creative, sense of what our ends might be. "How shall we live?" is, for Socrates, the fundamental question of human existence—and the attempt to answer that question is, for him, what makes human life worthwhile. And it is Plato and Shakespeare, Proust, Nietzsche and, most recently, Freud who complicated the issue by insisting that there are deep currents of meaning, often crosscurrents, running through the human soul which can at best be glimpsed through a glass darkly. This, if anything, is the Western tradition: not a specific set of values, but a belief that the human soul is too deep for there to be any easy answer to the question of how to live.

If one can dismiss Freud as a charlatan, one cannot only enjoy the sacrifice of a scapegoat, one can also evade troubling questions about the enigmatic nature of human motivation. Never mind that we are daily surrounded by events—from the assassination of Yitzhak Rabin to the war in Bosnia; from the murder of Nicole Simpson to the public fascination with it; from the government's burning of the Branch Davidian compound to the retaliation bombing in Oklahoma City—that cannot be understood in the terms that are standardly used to explain them. Philosophy, Aristotle said, begins in wonder. Psychoanalysis begins in wonder that the unintelligibility of the events that surround one do not cause more wonder.

4. Shrink Is In

There are two very different images of what humans must be like if democracy is to be a viable form of government. The prevalent one today treats humans as preference-expressing political atoms, and pays little attention to subatomic structure. Professional pollsters, political scientists and pundits portray society as an agglomeration of these atoms. The only irrationality they recognize is the failure of these preference-expressing monads to conform to the rules of rational choice theory. If one thinks that this is the only image of humanity that will sustain democracy, one will tend to view psychoanalysis as suspiciously anti-democratic.

Is there another, more satisfying, image of what humans are like which nevertheless makes it plausible that they should organize themselves and live in democratic societies? If we go back to the greatest participatory democracy the world has known—the polis of fifth-century Athens—we see that the flourishing of that democracy coincides precisely with the flowering of one of the world's great literatures: Greek tragedy. This coincidence is not mere coincidence. The tragic theater gave citizens the opportunity to retreat momentarily from the responsibility of making rational decisions for themselves and their society. At the same time, tragedy confronted them emotionally with the fact that they had to make their decisions in a world that was not entirely rational, in which rationality was sometimes violently disrupted, in which rationality itself could be used for irrational ends.

What, after all, is Oedipus's complex? That he killed his father and married his mother misses the point. Patricide and maternal incest are *consequences* of Oedipus's failure, not its source. Oedipus's fundamental mistake lies in his assumption that meaning is transparent to human reason. In horrified response to the Delphic oracle, Oedipus flees the people he (mistakenly) takes to be his parents. En route, he kills his actual father and propels himself into the arms of his mother. It is the classic scene of fulfilling one's fate in the very act of trying to escape it. But this scenario is only possible because Oedipus assumes he understands his situation, that the meaning of the oracle is immediately available to his conscious understanding. That is why he thinks he can respond to the oracle with a straightforward application of practical reason. Oedipus's mistake, in essence, is to ignore unconscious meaning.

For Sophocles, this was a sacrilegious crime, for he took this obscure meaning to flow from a divine source. But it is clear that, in Sophocles's vision, Oedipus attacks the very idea of unconscious meaning. In his angry confrontation with the prophet Tiresias, Oedipus boasts that it was his conscious reasoning, not any power of interpreting obscure meaning, which saved the city from the horrible Sphinx.

"Why, come, tell me, how can you be a true prophet? Why when the versifying hound was here did you not speak some word that could release the citizens? Indeed, her riddle was not one for the first comer to explain! It required prophetic skill, and you were exposed as having no knowledge from the birds or from the gods. No, it was I that came, Oedipus who knew nothing, and put a stop to her; I hit the mark by native wit, not by what I learned from birds."

What was Sophocles's message to the Athenian citizens who flocked to the theater? *You ignore the realm of unconscious meaning at your peril. Do so, and Oedipus's fate will be yours.* From this perspective, democratic citizens need to maintain a certain humility in the face of meanings which remain opaque to human reason. We need to be wary that what we take to be an exercise of reason will both hide and express an irrationality of which we remain unaware.

In all the recent attacks on Freud, can't one hear echoes of Oedipus's attack on Tiresias? Isn't the attack on Freud itself a repetition and re-enactment of Oedipus's complex, less an attack on the father than an attack on the very idea of repressed, unconscious meaning? One indication that this is so—a symptom, if you will—is that none of the attacks on Freud addresses the problems of human existence to which psychoanalysis is a response. From a psychoanalytic perspective, human irrationality is not merely a failure to make a coherent set of choices. Sometimes it is an unintelligible intrusion that overwhelms reason and blows it apart. Sometimes it is method in madness. But how could there be *method* in *madness*? Even if Freud did botch this case or ambitiously pursue that end, we still need to account for the pervasive manifestations of human irrationality. This is the issue, and it is one which the attacks on Freud ignore.

The real question is whether, and how, responsible autonomy is possible. In the development of the human self-image from Sophocles to Freud, there has been a shift in the locus of hidden meaning from a divine to the all-too-human realm. At first, it might look as though the recognition of a dark strain running through the human soul might threaten the viability of democratic culture. Certainly, the twentieth-century critiques of Enlightenment optimism, with the corresponding emphasis on human irrationality, also question or even pour scorn on the democratic ideal. It is in this context that Freud comes across as a much more ambiguous figure than he is normally taken to be. In one way, he is the advocate of the unconscious; in another, he is himself filled with Enlightenment optimism that the problems posed by the unconscious can be solved; in yet another, he is wary of the dark side of the human soul and pessimistic about doing much to alleviate psychological pain. He is Tiresias and Oedipus and Sophocles rolled into one.

If, for the moment, we concentrate on the optimism, we see a vision emerge of how one might both take human irrationality seriously and participate in a democratic ideal. If the source of irrationality lies within, rather than outside, the human realm, the pos-

1. BECOMING A PERSON: SEEKING SELF-IDENTITY

sibility opens up of a responsible engagement with it. Psychoanalysis is, in its essence, the attempt to work out just such an engagement. It is a technique that allows dark meanings and irrational motivations to rise to the surface of conscious awareness. They can then be taken into account; they can be influenced by other considerations; and they become less liable to disrupt human life in violent and incomprehensible ways. Critics of psychoanalysis complain that it is a luxury of the few. But, from the current perspective, no thinker has made creativity and imagination more democratically available than Freud. This is one of the truly important consequences of locating the unconscious inside the psyche. Creativity is no longer the exclusive preserve of the divinely inspired, or the few great poets. From a psychoanalytic point of view, everyone is poetic; everyone dreams in metaphor and generates symbolic meaning in the process of living. Even in their prose, people have unwittingly been speaking poetry all along.

And the question now is: To what poetic use are we going to put Freud? Freud *is* dead. He died in 1939, after an extraordinarily productive and creative life. Beneath the continued attacks upon him, ironically, lies an unwillingness to let him go. It is Freud who taught that only after we accept the actual death of an important person in our lives can we begin to mourn. Only then can he or she take on full symbolic life for us. Obsessing about Freud *the man* is a way of keeping Freud *the meaning* at bay. Freud's meaning, I think, lies in the recognition that humans make more meaning than they grasp, that this meaning can be painful and disruptive, but that humans need not be passive in the face of it. Freud began a process of dealing with unconscious meaning, and it is important not to get stuck on him, like some rigid symptom, either to idolize or to denigrate him. The many attacks on him, even upon psychoanalysis, refuse to recognize that Freud gave birth to a psychoanalytic movement which in myriad ways has moved beyond him. If Freud is alive anywhere, it is in a tradition which in its development of more sensitive techniques, and more sophisticated ways of thinking about unconscious motivation, has rendered some of the particular things Freud thought or did irrelevant. Just as democracy requires the recognition that the king is dead, both as an individual and as an institution, so the democratic recognition that each person is the maker of unconscious, symbolic meaning requires the acceptance of Freud's death. What matters, as Freud himself well understood, is what we are able to do with the meanings we make.

HOW USEFUL IS *Fantasy?*

Daydreams can help us prepare for future events by keeping us aware of unfinished business

Paul M. Insel, Ph.D.

Dr. Insel, Editor-in-Chief of HEALTHLINE, is Clinical Associate Professor of Psychiatry at the Stanford University School of Medicine.

EVERYONE DAYDREAMS, ESPECIALLY THOSE of us who are fantasy-prone, and particularly at times when we are tired of focusing on tasks that are tedious or intense. Daydreaming, or fantasizing, can be adaptive: it can help prepare us for future events. It can also substitute for impulsive behavior and help us get past a frustrating or anger-provoking experience.

Here's an example of one use of fantasy: Ralph Thomas, a mild-mannered bank clerk, pulls into the parking lot at work and finds that his parking space is taken by one of the senior bank managers, who is both aggressive and unfriendly. Instead of confronting the manager, Ralph fantasizes about walking up to him, grabbing him by the scruff of the neck in front of admiring onlookers, and yelling at him about his inconsiderate and callous behavior. Although he never says a thing to the manager, he nevertheless feels better about the situation, at least for the moment. If it happens again he still is unlikely to assertively confront the manager, but he may be prompted to at least mention his frustration to the manager or another employee.

Through extensive interviews and questionnaires, psychologist Jerome Singer has found that almost everyone has daydreams, or waking fantasies, every day—on the train, on the job, in the elevator, or walking down the street; in fact, we daydream almost anywhere, at any time. Young adults spend more time daydreaming and admit to more sexual fantasies than do older adults.

In *The Secret Life of Walter Mitty*, a classic story by James Thurber, Mitty seasons a rather bland life with heroic fantasies, imagining himself as the hero in a variety of scenes played out in his mind's eye. He returns triumphant at the head of an army to the acclaim of the crowd. As he drives past a hospital, Dr. Mitty astounds renowned specialists with his surgical skill. In one fantasy after another he is courageous and valiant, reaching unending pinnacles of heroism.

Not all fantasy is escapist or dramatic. Mostly people daydream about the details of their lives, such as imagining an alternative approach to a task they are performing, picturing themselves explaining to the boss why they are late, or replaying "mind tapes" about personal encounters they either savor or wish had gone differently.

According to one study, close to 4 percent of the population has fantasy-prone personalities. As children, they had enjoyed intense make-believe play with their dolls, stuffed animals, or imaginary companions. As adults, they reported spending more than half their time fantasizing. They would relive experiences or imagine scenes so vividly that occasionally they later had trouble differentiating remembered fantasies from their memories of actual events. Most of the women with fantasy-prone personalities were able to experience orgasm solely through sexual fantasy.

Are the many hours we spend in fantasy merely a way of escaping reality, or can this daydreaming serve another purpose? Studies of children have shown that daydreaming in the form of imaginative play has been shown to play an important role in social and cognitive development. Playful fantasies also enhance the creativity of scientists, writers, and artists. Albert Einstein felt this way about fantasy: *When I examined myself, and my methods of thought, I came to the conclusion that the gift of fantasy has meant more to me than my talent for absorbing positive knowledge.*

For many of us, fantasy is adaptive and useful. Daydreams can help us prepare for future events by keeping us aware of unfinished business. This unique kind of mind process can help us rehearse upcoming events, observe potential problems in our behavior, and resolve them before the event is experienced. Behavior therapy makes use of mental rehearsal to help us safely experience frightening thoughts or ideas.

Therapists use imagery, a kind of fantasy, to strip encounters that are intimidating or anxiety-producing of their fearful aspects. One woman dreaded appearing in court because she was intimidated by the authority of lawyers and judges. She was able to overcome this fear by imagining these authorities in tennis shorts and polo shirts with funny sayings on them. The use of imagery has been successful with people who suffer from test or performance anxiety by

1. BECOMING A PERSON: SEEKING SELF-IDENTITY

helping them to see themselves as feeling confident and accomplished when taking tests.

Can fantasy also substitute for impulsive and aggressive behavior? Dr. Singer has suggested that people who are prone to delinquency and violence, or who seek the artificial highs of dangerous drugs have fewer vivid fantasies than average. Psychologist Seymour Feshbach from the University of California tested the theory that fantasy works to reduce subsequent aggression. He set up his experiment with students who were insulted by their instructor. Half of the students were given the opportunity to write imaginative stories about aggression, while the other half were not given the opportunity. There was also a control group of students who were not insulted. Feshbach's results showed that people who had been given the opportunity to write stories about aggression were less aggressive than those who were not given the opportunity. Both groups of insulted students were more aggressive than the control group of students who were not insulted at all.

A fantasy can be a map or a navigational path that steers us safely between the reefs and shoals of anger, guilt, frustration, anxiety, and inhibition; it can help prepare us for future events; and it can add spice and excitement to an otherwise dull existence.

The Rewards of Learning

To teach without using extrinsic rewards is analogous to asking our students to learn to draw with their eyes closed, Mr. Chance maintains. Before we do that, we should open our own eyes.

Paul Chance

Paul Chance (Eastern Shore Maryland Chapter) is a psychologist, writer, and teacher. He is the author of Thinking in the Classroom *(Teachers College Press, 1986) and teaches at James H. Groves Adult High School in Georgetown, Del.*

A man is seated at a desk. Before him lie a pencil and a large stack of blank paper. He picks up the pencil, closes his eyes, and attempts to draw a four-inch line. He makes a second attempt, a third, a fourth, and so on, until he has made well over a hundred attempts at drawing a four-inch line, all without ever opening his eyes. He repeats the exercise for several days, until he has drawn some 3,000 lines, all with his eyes closed. On the last day, he examines his work. The question is, How much improvement has there been in his ability to draw a four-inch line? How much has he learned from his effort?

E. L. Thorndike, the founder of educational psychology and a major figure in the scientific analysis of learning, performed this experiment years ago, using himself as subject.[1] He found no evidence of learning. His ability to draw a four-inch line was no better on the last day than it had been on the first.

The outcome of this experiment may seem obvious to us today, but it was an effective way of challenging a belief widely held earlier in this century, a belief that formed the very foundation of education at the time: the idea that "practice makes perfect."

It was this blind faith in practice that justified countless hours of rote drill as a standard teaching technique. Thorndike's experiment demonstrated that practice in and of itself is not sufficient for learning. Based on this and other, more formal studies, Thorndike concluded that practice is important only insofar as it provides the opportunity for reinforcement.

To reinforce means to strengthen, and among learning researchers *reinforcement* refers to a procedure for strengthening behavior (that is, making it likely to be repeated) by providing certain kinds of consequences.[2] These consequences, called *reinforcers,* are usually events or things a person willingly seeks out. For instance, we might teach a person to draw a four-inch line with his eyes closed merely by saying "good" each time the effort is within half an inch of the goal. Most people like to succeed, so this positive feedback should be an effective way of reinforcing the appropriate behavior.

Hundreds of experimental studies have demonstrated that systematic use of reinforcement can improve both classroom conduct and the rate of learning. Yet the systematic use of reinforcement has never been widespread in American schools. In *A Place Called School*, John Goodlad reports that, in the elementary grades, an average of only 2% of class time is devoted to reinforcement; in the high schools, the figure falls to 1%.[3]

THE COSTS OF REWARD

There are probably many reasons for our failure to make the most of reinforcement. For one thing, few schools of education provide more than cursory instruction in its use. Given Thorndike's finding about the role of practice in learning, it is ironic that many teachers actually use the term *reinforcement* as a synonym for *practice*. ("We assign workbook exercises for reinforcement.") If schools of education do not teach future teachers the nature of reinforcement and how to use it effectively, teachers can hardly be blamed for not using it.

The unwanted effects of misused reinforcement have led some teachers to shy away from it. The teacher who sometimes lets a noisy class go to recess early will find the class getting noisier before recess. If high praise is reserved for long-winded essays, students will develop wordy and redundant writing styles. And it should surprise no one if students are seldom original in classrooms where only conventional work is admired or if they are uncooperative in classrooms where one can earn recognition only through competition. Reinforcement is powerful stuff, and its misuse can cause problems.

Another difficulty is that the optimal use of reinforcement would mean teaching in a new way. Some studies suggest that maximum learning in elementary and middle schools might require very high rates of reinforcement, perhaps with teachers praising someone in the class an average of once every 15 seconds.[4] Such a requirement is clearly incompatible with traditional teaching practices.

Systematic reinforcement can also mean more work for the teacher. Reinforcing behavior once every 15 seconds means 200 reinforcements in a 50-minute period — 1,000 reinforcements in a typical school day. It also implies that, in order to spot behavior to reinforce, the teacher must be moving about the room, not sitting at a desk marking papers. That may be too much to ask. Some studies have found that teachers who have been taught how to make good use of reinforcement often revert to their old style of teaching. This is so even though the teachers acknowledge that increased use of reinforcement means fewer discipline problems and a much faster rate of learning.[5]

Reinforcement also runs counter to our Puritan traditions. Most Americans have

1. BECOMING A PERSON: SEEKING SELF-IDENTITY

always assumed — occasional protestations to the contrary notwithstanding — that learning should be hard work and at least slightly unpleasant. Often the object of education seems to be not so much to teach academic and social skills as to "build character" through exposure to adversity. When teachers reinforce students at a high rate, the students experience a minimum of adversity and actually enjoy learning. Thus some people think that reinforcement is bad for character development.

All of these arguments against reinforcement can be countered effectively. Schools of education do not provide much instruction in the practical use of reinforcement, but there is no reason why they cannot do so. Reinforcement can be used incorrectly and with disastrous results, but the same might be said of other powerful tools. Systematic use of reinforcement means teaching in a new way, but teachers can learn to do so.[6] A great deal of reinforcement is needed for optimum learning, but not all of the reinforcement needs to come from the teacher. (Reinforcement can be provided by computers and other teaching devices, by teacher aides, by parents, and by students during peer teaching and cooperative learning.) No doubt people do sometimes benefit from adversity, but the case for the character-building properties of adversity is very weak.[7]

However, there is one argument against reinforcement that cannot be dismissed so readily. For some 20 years, the claim has been made that systematic reinforcement actually undermines student learning. Those few teachers who make extensive use of reinforcement, it is claimed, do their students a disservice because reinforcement reduces interest in the reinforced activity.

Not all forms of reinforcement are considered detrimental. A distinction is made between reinforcement involving intrinsic reinforcers — or rewards, as they are often called — and reinforcement involving extrinsic rewards.[8] Only extrinsic rewards are said to be harmful. An *intrinsic reward* is ordinarily the natural consequence of behavior, hence the name. We learn to throw darts by seeing how close the dart is to the target; learn to type by seeing the right letters appear on the computer screen; learn to cook from the pleasant sights, fragrances, and flavors that result from our culinary efforts; learn to read from the understanding we get from the printed word; and learn to solve puzzles by finding solutions. The Japanese say, "The bow teaches the archer." They are talking about intrinsic rewards, and they are right.

Extrinsic rewards come from an outside source, such as a teacher. Probably the most ubiquitous extrinsic reward (and one of the most effective) is praise. The teacher reinforces behavior by saying "good," "right," "correct," or "excellent" when the desired behavior occurs. Other extrinsic rewards involve nonverbal behavior such as smiles, winks, thumbs-up signs, hugs, congratulatory handshakes, pats on the back, or applause. Gold stars, certificates, candy, prizes, and even money have been used as rewards, but they are usually less important in teaching — and even in the maintenance of good discipline — than those mentioned earlier.

The distinction between intrinsic and extrinsic rewards is somewhat artificial. Consider the following example. You put money into a vending machine and retrieve a candy bar. The behavior of inserting money into a vending machine has been reinforced, as has the more general behavior of interacting with machines. But is the food you receive an intrinsic or an extrinsic reward? On the one hand, the food is the automatic consequence of inserting money and pressing buttons, so it would appear to be an intrinsic reward. On the other hand, the food is a consequence that was arranged by the designer of the machine, so it would seem to be an extrinsic reward.[9]

Though somewhat contrived, the distinction between intrinsic and extrinsic rewards has been maintained partly because extrinsic rewards are said to be damaging.[10] Are they? First, let us be clear about the charge. The idea is that — if teachers smile, praise, congratulate, say "thank you" or "right," shake hands, hug, give a pat on the back, applaud, provide a certificate of achievement or attendance, *or in any way provide a positive consequence (a reward) for student behavior* — the student will be less inclined to engage in that behavior when the reward is no longer available.

For example, teachers who offer prizes to students for reading books will, it is said, make the children less likely to read when prizes are no longer available. The teacher who reads a student's story aloud to the class as an example of excellent story writing actually makes the student less likely to write stories in the future, when such public approval is not forthcoming. When teachers (and students) applaud a youngster who has given an excellent talk, they make that student disinclined to give talks in the future. The teacher who comments favorably on the originality of a painting steers the young artist away from painting. And so on. This is the charge against extrinsic rewards.

No one disputes the effectiveness of extrinsic rewards in teaching or in maintaining good discipline. Some might therefore argue that extrinsic rewards should be used, even if they reduce interest in learning. Better to have students who read only when required to do so, some might say, than to have students who cannot read at all.

But if rewards do reduce interest, that fact is of tremendous importance. "The teacher may count himself successful," wrote B. F. Skinner, "when his students become engrossed in his field, study conscientiously, and do more than is required of them, but *the important thing is what they do when they are no longer being taught*" (emphasis added).[11] It is not enough for students to learn the three R's and a little science and geography; they must be prepared for a lifetime of learning. To reduce their interest in learning would be a terrible thing — even if it were done in the interest of teaching them effectively.

The question of whether rewards adversely affect motivation is not, then, of merely academic or theoretical importance. It is of great practical importance to the classroom teacher.

Extrinsic rewards are said to be damaging. Are they? First, let us be clear about the charge.

6. Rewards of Learning

More than 100 studies have examined this question.[12] In a typical experiment, Mark Lepper and his colleagues observed 3- to 5-year-old nursery school children playing with various kinds of toys.[13] The toys available included felt tip pens of various colors and paper to draw on. The researchers noted the children's inclination to draw during this period. Next the researchers took the children aside and asked them to draw with the felt tip pens. The researchers promised some children a "Good Player Award" for drawing. Other children drew pictures without receiving an award.

Two weeks later, the researchers returned to the school, provided felt tip pens and paper, and observed the children's inclination to draw. They found that children who had been promised an award spent only half as much time drawing as they had originally. Those students who had received no award showed no such decline in interest.

Most studies in this area follow the same general outline: 1) students are given the opportunity to participate in an activity without rewards; 2) they are given extrinsic rewards for participating in the activity; and 3) they are again given the opportunity to participate in the activity without rewards.

The outcomes of the studies are also fairly consistent. Not surprisingly, there is usually a substantial increase in the activity during the second stage, when extrinsic rewards are available. And, as expected, participation in the activity declines sharply when rewards are no longer available. However, interest sometimes falls below the initial level, so that students are less interested in the activity than they had been before receiving rewards. It is this net loss of motivation that is of concern.

Researchers have studied this decline in motivation and found that it occurs only under certain circumstances. For example, the effect is most likely to occur when the initial interest in the activity is very high, when the rewards used are *not* reinforcers, and when the rewards are held out in advance as incentives.[14]

But perhaps the best predictor of negative effects is the nature of the "reward contingency" involved. (The term *reward contingency* has to do with the nature of the relationship between behavior and its reward.) Alyce Dickinson reviewed the research literature in this area and identified three kinds of reward contingency:[15]

Task-contingent rewards are available for merely participating in an activity, without regard to any standard of performance. Most studies that find a decline in interest in a rewarded activity involve task-contingent rewards. In the Lepper study described above, for instance, children received an award for drawing *regardless of how they drew*. The reward was task-contingent.

Performance-contingent rewards are available only when the student achieves a certain standard. Performance-contingent rewards sometimes produce negative results. For instance, Edward Deci offered college students money for solving puzzles, $1 for each puzzle solved. The rewarded students were later less inclined to work on the puzzles than were students who had not been paid. Unfortunately, these results are difficult to interpret because the students sometimes failed to meet the reward standard, and failure itself is known to reduce interest in an activity.[16]

Success-contingent rewards are given for good performance and might reflect either success or progress toward a goal. Success-contingent rewards do not have negative effects; in fact, they typically *increase* interest in the rewarded activity. For example, Ross Vasta and Louise Stirpe awarded gold stars to third- and fourth-graders each time they completed a kind of math exercise they enjoyed. After seven days of awards, the gold stars stopped. Not only was there no evidence of a loss in interest, but time spent on the math activity actually increased. Nor was there any decline in the quality of the work produced.[17]

Dickinson concludes that the danger of undermining student motivation stems not from extrinsic rewards, but from the use of inappropriate reward contingencies. Rewards reduce motivation when they are given without regard to performance or when the performance standard is so high that students frequently fail. When students have a high rate of success and when those successes are rewarded, the rewards *do not have negative effects*. Indeed, success-contingent rewards tend to increase interest in the activity. This finding, writes Dickinson, "is robust and consistent." She adds that "even strong opponents of contingent rewards recognize that success-based rewards do not have harmful effects."[18]

The evidence, then, shows that extrinsic rewards can either enhance or reduce interest in an activity, depending on how they are used. Still, it might be argued that, because extrinsic rewards *sometimes* cause problems, we might be wise to avoid their use altogether. The decision not to use extrinsic rewards amounts to a decision to rely on alternatives. What are those alternatives? And are they better than extrinsic rewards?

ALTERNATIVES TO REWARDS

Punishment and the threat of punishment are — and probably always have been — the most popular alternatives to extrinsic rewards. Not so long ago, lessons were "taught to the tune of a hickory stick," but the tune was not merely tapped on a desk. Students who did not learn their lessons were not only beaten; they were also humiliated: they sat on a stool (up high, so everyone could see) and wore a silly hat.

Gradually, more subtle forms of punishment were used. "The child at his desk," wrote Skinner, "filling in his workbook, is behaving primarily to escape from the threat of a series of minor aversive events — the teacher's displeasure, the criticism or ridicule of his classmates, an ignominious showing in a competition, low marks, a trip to the office 'to be talked to' by the principal, or a word to the parent who may still resort to the birch rod."[19] Skinner spent a lifetime inveighing against the use of such "aversives," but his efforts were largely ineffective. While extrinsic rewards have been condemned, punishment and the threat of punishment are widely sanctioned.

Punishment is popular because, in the short run at least, it gets results. This is illustrated by an experiment in which Deci and Wayne Cascio told students that, if they did not solve problems correctly within a time limit, they would be exposed to a loud, unpleasant sound. The threat worked: all the students solved all the problems within the time limit, so the threat never had to be fulfilled. Students who were merely rewarded for correct solutions did not do nearly as well.[20]

But there are serious drawbacks to the use of punishment. For one thing, although punishment motivates students to learn, it does not teach them. Or, rather, it teaches them only what *not* to do, not what *to* do. "We do not teach [a student] to learn quickly," Skinner observed, "by punishing him when he learns slowly, or to recall what he has learned by punishing him when he forgets, or to

1. BECOMING A PERSON: SEEKING SELF-IDENTITY

think logically by punishing him when he is illogical."[21]

Punishment also has certain undesirable side effects.[22] To the extent that punishment works, it works by making students anxious. Students get nervous before a test because they fear a poor grade, and they are relieved or anxious when they receive their report card depending on whether or not the grades received will result in punishment from their parents.[23] Students can and do avoid the anxiety caused by such punishment by cutting classes and dropping out of school. We do the same thing when we cancel or "forget" a dental appointment.

Another response to punishment is aggression. Students who do not learn easily — and who therefore cannot readily avoid punishment — are especially apt to become aggressive. Their aggression often takes the form of lying, cheating, stealing, and refusing to cooperate. Students also act out by cursing, by being rude and insulting, by destroying property, and by hitting people. Increasingly, teachers are the objects of these aggressive acts.

Finally, it should be noted that punishment has the same negative impact on intrinsic motivation as extrinsic rewards are alleged to have. In the Deci and Cascio study just described, for example, when students were given the chance to work on puzzles with the threat of punishment removed, they were less likely to do so than were students who had never worked under the threat of punishment.[24] Punishment in the form of criticism of performance also reduces interest in an activity.[25]

Punishment is not the only alternative to the use of extrinsic rewards. Teachers can also encourage students. Encouragement consists of various forms of behavior intended to induce students to perform. We encourage students when we urge them to try, express confidence in their ability to do assignments, and recite such platitudes as "A winner never quits and a quitter never wins."[26]

In encouraging students, we are not merely urging them to perform, however; we are implicitly suggesting a relationship between continued performance and certain consequences. "Come on, Billy — you can do it" means, "If you persist at this task, you will be rewarded with success." The power of encouragement is ultimately dependent on the occurrence of the implied consequences. If the teacher tells Billy he can do it and if he tries and fails, future urging by the teacher will be less effective.

Another problem with encouragement is that, like punishment, it motivates but does not teach. The student who is urged to perform a task is not thereby taught how to perform it. Encouragement is a safer procedure than punishment, since it is less likely to provoke anxiety or aggression. Students who are repeatedly urged to do things at which they ultimately fail do, however, come to distrust the judgment of the teacher. They also come to believe that they cannot live up to the expectations of teachers — and therefore must be hopelessly stupid.

Intrinsic rewards present the most promising alternative to extrinsic rewards. Experts on reinforcement, including defenders of extrinsic rewards, universally sing the praises of intrinsic rewards. Unlike punishment and encouragement, intrinsic rewards actually teach. Students who can see that they have solved a problem correctly know how to solve other problems of that sort. And, unlike extrinsic rewards, intrinsic rewards do not depend on the teacher or some other person.

But there are problems with intrinsic rewards, just as there are with extrinsic ones. Sometimes students lack the necessary skills to obtain intrinsic rewards. Knowledge, understanding, and the aesthetic pleasures of language are all intrinsic rewards for reading, but they are not available to those for whom reading is a difficult and painful activity.

Often, intrinsic rewards are too remote to be effective. If a student is asked to add 3 + 7, what is the intrinsic reward for answering correctly? The student who learns to add will one day experience the satisfaction of checking the accuracy of a restaurant bill, but this future reward is of no value to the youngster just learning to add. Though important in maintaining what has been learned, intrinsic rewards are often too remote to be effective reinforcers in the early stages of learning.

One problem that often goes unnoticed is that the intrinsic rewards for academic work are often weaker than the rewards available for other behavior. Students are rewarded for looking out the window, daydreaming, reading comic books, taking things from other students, passing notes, telling and listening to jokes, moving about the room, fighting, talking back to the teacher, and for all sorts of activities that are incompatible with academic learning. Getting the right answer to a grammar question might be intrinsically rewarding, but for many students it is considerably less rewarding than the laughter of one's peers in response to a witty remark.

While intrinsic rewards are important, then, they are insufficient for efficient learning.[27] Nor will encouragement and punishment fill the gap. The teacher must supplement intrinsic rewards with extrinsic rewards. This means not only telling the student when he or she has succeeded, but also praising, complimenting, applauding, and providing other forms of recognition for good work. Some students may need even stronger reinforcers, such as special privileges, certificates, and prizes.

REWARD GUIDELINES

Yet we cannot ignore the fact that extrinsic rewards can have adverse effects on student motivation. While there seems to be little chance of serious harm, it behooves us to use care. Various experts have suggested guidelines to follow in using extrinsic rewards.[28] Here is a digest of their recommendations:

1. Use the weakest reward required to strengthen a behavior. Don't use money if a piece of candy will do; don't use candy if praise will do. The good effects of reinforcement come not so much from the reward itself as from the reward contingency: the relationship between the reward and the behavior.

2. When possible, avoid using rewards as incentives. For example, don't say, "If you do X, I'll give you Y." Instead, ask the student to perform a task and then provide a reward for having completed it. In most cases, rewards work best if they are pleasant surprises.

3. Reward at a high rate in the early stages of learning, and reduce the frequency of rewards as learning progresses. Once students have the alphabet down pat, there is no need to compliment them each time they print a letter correctly. Nor is there much need to reward behavior that is already occurring at a high rate.

4. Reward only the behavior you want repeated. If students who whine and complain get their way, expect to see a lot of whining and complaining. Similarly, if you provide gold stars only for the three best papers in the class, you are rewarding competition and should not be surprised if students do not cooperate

with one another. And if "spelling doesn't count," don't expect to see excellent spelling.

5. Remember that what is an effective reward for one student may not work well with another. Some students respond rapidly to teacher attention; others do not. Some work well for gold stars; others don't. Effective rewards are ordinarily things that students seek — positive feedback, praise, approval, recognition, toys — but ultimately a reward's value is to be judged by its effect on behavior.

6. Reward success, and set standards so that success is within the student's grasp. In today's heterogeneous classrooms, that means setting standards for each student. A good way to do this is to reward improvement or progress toward a goal. Avoid rewarding students merely for participating in an activity, without regard for the quality of their performance.

7. Bring attention to the rewards (both intrinsic and extrinsic) that are available for behavior from sources *other than the teacher*. Point out, for example, the fun to be had from the word play in poetry or from sharing a poem with another person. Show students who are learning computer programming the pleasure in "making the computer do things." Let students know that it's okay to applaud those who make good presentations so that they can enjoy the approval of their peers for a job well done. Ask parents to talk with their children about school and to praise them for learning. The goal is to shift the emphasis from rewards provided by the teacher to those that will occur even when the teacher is not present.[29]

Following these rules is harder in practice than it might seem, and most teachers will need training in their implementation. But reinforcement is probably the most powerful tool available to teachers, and extrinsic rewards are powerful reinforcers. To teach without using extrinsic rewards is analogous to asking our students to learn to draw with their eyes closed. Before we do that, we should open our own eyes.

---

1. The study is described in E. L. Thorndike, *Human Learning* (1931; reprint ed., Cambridge, Mass.: MIT Press, 1966).
2. There are various theories (cognitive, neurological, and psychosocial) about why certain consequences reinforce or strengthen behavior. The important thing for our purposes is that they do.
3. John I. Goodlad, *A Place Called School: Prospects for the Future* (New York: McGraw-Hill, 1984). Goodlad complains about the "paucity of praise" in schools. In doing so, he echoes B. F. Skinner, who wrote that "perhaps the most serious criticism of the current classroom is the relative infrequency of reinforcement." See B. F. Skinner, *The Technology of Teaching* (Englewood Cliffs, N.J.: Prentice-Hall, 1968), p. 17.
4. Bill L. Hopkins and R. J. Conard, "Putting It All Together: Superschool," in Norris G. Haring and Richard L. Schiefelbusch, eds., *Teaching Special Children* (New York: McGraw-Hill, 1975), pp. 342-85. Skinner suggests that mastering the first four years of arithmetic instruction efficiently would require something on the order of 25,000 reinforcements. See Skinner, op. cit.
5. See, for example, Bill L. Hopkins, "Comments on the Future of Applied Behavior Analysis," *Journal of Applied Behavior Analysis*, vol. 20, 1987, pp. 339-46. In some studies, students learned at double the normal rate, yet most teachers did not continue reinforcing behavior at high rates after the study ended.
6. See, for example, Hopkins and Conard, op. cit.
7. For example, Mihaly Csikszentmihalyi found that adults who are successful and happy tend to have had happy childhoods. See Tina Adler, "Support and Challenge: Both Key for Smart Kids," *APA Monitor*, September 1991, pp. 10-11.
8. The terms *reinforcer* and *reward* are often used interchangeably, but they are not really synonyms. A reinforcer is defined by its effects: an event that strengthens the behavior it follows is a reinforcer, regardless of what it was intended to do. A reward is defined by social convention as something desirable; it may or may not strengthen the behavior it follows. The distinction is important since some studies that show negative effects from extrinsic rewards use rewards that are *not* reinforcers. See Alyce M. Dickinson, "The Detrimental Effects of Extrinsic Reinforcement on 'Intrinsic Motivation,'" *The Behavior Analyst*, vol. 12, 1989, pp. 1-15.
9. John Dewey distrusted the distinction between extrinsic and intrinsic rewards. He wrote that "what others do to us when we act is as natural a consequence of our action as what the fire does to us when we plunge our hands in it." Quoted in Samuel M. Deitz, "What Is Unnatural About 'Extrinsic Reinforcement'?," *The Behavior Analyst*, vol. 12, 1989, p. 255.
10. Dickinson writes that "several individuals have demanded that schools abandon reinforcement procedures for fear that they may permanently destroy a child's 'love of learning.'" See Alyce M. Dickinson, "Exploring New Vistas," *Performance Management Magazine*, vol. 9, 1991, p. 28. It is interesting to note that no one worries that earning a school letter will destroy a student's interest in sports. Nor does there seem to be much fear that people who win teaching awards will suddenly become poor teachers. For the most part, only the academic work of students is said to be put at risk by extrinsic rewards.
11. Skinner, p. 162.
12. For reviews of this literature, see Edward L. Deci and Richard M. Ryan, *Intrinsic Motivation and Self-Determination in Human Behavior* (New York: Plenum, 1985); Dickinson, "The Detrimental Effects"; and Mark R. Lepper and David Greene, eds., *The Hidden Costs of Reward: New Perspectives on the Psychology of Human Motivation* (Hillsdale, N.J.: Erlbaum, 1978).
13. Mark R. Lepper, David Greene, and Richard E. Nisbett, "Undermining Children's Intrinsic Interest with Extrinsic Rewards," *Journal of Personality and Social Psychology*, vol. 28, 1973, pp. 129-37.
14. See, for example, Dickinson, "The Detrimental Effects"; and Mark Morgan, "Reward-Induced Decrements and Increments in Intrinsic Motivation," *Review of Educational Research*, vol. 54, 1984, pp. 5-30. Dickinson notes that studies producing negative effects are often hard to interpret since other variables (failure, deadlines, competition, and so on) could account for the findings. By way of example, she cites a study in which researchers offered a $5 reward to top performers. The study was thus contaminated by the effects of competition, yet the negative results were attributed to extrinsic rewards.
15. Dickinson, "The Detrimental Effects."
16. Edward L. Deci, "Effects of Externally Mediated Rewards on Intrinsic Motivation," *Journal of Personality and Social Psychology*, vol. 18, 1971, pp. 105-15.
17. Ross Vasta and Louise A. Stirpe, "Reinforcement Effects on Three Measures of Children's Interest in Math," *Behavior Modification*, vol. 3, 1979, pp. 223-44.
18. Dickinson, "The Detrimental Effects," p. 9. See also Morgan, op. cit.
19. Skinner, p. 15.
20. Edward L. Deci and Wayne F. Cascio, "Changes in Intrinsic Motivation as a Function of Negative Feedback and Threats," paper presented at the annual meeting of the Eastern Psychological Association, Boston, May 1972. This paper is summarized in Edward L. Deci and Joseph Porac, "Cognitive Evaluation Theory and the Study of Human Motivation," in Lepper and Greene, pp. 149-76.
21. Skinner, p. 149.
22. For more on the problems associated with punishment, see Murray Sidman, *Coercion and Its Fallout* (Boston: Authors Cooperative, Inc., 1989).
23. Grades are often referred to as rewards, but they are more often punishments. Students study not so much to receive high grades as to avoid receiving low ones. Deci and Cascio, op. cit.
24. Deci and Cascio, op. cit.
25. See, for example, Edward L. Deci, Wayne F. Cascio, and Judy Krusell, "Sex Differences, Positive Feedback, and Intrinsic Motivation," paper presented at the annual meeting of the Eastern Psychological Association, Washington, D.C., May 1973. This paper is summarized in Deci and Porac, op. cit.
26. It should be noted that encouragement often closely resembles reinforcement in form. One teacher may say, "I know you can do it, Mary," as Mary struggles to answer a question; another teacher may say, "I knew you could do it, Mary!" when Mary answers the question correctly. The first teacher is encouraging; the second is reinforcing. The difference is subtle but important.
27. Intrinsic rewards are more important to the maintenance of skills once learned. An adult's skill at addition and subtraction is not ordinarily maintained by the approval of peers but by the satisfaction that comes from balancing a checkbook.
28. See, for example, Jere Brophy, "Teacher Praise: A Functional Analysis," *Review of Educational Research*, vol. 51, 1981, pp. 5-32; Hopkins and Conard, op. cit.; and Dickinson, "The Detrimental Effects."
29. "Instructional contingencies," writes Skinner, "are usually contrived and should always be temporary. If instruction is to have any point, the behavior it generates will be taken over and maintained by contingencies in the world at large." See Skinner, p. 144.

The Stability of Personality: Observations and Evaluations

Robert R. McCrae and Paul T. Costa, Jr.

Robert R. McCrae is Research Psychologist and **Paul T. Costa, Jr.,** is Chief, Laboratory of Personality and Cognition, both at the Gerontology Research Center, National Institute on Aging, National Institutes of Health. Address correspondence to Robert R. McCrae, Personality, Stress and Coping Section, Gerontology Research Center, 4940 Eastern Ave., Baltimore, MD 21224.

"There is an optical illusion about every person we meet," Ralph Waldo Emerson wrote in his essay on "Experience":

In truth, they are all creatures of given temperament, which will appear in a given character, whose boundaries they will never pass: but we look at them, they seem alive, and we presume there is impulse in them. In the moment it seems impulse; in the year, in the lifetime, it turns out to be a certain uniform tune which the revolving barrel of the music-box must play.[1]

In this brief passage, Emerson anticipated modern findings about the stability of personality and pointed out an illusion to which both laypersons and psychologists are prone. He was also perhaps the first to decry personality stability as the enemy of freedom, creativity, and growth, objecting that "temperament puts all divinity to rout." In this article, we summarize evidence in support of Emerson's observations but offer arguments against his evaluation of them.[2]

EVIDENCE FOR THE STABILITY OF ADULT PERSONALITY

Emerson used the term *temperament* to refer to the basic tendencies of the individual, dispositions that we call *personality traits*. It is these traits, measured by such instruments as the Minnesota Multiphasic Personality Inventory and the NEO Personality Inventory, that have been investigated in a score of longitudinal studies over the past 20 years. Despite a wide variety of samples, instruments, and designs, the results of these studies have been remarkably consistent, and they are easily summarized.

1. The mean levels of personality traits change with development, but reach final adult levels at about age 30. Between 20 and 30, both men and women become somewhat less emotional and thrill-seeking and somewhat more cooperative and self-disciplined—changes we might interpret as evidence of increased maturity. After age 30, there are few and subtle changes, of which the most consistent is a small decline in activity level with advancing age. Except among individuals with dementia, stereotypes that depict older people as being withdrawn, depressed, or rigid are unfounded.

2. Individual differences in personality traits, which show at least some continuity from early childhood on, are also essentially fixed by age 30. Stability coefficients (test-retest correlations over substantial time intervals) are typically in the range of .60 to .80, even over intervals of as long as 30 years, although there is some decline in magnitude with increasing retest interval. Given that most personality scales have short-term retest reliabilities in the range from

.70 to .90, it is clear that by far the greatest part of the reliable variance (i.e., variance not due to measurement error) in personality traits is stable.

3. Stability appears to characterize all five of the major domains of personality—neuroticism, extraversion, openness to experience, agreeableness, and conscientiousness. This finding suggests that an adult's personality profile as a whole will change little over time, and studies of the stability of configural measures of personality support that view.

4. Generalizations about stability apply to virtually everyone. Men and women, healthy and sick people, blacks and whites all show the same pattern. When asked, most adults will say that their personality has not changed much in adulthood, but even those who claim to have had major changes show little objective evidence of change on repeated administrations of personality questionnaires. Important exceptions to this generalization include people suffering from dementia and certain categories of psychiatric patients who respond to therapy, but no moderators of stability among healthy adults have yet been identified.[3]

When researchers first began to publish these conclusions, they were greeted with considerable skepticism—"I distrust the facts and the inferences" Emerson had written—and many studies were designed to test alternative hypotheses. For example, some researchers contended that consistent responses to personality questionnaires were due to memory of past responses, but retrospective studies showed that people could not accurately recall how they had previously responded even when instructed to do so. Other researchers argued that temporal consistency in self-reports merely meant that individuals had a fixed idea of themselves, a crystallized self-concept that failed to keep pace with real changes in personality. But studies using spouse and peer raters showed equally high levels of stability.[4]

The general conclusion that personality traits are stable is now widely accepted. Some researchers continue to look for change in special circumstances and populations; some attempt to account for stability by examining genetic and environmental influences on personality. Finally, others take the view that there is much more to personality than traits, and seek to trace the adult developmental course of personality perceptions or identity formation or life narratives.

These latter studies are worthwhile, because people undoubtedly do change across the life span. Marriages end in divorce, professional careers are started in mid-life, fashions and attitudes change with the times. Yet often the same traits can be seen in new guises: Intellectual curiosity merely shifts from one field to another, avid gardening replaces avid tennis, one abusive relationship is followed by another. Many of these changes are best regarded as variations on the "uniform tune" played by individuals' enduring dispositions.

ILLUSORY ATTRIBUTIONS IN TEMPORAL PERSPECTIVE

Social and personality psychologists have debated for some time the accuracy of attributions of the causes of behavior to persons or situations. The "optical illusion" in person perception that Emerson pointed to was somewhat different. He felt that people attribute behavior to the live and spontaneous person who freely creates responses to the situation, when in fact behavior reveals only the mechanical operation of lifeless and static temperament. We may (and we will!) take exception to this disparaging, if common, view of traits, but we must first concur with the basic observation that personality processes often appear different when viewed in longitudinal perspective: "The years teach much which the days never know."

Consider happiness. If one asks individuals why they are happy or unhappy, they are almost certain to point to environmental circumstances of the moment: a rewarding job, a difficult relationship, a threat to health, a new car. It would seem that levels of happiness ought to mirror quality of life, and that changes in circumstances would result in changes in subjective well-being. It would be easy to demonstrate this pattern in a controlled laboratory experiment: Give subjects $1,000 each and ask how they feel!

But survey researchers who have measured the objective quality of life by such indicators as wealth, education, and health find precious little association with subjective well-being, and longitudinal researchers have found surprising stability in individual differences in happiness, even among people whose life circumstances have changed markedly. The explanation is simple: People adapt to their circumstances rapidly, getting used to the bad and taking for granted the good. In the long run, happiness is largely a matter of enduring personality traits.[5] "Temper prevails over everything of time, place, and condition, and . . . fix[es] the measure of activity and of enjoyment."

A few years ago, William Swann and Craig Hill provided an ingenious demonstration of the errors to which too narrow a temporal perspective can lead. A number of experiments had shown that it was relatively easy to induce changes in the self-concept by providing self-discrepant feedback. Introverts told that they were really extraverts rated themselves higher in extraversion than they had before. Such studies supported the view that the self-concept is highly malleable, a mirror of the evaluation of the immediate environment.

1. BECOMING A PERSON: SEEKING SELF-IDENTITY

Swann and Hill replicated this finding, but extended it by inviting subjects back a few days later. By that time, the effects of the manipulation had disappeared, and subjects had returned to their initial self-concepts. The implication is that any one-shot experiment may give a seriously misleading view of personality processes.[6]

The relations between coping and adaptation provide a final example. Cross-sectional studies show that individuals who use such coping mechanisms as self-blame, wishful thinking, and hostile reactions toward other people score lower on measures of well-being than people who do not use these mechanisms. It would be easy to infer that these coping mechanisms detract from adaptation, and in fact the very people who use them admit that they are ineffective. But the correlations vanish when the effects of prior neuroticism scores are removed; an alternative interpretation of the data is thus that individuals who score high on this personality factor use poor coping strategies and also have low well-being: The association between coping and well-being may be entirely attributable to this third variable.[7]

Psychologists have long been aware of the problems of inferring causes from correlational data, but they have not recognized the pervasiveness of the bias that Emerson warned about. People tend to understand behavior and experience as the result of the immediate context, whether intrapsychic or environmental. Only by looking over time can one see the persistent effects of personality traits.

THE EVALUATION OF STABILITY

If few findings in psychology are more robust than the stability of personality, even fewer are more unpopular. Gerontologists often see stability as an affront to their commitment to continuing adult development; psychotherapists sometimes view it as an alarming challenge to their ability to help patients;[8] humanistic psychologists and transcendental philosophers think it degrades human nature. A popular account in *The Idaho Statesman* ran under the disheartening headline "Your Personality—You're Stuck With It."

In our view, these evaluations are based on misunderstandings: At worst, stability is a mixed blessing. Those individuals who are anxious, quarrelsome, and lazy might be understandably distressed to think that they are likely to stay that way, but surely those who are imaginative, affectionate, and carefree at age 30 should be glad to hear that they will probably be imaginative, affectionate, and carefree at age 90.

Because personality is stable, life is to some extent predictable. People can make vocational and retirement choices with some confidence that their current interests and enthusiasms will not desert them. They can choose friends and mates with whom they are likely to remain compatible. They can vote on the basis of candidates' records, with some assurance that future policies will resemble past ones. They can learn which co-workers they can depend on, and which they cannot. The personal and social utility of personality stability is enormous.

But it is precisely this predictability that so offends many critics. ("I had fancied that the value of life lay in its inscrutable possibilities," Emerson complained.) These critics view traits as mechanical and static habits and believe that the stability of personality traits dooms human beings to lifeless monotony as puppets controlled by inexorable forces. This is a misunderstanding on several levels.

First, personality traits are not repetitive habits, but inherently dynamic dispositions that interact with the opportunities and challenges of the moment.[9] Antagonistic people do not yell at everyone; some people they flatter, some they scorn, some they threaten. Just as the same intelligence is applied to a lifetime of changing problems, so the same personality traits can be expressed in an infinite variety of ways, each suited to the situation.

Second, there are such things as spontaneity and impulse in human life, but they are stable traits. Individuals who are open to experience actively seek out new places to go, provocative ideas to ponder, and exotic sights, sounds, and tastes to experience. Extraverts show a different kind of spontaneity, making friends, seeking thrills, and jumping at every chance to have a good time. People who are introverted and closed to experience have more measured and monotonous lives, but this is the kind of life they choose.

Finally, personality traits are not inexorable forces that control our fate, nor are they, in psychodynamic language, ego alien. Our traits characterize us; they are our very selves;[10] we act most freely when we express our enduring dispositions. Individuals sometimes fight against their own tendencies, trying perhaps to overcome shyness or curb a bad temper. But most people acknowledge even these failings as their own, and it is well that they do. A person's recognition of the inevitability of his or her one and only personality is a large part of what Erik Erikson called *ego integrity*, the culminating wisdom of a lifetime.

Notes

1. All quotations are from "Experience," in *Essays: First and Second Series*, R.W. Emerson (Vintage, New York, 1990) (original work published 1844).

2. For recent and sometimes divergent treatments of this topic, see R.R. McCrae and P.T. Costa, Jr., *Personality in Adulthood* (Guilford, New York, 1990); D.C. Funder, R.D. Parke, C. Tomlinson-Keasey, and K. Widaman, Eds., *Studying Lives Through Time: Personality and Development* (American Psychological Association, Washington, DC, 1993); T. Heatherton and J. Weinberger, *Can Personality Change?* (American Psychological Association, Washington, DC, 1994).

3. I.C. Siegler, K.A. Welsh, D.V. Dawson, G.G. Fillenbaum, N.L. Earl, E.B. Kaplan, and C.M. Clark, Ratings of personality change in patients being evaluated for memory disorders, *Alzheimer Disease and Associated Disorders*, 5, 240–250 (1991); R.M.A.

Hirschfeld, G.L. Klerman, P. Clayton, M.B. Keller, P. McDonald-Scott, and B. Larkin, Assessing personality: Effects of depressive state on trait measurement, *American Journal of Psychiatry, 140,* 695–699 (1983); R.R. McCrae, Moderated analyses of longitudinal personality stability, *Journal of Personality and Social Psychology, 65,* 577–585 (1993).

4. D. Woodruff, The role of memory in personality continuity: A 25 year follow-up, *Experimental Aging Research, 9,* 31–34 (1983); P.T. Costa, Jr., and R.R. McCrae, Trait psychology comes of age, in *Nebraska Symposium on Motivation: Psychology and Aging,* T.B. Sonderegger, Ed. (University of Nebraska Press, Lincoln, 1992).

5. P.T. Costa, Jr., and R.R. McCrae, Influence of extraversion and neuroticism on subjective well-being: Happy and unhappy people, *Journal of Personality and Social Psychology, 38,* 668–678 (1980).

6. The study is summarized in W.B. Swann, Jr., and C.A. Hill, When our identities are mistaken: Reaffirming self-conceptions through social interactions, *Journal of Personality and Social Psychology, 43,* 59–66 (1982). Dangers of single-occasion research are also discussed in J.R. Council, Context effects in personality research, *Current Directions in Psychological Science, 2,* 31–34 (1993).

7. R.R. McCrae and P.T. Costa, Jr., Personality, coping, and coping effectiveness in an adult sample, *Journal of Personality, 54,* 385–405 (1986).

8. Observations in nonpatient samples show what happens over time under typical life circumstances; they do not rule out the possibility that psychotherapeutic interventions can change personality. Whether or not such change is possible, in practice much of psychotherapy consists of helping people learn to live with their limitations, and this may be a more realistic goal than "cure" for many patients. See P.T. Costa, Jr., and R.R. McCrae, Personality stability and its implications for clinical psychology, *Clinical Psychology Review, 6,* 407–423 (1986).

9. A. Tellegen, Personality traits: Issues of definition, evidence and assessment, in *Thinking Clearly About Psychology: Essays in Honor of Paul E. Meehl,* Vol. 2, W. Grove and D. Cicchetti, Eds. (University of Minnesota Press, Minneapolis, 1991).

10. R.R. McCrae and P.T. Costa, Jr., Age, personality, and the spontaneous self-concept, *Journals of Gerontology: Social Sciences, 43,* S177–S185 (1988).

Determinants of Behavior: Motivation, Environment, and Physiology

On the front pages of every newspaper, in practically every televised newscast, and on many magazine covers the problems of substance abuse in America haunt us. Innocent children are killed when caught in the crossfire of the guns of drug lords. Prostitutes selling their bodies for drug money spread the deadly AIDS virus. The white-collar middle manager loses his job because he embezzled company money to support his cocaine habit.

Why do people turn to drugs? Why doesn't all of the publicity about the ruining of human lives diminish the drug problem? Why can some people consume two cocktails and stop, while others feel helpless against the inebriating seduction of alcohol? Why do some people crave heroin as their drug of choice, while others choose marijuana?

The causes of individual behavior such as drug and alcohol abuse are the focus of this section. If physiology, either biochemistry or genes, is the determinant of our behavior, then solutions to such puzzles as alcoholism lie in the field of *psychobiology* (the study of behavior in relation to biological processes). However, if experience as a function of our environment and learning histories creates personality and coping ability and thus causes subsequent behavior, normal or not, then researchers must take a different tack and explore features of the environment responsible for certain behaviors. A third explanation is that ability to adjust to change is produced by some complex interaction or interplay between experience and biology. If this interaction accounts for individual differences in personality and ability to cope, scientists then have a very complicated task ahead of them.

Conducting research designed to unravel the determinants of behavior is difficult. Scientists must call upon their best design skills to develop studies that will yield useful and replicable findings. A researcher hoping to examine the role of experience in personal growth and behavior needs to be able to isolate one or two stimuli or environmental features that seem to control a particular behavior. Imagine trying to delimit the complexity of the world sufficiently so that only one or two events stand out as the cause of an individual's alcoholism. Likewise, researchers interested in psychobiology also need refined, technical knowledge. Suppose a scientist hopes to show that a particular form of mental illness is inherited. She cannot merely examine family genetic histories, because family members can also learn maladaptive behaviors from one another. The researcher's ingenuity will be challenged; she must use intricate techniques such as comparing children to their adoptive as well to their biological parents. Volunteer subjects may be difficult to find, and even then, the data may be hard to interpret.

This unit is meant to familiarize you with a variety of hypothesized determinants of behavior. "Nature, Nurture, Brains and Behavior," discusses the age-old issue of biology vs. environment as contributors to our psychological makeup. In examining the *nature-nurture* controversy, the article provides an overview for the rest of this unit.

The next two articles collectively examine the nature-nurture controversy with an eye to specific components, especially physiological components. In "Unraveling the Mystery of Life," Mariette DiChristina discusses the explosion of modern genome research, which is helping us understand the genetic bases of certain psychological and biological disorders. She provides a good overview of the reasons why genes and heredity are so important. In a companion piece, "The New Social Darwinists," the work of evolutionary psychologists is discussed. Their work on stepparents' murdering their stepchildren is particularly intriguing as it relates to genetic motives for such murders.

The subsequent articles concern the nervous system. "Revealing the Brain's Secrets" describes the nervous system and how it is responsible for influencing our behaviors. More importantly, it explains various brain disorders such as Alzheimer's disease. Understanding the neuronal bases of such disorders is the beginning of finding a treatment for them. In a companion article, Gina Kolata discusses how scientists using magnetic resonance imaging are discovering that men's and women's brains differ. Such differences point to the underlying reasons for cognitive, behavioral, and emotional differences between the sexes.

The third article in this series about the brain is "Kernel of Fear." Mark Caldwell describes the role the amygdala plays in fear and in posttraumatic stress disorder. This small piece of brain tissue can create major problems of adjustment for afflicted individuals. Scientists have also discovered that various other emotions are found in dif-

UNIT 2

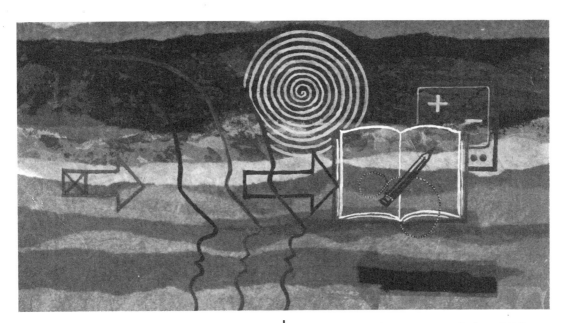

fering parts of the brain. In fact, some of these emotions have always been thought of as opposites, yet they are not centered in the same specific area of the brain. This new and startling discovery is revealed in "The Brain Manages Happiness and Sadness in Different Centers."

In the final article in this unit, we stray far from laboratory and hospital research. In "Faith and Healing," Claudia Wallis discloses that people are turning more and more to forms of healing other than medical treatment. Some individuals turn to religion; others look inward and examine their feelings and attitudes. In any event, astonishing new research is demonstrating that there is indeed a mind-body connection, finding that those who turn to religion, for example, are healthier than those who do not.

In summary, this unit covers factors that determine our behavior, whether the factors are internal, as in genetics, physiology, and our own private thoughts, or external, such as our environment and those around us or some combination of the two.

Looking Ahead: Challenge Questions

Based on your experience observing children, what would you say most contributes to their personal growth: physiological or environmental factors? Explain why you think that different aspects of our behaviors and personalities are accounted for by physiology, experience, or some interaction between the two.

Why is it important to study genetics? How is genome research conducted, and why is it important? If we knew that a certain form of cancer was inherited, what could we do about it? Would your answer be the same if asked what we should do about a certain kind of inherited mental illness?

What is evolutionary psychology? Why are evolutionary psychologists interested in studying human behavior? What human behaviors are they busy studying? What data do they provide to support their contentions?

How can we map the brain? What are the various parts of the brain? Explain whether or not you can ascribe certain behaviors to certain parts of the brain. What brain disorders are being studied with modern scientific techniques? Why are we studying these already disordered brains; why not concentrate on normal brains?

Name some bona fide brain differences between the sexes that have been discovered by neuroscientists. What perceived differences are due to stereotypes and therefore untrue? Where do these differences originate? Do you think the sexes are more similar than they are different? Why or why not?

Besides sex differences can you think of other psychological phenomena that would be interesting or worth examining to determine what factors contribute to them or to detect individual differences? Name some. What utility or practical application does searching for causes of individual differences in behaviors have?

Where is the amygdala? What role does it play in emotions? What is posttraumatic stress syndrome? How can we help people who suffer from this syndrome?

By mapping the brain, we have discovered where certain emotions are centered. Where are various emotions found in the brain? What are the implications of the fact that happiness and sadness are not centered in the same part of the brain?

How can our minds affect our physical health? Offer data to support your position. If the mind does affect the body, what can we do to keep ourselves mentally and physically well?

Nature, Nurture, Brains, and Behavior

Scientists are beginning to unravel the complex processes by which genetics and environment interact to determine brain development and human potential.

Kenneth J. Mack

Kenneth J. Mack is a child neurologist and molecular biologist at the Waisman Center on Mental Retardation, University of Wisconsin, Madison. His research interests deal with how seizures and learning affect gene expression.

The genetic makeup of a child seems to have a direct effect on that child's development. Yet anyone who has spent time around children has to acknowledge that the environment also has a large impact on development. The question that has puzzled many a researcher, philosopher, psychologist, and parent is, what role does each factor play, and how do these two factors interact to determine our brain development?

Advances in understanding how genes affect neural development offer the hope that science may one day be able to explain how genes affect behavior, and conversely, how environment and behavior affect genes.

Genetic effects on nervous-system development

Our genes are coded instructions for making a rich variety of protein molecules, with one gene corresponding roughly to one protein. These genetic instructions are contained in a DNA language consisting of bits of nucleic acids called basepairs. The human genome, containing approximately 3.3 billion basepairs, is transcribed or expressed into about 100,000 different units of messenger RNA, which in turn are used to generate about 100,000 different proteins. Hence we say that the human genome consists of about 100,000 different genes.

Some researchers have estimated that approximately 30,000–50,000 of these genes are expressed in the central nervous system, and about two-thirds of these are expressed only in the brain. The specific RNA messages that a cell expresses will help determine its structure, function, and activity level. A nerve cell's specific pattern of gene expression, for example, may help make it unique among the nervous system's one trillion total cells.

In simplified form, gene expression may be thought of as a two-step process in which the message contained within the DNA is first "transcribed" into another nucleic-acid language, an RNA form. In the second step, the RNA message is "translated" into protein. Most gene expression is controlled at the level of transcription. Proteins known as transcription factors bind to a gene's regulatory region at the front end of a gene and either promote or repress transcription. Typically, a single transcription factor is not enough to start transcription. Oftentimes the combined action of three or more factors is needed to promote transcription. Hence these transcription factors help determine which of our genes are expressed and to what degree.

It is estimated that there are approximately 5,000 transcription factors in humans, and these are classified into at least 12 different families based on their protein structure. Some families of transcription factors, such as homeodomains and paired boxes, have been implicated in development, whereas transcription factors of the leucine-zipper and zinc-finger type have roles in learning.

In the nervous system, much of gene expression is preprogrammed and independent of environment. An example of this preprogrammed process is the determination of whether a cell will survive through development

8. Nature, Nurture, Brains, and Behavior

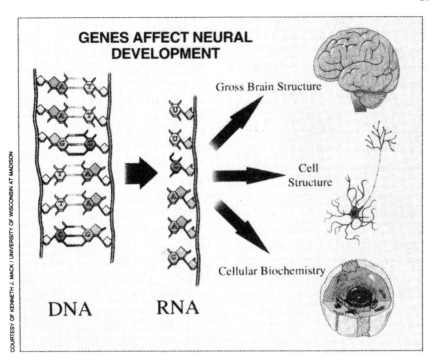

■ Genes affect nervous-system development at many different levels via a two-step process. First, the genetic codes of DNA are "transcribed" into RNA, which is then "translated" into protein molecules that perform myriad functions.

or undergo a process called "programmed cell death." For instance, the nematode *C. elegans* (a type of wormlike creature) produces exactly 1,090 cells during its growth to adulthood. Of these 1,090 cells, exactly 131 are destined to die as part of the animal's normal development. Most (80 percent) of the cells "destined to die" are nerve cells.

Cells that express programmed-cell-death genes undergo an active process of suicide unless these cells also express genes that specifically protect them from programmed cell death. This normal developmental process also occurs in humans. However, many researchers now believe that aberrations in programmed cell death may be responsible for diseases such as amyotrophic lateral sclerosis (Lou Gehrig's disease) and certain muscular diseases of childhood.

Across many animal species, certain transcription factors produced by key developmental genes determine the formation of specific brain regions. Present also in humans, these genes include those of the homeobox (Hox), homeodomain, zinc finger, and paired box (Pax) families. Many of these genes are specifically expressed in certain brain regions and have an important role in determining the structure of that region. For example, studies in the embryonic development of the mouse have revealed that the Pax and the Hox genes are expressed in spatially and temporarily restricted patterns during the development of the nervous system. Pax transcription factors seem to play a role in the dorsal-ventral (back to front) positioning of cells, whereas Hox genes are more likely to play a role in the positioning along the rostral-caudal (head to toe) axis. Hence these transcription factors specify the position for the cell in the nervous system.

Pax and Hox genes producing Pax and Hox transcription factors are examples of how structural aspects of brain development are genetically determined. Mutations in these developmental genes have already been identified in human clinical syndromes of developmental abnormalities. Craniosynostosis is a condition where premature closure of an infant's skull sutures occurs. Recently this abnormality has been associated with Pax-2 mutations in one family. Pax-3 mutations are found in patients with Waardenburg's syndrome, which consists of deafness and partial albinism. Pax-6 mutations are found in aniridia (complete or partial absence of the iris) in humans.

Regulatory genes may assist in determining not only the position of the cell but also the specific attributes of the cell. The Hox-type gene Gtx is specifically expressed in glial cells (support cells in the nervous system). The gene for transcription factor SCIP is expressed in layer 5 pyramidal neurons. These genes demonstrate the cell-type specificity of many of these factors. Certainly, what genes a cell expresses will predetermine whether it will survive development and what type of cell it will become.

Importance of gene expression in intelligence

Most of us are born with "normal" intelligence. Of the 30,000–50,000 genes that are expressed in our nervous system, most seem to function well and allow us to survive in a complex world. Our environment can presumably help, or hinder, our genetic substrate and determine our current intellect. Perhaps the clearest examples of environmental influences on intellect are demonstrated in disease states or in extreme conditions.

Three percent of all children are mentally retarded. The roles of environment and education become critical to optimize their final developmental level. Mental retardation can result from

2. DETERMINANTS OF BEHAVIOR: MOTIVATION, ENVIRONMENT, AND PHYSIOLOGY

more than 500 genetic conditions, as well as innumerable "acquired" mental-retardation syndromes, such as head trauma and prematurity. Although the molecular etiology of many mental-retardation syndromes is diverse, a basic problem to all these syndromes is the difficulty in learning. In some forms of mental retardation, the neural substrates of learning—the cerebral cortex and the hippocampus—may be absent or severely malformed. In other conditions, the basic neuronal architecture and connections seem to be present, and the mechanisms for the cognitive problems remain more elusive.

How can one make learning more efficient and effective? Part of the difficulty in answering this question is that only a superficial understanding of the mechanisms of learning is known. In animal models, multiple biochemical and structural changes occur after learning and during critical periods in development. It is generally believed that many important aspects of learning take place in the connections between nerve cells, called synapses, and many of these changes are dependent on gene expression. A more focused question then becomes, how does learning cause changes in gene expression?

Does experience affect nervous-system development?

Despite a beautifully complex and exact role for predetermined gene regulation in neuronal development, environment also plays a major role. Yet, at a scientific level, it is difficult to ask directly how environmental influences change the circuitry and molecular biology of the brain. Some researchers maintain that a complex environment that promotes learning will excite specific groups of nerve cells, resulting in changes specific to learning. Thus, investigators often study nerve-cell excitation as a model of learning.

One important function of neuronal excitation is to support the survival of developing neurons. In a fetus, the number of nerve cells, as well as the number of connections or "synapses" between cells, continues to expand. However, starting after infancy, the number of nerve cells and synapses decreases as a normal part of development. As mentioned above, much of this "programmed cell death" is determined genetically. Yet studies have shown that whenever cells are excited, or "depolarized," they are much less likely to die. When excitation is blocked, the nerve cells are more likely to die. One may infer from these studies that neuronal activity will promote neuronal cell survival. The nervous system almost seems to follow a "use it or lose it" rule during development.

Prevention of programmed cell death in the central nervous system of a young animal or human is important. In the visual system, the blocking of optic-nerve activity from the eye leads to increased cell death in visual areas of the brain. Restoration of this visual activity is followed by decreased cell death.

Perhaps some of the most compelling examples of the effects of experience on gene expression come from observations made in the behavioral sciences. In the 1940s, Rene Spitz observed two groups of orphans. One group was taken care of in a foundling home, with one nurse per seven children. These children were kept relatively isolated in a crib with a white sheet over it. A second group of orphans was raised in a nurs-

■ "Use it or lose it" seems to be the guideline for neuronal development in the preschool child. The cell's existence and its unique configuration of dendritic connections (synapses) with other neurons are strongly influenced by environmental stimulation, or the lack of it.

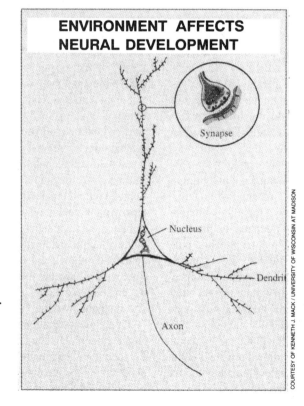

ENVIRONMENT AFFECTS NEURAL DEVELOPMENT

ing home attached to a women's prison. These orphans received more "one on one" attention from the women prisoners and were raised in cribs where they could see more of their environment.

At 4 months of age, the foundling infants were slightly more advanced than the nursing-home infants. However, at 2 years of age, the nursing-home infants were significantly more advanced than the foundling infants. The nursing-home infants were normal, while only 2 of 26 foundling infants could walk by 24 months (normally children walk before 15 months of age). Most of the foundling infants used very few words at this age, while many normal infants use 100 or more words. These studies show that an impoverished environment can result in long-term developmental delays.

Related observations in a more controlled animal experiment were made by Harry Harlow and coworkers at the University of Wisconsin in the late 1950s. Harlow observed that if monkeys were raised in isolation (typical laboratory conditions for that time), they showed poor social interaction as adults. However, the presence of a mother, or other peer monkeys, would increase the skills of the observed monkeys. Harlow's studies suggested that early experience may have a permanent effect on behavior.

What are the structural and biochemical changes that underlie the behavioral changes? The visual system has been a useful model in trying to sort out these effects. As early as 1932, Marius von Senden noted that children with cataracts removed at 10–20 years of age would be able to recognize color but had difficulty recognizing form. Presumably some early activation of specific visual pathways was necessary to develop this pattern recognition.

If deprivation can cause a decrease in gene expression, then can an increase in activity cause an increase in gene expression?

Nobel laureates David Hubel and Torsten Weisel of Harvard University, in a set of now classic studies, were able to demonstrate that connections from the thalamus (a relay nucleus for visual input) to the primary visual cortex (where basic visual perception is perceived) were arranged in columns, with input from each eye controlling alternate columns of cells. If the vision from one eye were disrupted during development, then the relative size of its representation in the cortex would change. It is now well known that early visual deprivation will produce gross alterations in visual cortex organization. Hubel and Weisel's experiments helped demonstrate that experience affects the gross morphology of the brain.

William Greenough at the University of Illinois has asked if experience can affect the structure of individual nerve cells. In Greenough's experiments, rats were raised in an either "enriched" or "impoverished" environment. These experiments focused on a part of the neuron called a dendrite, whose function is to receive input from other cells. Greenough noted that the complexity of dendrites is positively correlated with experience, with the more experienced animals having a much more complex and elegant dendritic system. Interestingly, a parallel observation occurs in humans with mental retardation. Individuals with some forms of mental retardation have a much simpler set of dendrites than do normal subjects.

Experience affects gene expression

The above studies suggest that visual experience during development affects the viability and structure of the nerve cell. However, experience affects not only the morphology of nerve cells but also their molecular biology. Stewart Hendry and Edward Jones, of the University of California at Irvine, have looked at how visual experience affects expression of the protein glutamic acid decarboxylase (GAD), the rate-limiting enzyme involved in the synthesis of the neurotransmitter GABA. Hendry and Jones demonstrated that depriving a visual system of input would cause a decrease in its GAD levels. In contrast, restoring visual activity to the system leads to restoration of GAD expression.

If deprivation can cause a decrease in gene expression, then can an increase in activity cause an increase in gene expression? To answer this question, multiple investigators have studied the rodent barrel cortex system, another excellent model for studying the effects of experience. The barrel cortex receives information from the animal's whiskers, or vibrissae. Many animals use their whiskers in the same way humans use their fingers to touch and explore objects. The information encoded in the barrel cortex seems not to represent simple touch but rather information about the form of an object. A rodent uses this barrel information to understand if a touched object is food, another animal, or some structure. It is superficially comparable to stereognosis in humans, where an individual is able to recognize an object (such as a coin, paper clip, or rock) by form.

Hendrik VanderLoos and colleagues of the University of Lausanne, Switzerland, used the barrel cortex to ask if new experience can result in an increase in gene expression. They observed that stimulating a rat's whiskers resulted in an increase of GAD expression, suggesting that environmental stimuli are important for maintaining GAD expression by nerve cells. More sensory experience increases the levels of this synaptic protein, whereas deprivation decreases this level. Since GAD is regulated in an experience-dependent manner, and since GAD-containing neurons constitute 25–30 percent of the neuronal population in the cortex, it has been suggested that this system plays a major role in cortical plasticity and learning.

My own research at the University of Wisconsin has asked what biochemical steps occur between a learning type of experience and the final synaptic changes that take place in nerve cells. After a learning experience, nerve cells are "excited," or activated, and they express many of the same transcription factors seen in development. These factors can then interact with the regulatory regions of genes for several synaptic proteins, including GAD. The end result of these changes is seen in the biochemistry and structure of the synapse, where learning is presumed to be based. Anatomical studies looking at synaptic morphology would suggest that experience results in long-lasting biochemical and structural changes.

Opportunities for gene therapy

If we can identify molecular pathways that are involved in experience and learning, then can we effectively change these pathways? Can one make these pathways more efficient and thereby facilitate learning? Unfortunately, the answer is probably not, given the technology of 1996.

In the best scenario, one could envision that the addition of a single gene (such as the gene for a transcription factor specific to learning) could optimize "learning" and therefore improve the lot of the mentally retarded, or even of normal children. Unfortunately, gene therapeutic approaches for single gene/protein defects have been wanting. Even in the area of Parkinson's disease, where the pathology is relatively limited and the biochemistry is relatively well understood, gene-therapy techniques have not been able to facilitate upregulation of tyrosine hydroxylase (the deficit involved in Parkinson's disease) in a long-term and side effect–free manner.

Some researchers have speculated on a pharmaceutical approach to gene transcription. It is theoretically possible to have compounds that directly interact with transcription factors. These pharmaceutical compounds may then specifically up-or down-regulate gene transcription. Transcription factors are prime candidates for this type of pharmaceutical development, because of their specificity, diversity, and importance in human disease.

A third approach may be to optimize the benefits obtained from a learning experience. Given the molecular complexity of developmental plasticity and learning, it may be wisest to use the neuronal pathways that are already in place. Although technically not very exciting, this relies on the beautifully complex nature of the nervous system to reinforce itself. The combination of a well-structured educational approach, as well as medically keeping these children healthy (free of seizure activity, and well nourished), may be the most efficacious "molecular" approach we have to facilitate learning in the normal as well as mentally retarded child.

Programs that facilitate experience in young children

The largest experiment to optimize human potential within developing children is certainly the Head Start program. Started in the 1960s, this program has allowed children from disadvantaged backgrounds to improve their educational experience and optimize their potential. Many investigators have studied the results of Head Start, and the summary of its effectiveness is certainly controversial. It seems that children who go through the program show gains in achievement through at least the early elementary years, but beyond that the achievements are harder to document. In a more comprehensive early intervention program, the Perry Preschool Project, researchers were able to demonstrate benefits of the program into young adulthood.

For children at risk for cognitive disabilities, federally mandated early intervention programs are provided by local school districts. From zero to three years of age, the children are provided with a variety of positive interventions, including physical therapy, occupational therapy, and speech therapy. The children then go into a classroom situation from age three until kindergarten. Studies have shown benefits in measures of development and IQ in select populations. Anecdotally, parents seem to be extremely supportive of the role that these programs play in their children's education.

Perhaps the most interesting long-term effect of childhood education is evidenced by a study from Shanghai, China. This study provided evidence that education may help prevent Alzheimer's disease. People who were formally educated through only early grade school years are almost 10 times more likely to develop Alzheimer's than people who were educated through at least high school. An additional positive effect is seen with further postsecondary education. Although the purpose of early education programs is not to prevent Alzheimer's disease, these data do point out that early education results in long-lasting changes in the central nervous system.

The challenges for researchers in this area are innumerable. The specific genetics of neuronal development, and the effects of learning on gene expression, are at best superficially understood. Even if we can identify single gene abnormalities that result in poor learning, medicine is years to decades away from developing effective gene-therapy approaches for neurological diseases. The challenge for behavioral scientists is to understand when an educational approach will make a difference. For example, should structured educational situations be offered for all four-year-olds? For infants? Even those from nondisadvantaged backgrounds? Perhaps an even more formidable challenge is to understand what type of educational approach is optimal. We haven't yet answered that question for most elementary or secondary education.

Conclusion

Like a complex musical score, the nervous system exhibits an intricate program of gene expression during development. However, similar to the way a conductor directs that musical score, the environment exerts a strong influence on how that genetic potential is expressed. It is still too early to incorporate the above information into specific useful suggestions for educators and parents. In general, however, it seems that positive interpersonal interactions encourage positive developmental and behavioral changes in children. Additionally, exposure to learning situations in the early childhood years results in long-term effects on brain growth, development, and achievement.

A study from Shanghai, China, provided evidence that education may help prevent Alzheimer's disease.

Unraveling the Mystery of Life

Boston University researchers, in collaboration with other medical science teams, continue to make significant contributions with their discoveries in the field of genetic knowledge.

Mariette DiChristina

Mariette DiChristina (COM '86) *is a senior editor at* Popular Science.

"EACH OF THESE SAMPLES HOLDS A PIECE OF genetic code," says Chris Amemiya, Ph.D., his scarlet and navy paisley tie and khakis poking out from a long white lab coat. In tiny breakers resting atop a black ice bucket like shrimp cocktail, these crucial codes look surprisingly inconsequential—rather like simple tap water.

Yet codes like these have awesome power over human destiny. They determine whether you are tall or short, have blue eyes or brown, curly hair or straight. And more important, they may tell whether you will get sick someday, and from what. There are perhaps 3,000 to 4,000 ailments caused by genetic defects.

In this tidy, well-lit lab, Amemiya, an assistant professor at the Center for Human Genetics at the Boston University School of Medicine, and others are working to help figure out, or characterize, sequences of these genetic codes. Their efforts are just one small part of the impressive ongoing genetic research at the University.

Individually as well as in collaboration with other medical science teams, BU scientists have contributed to many nationally recognized achievements in the complex arena of genetic research. Their work covers the spectrum of discovery—from persevering with pipettes in the lab to number-crunching reams of data with computers to dealing with the human consequences of the search for greater genetic knowledge.

On the world stage, genome research has seen some remarkable advances. So far, some two dozen genes have been linked to human diseases. The past year alone has seen the discovery of a gene commonly implicated in many varieties of cancer, as well as ones for breast cancer, obesity, a form of youth-onset Alzheimer's, even the general site of a gene linked with persistent bed-wetting in children.

Not so long ago, no one even knew what a gene was. Since Gregor Mendel's famous work with peas, scientists have known the importance of heritage. But it wasn't until 1952 that scientists discovered that DNA is the basic stuff of heredity. Short for deoxyribonucleic acid, DNA is a long thread-like molecule that is part of a gene (see "A Genetic Dictionary"). Today we know that DNA acts like a biological computer program some three billion bits long. This program spells out the key instructions for making proteins, the basic building blocks of life. If you could print it out, the entire human genome—the blueprint that makes each of us a unique individual—would fill a thousand 1,000-page telephone books.

The genome is so large and the work to decipher it so painstaking that fewer than 5 percent of these genetic codes have been sequenced. To explain why this is so, many researchers cite the example of the landmark 1989 discovery of the gene for cystic fibrosis. The many independent groups that worked simultaneously on the project often duplicated one another's efforts, and the total cost probably exceeded $120 million.

5,000 Genes a Year

Enter the Human Genome Project. Launched in 1990, the massive, multibillion-dollar project seeks to identify an estimated 50,000 to 100,000 human genes by the year 2005. An international effort involving hundreds of scientists at dozens of universities and medical institutions, the project is supported in the United States by the National Institutes of Health and the Department of Energy.

A pioneer was Charles DeLisi, Ph.D., who initiated the project in the 1980s as a director of the Department of Energy's health and environment research programs. An internationally recognized researcher in molecular structure and function, DeLisi is now professor of biomedical engineering and dean of BU's College of Engineering.

Among those continuing in the wake of DeLisi's efforts are scientists at the BU Center for Advanced Biotechnology, on the Charles River Campus. Charles Cantor, Ph.D., the center's director and a member of the National Academy of Sciences, says a key goal of the researchers is to reduce the tremendous cost and time involved in genetic research.

Shortcuts

To ease the arduous task of sifting through forty-six human chromosomes of marvelous complexity, many scientists seek to create some basic road maps. Cassandra L. Smith, Ph.D., deputy director of the Center for Advanced Biotechnology, is one researcher who focuses on new methods of faster DNA mapping and sequencing.

"The technical problem is that the genome is very large and you can't look at the whole genome at one time with current technology," says Smith. "So we've developed methods of looking at subsets of the genome that are likely to have changes that might cause diseases. When a gene falls into such a region, you already might have a lot of the resources to help pinpoint it."

To explain the point, Smith offers an analogy. Imagine you're looking for a certain house in a city. You could start at any random street and then search block by block. Or you could look at an overall map of the city and get a general idea of where to begin. Having the genetic markers, she says, "is like having a map of the city."

One marking technique is to use restriction enzymes, which chemically clip DNA at places where the enzymes recognize specific base sequences. Eventually gene mappers would like to create a regularly spaced set of markers at close intervals. Using these markers as signposts for genetic "neighborhoods" on the imaginary city map, scientists can then find the important "streets" and "houses." When there are differences around these markers in family members who have a genetic disease — but not in disease-free members — scientists can locate the genetic cause.

This method of gene hunting has produced some notable successes at BU: location of the genes for Waardenburg's syndrome as well as for Huntington's disease.

In 1992 a team led by Clinton T. Baldwin, Ph.D., an associate professor of pediatrics and the director of molecular genetics research at the Center for Human Genetics, found the genetic cause of a form of deafness called Waardenburg's syndrome. Waardenburg's, which is accompanied by pigment disorders of the skin, eyes, and hair, causes about 3 percent of all cases of congenital deafness.

"We determined the [key part of a] DNA sequence of an individual with the disease, compared it to a person without the disease, and found a single base change that resulted in a single amino acid change," explains Baldwin. "This was sufficient to destroy the ability of the protein to function." Using earlier research done on the genetics of mice and fruit flies — which have some genes similar to human genes — also helped the researchers understand the genes involved.

The gene for Huntington's was also located with this search technique. Huntington's is a deadly neurodegenerative disease whose best known victim was folksinger Woodie Guthrie. Unlike Waardenburg's, Huntington's is not a single error. Rather, explains Richard Myers, Ph.D., of the BU Medical Center, it is a "stutter" flaw. There are too many repeats of one tiny bit of code, as if the genetic photocopier went haywire. Myers, who was part of the team that made the 1993 discovery of the Huntington's gene after a decade-long search, says the more copies of this gene a Huntington's patient has, the more severe the symptoms and the earlier the onset of the disease. Continuing in his research, Myers is exploring some puzzling differences in the complexity of nerve cells of Huntington's patients and those without the disease.

Another place scientists look for gene clues is in people whose relationship is even closer than most family members: identical twins. Because identical twins develop from the same fertilized egg, they have the same genetic material.

A Genetic Dictionary

DNA — Two yards of DNA are packed into each one of the 100 trillion cells in your body. A strand of DNA, or deoxyribonucleic acid, is more than 37,000 times thinner than a human hair. The DNA is on twenty-three pairs of chromosomes; you get one set of twenty-three chromosomes from each of your parents.

CHROMOSOME — Each of the forty-six human chromosomes contains the DNA for thousands of individual genes, the chemical units of heredity.

GENE — A gene is a snippet, or sequence, of DNA that holds the recipe for making a specific molecule, usually a protein. These recipes are spelled out in four chemical bases: adenine (A), thymine (T), guanine (G), and cytosine (C). The bases form interlocking pairs; A always pairs with T and G pairs with C. In some cases, genetic defects are caused by the substitution of just one base pair for another.

PROTEIN — Amino acids make up proteins, which are key components of all human organs and chemical activities in your body. Their function depends on their shape, which is determined by the 50,000 to 100,000 genes in the cell nucleus. — MD

2. DETERMINANTS OF BEHAVIOR: MOTIVATION, ENVIRONMENT, AND PHYSIOLOGY

Studies of gay men and their twin brothers by psychiatrists Richard Pillard of the BU School of Medicine and J. Michael Bailey of Northeastern University indicate that there is a heredity factor in homosexuality. When one brother is gay, they discovered, there is a far greater likelihood that the identical twin is gay too.

If one twin has a trait that the other doesn't have, this gives scientists a hint about where to look for the specific gene that causes that trait. For example, Cassandra Smith is conducting studies with twins in the search for genes responsible for schizophrenia. "I take identical twins who are discordants — that is, one has and one doesn't have schizophrenia — and compare the DNA to find the differences," she says. By doing so she seeks the triggers for this chronic disease.

A third way to shorten the search for genes is to differentiate between the 3 percent of DNA that creates coding and the 97 percent that is noncoding. Noncoding DNA is called *junk* because no one knows its purpose. "What could this 97 percent be doing?" asks H. Eugene Stanley, Ph.D., professor of physics and director of the Center for Polymer Studies at BU. "One idea is that it's just accumulated during evolution the way junk accumulates in my office," he says with a sweep of his arm taking in stacks of books and piles of paper.

Work by Stanley and colleagues at Boston University and Harvard indicates that the junk may be a language. One language feature in junk–a discovery led by team member S. Martina Ossadnik–is that it has correlations. That is, certain bits of information generally follow certain others–the way *u* follows *q* in English. Taking that a step further, Rosario Mantegna, then a BU graduate student and now a research associate in the physics department, computer-analyzed the junk, applying tests used by linguists. He found "word" repetitions, another common language feature. "Language is a structured thing," adds Stanley. "There is a lot of redundancy: I could leave out a word and you would understand me. A code is the opposite. It is very strict; you cannot make a mistake." Genetic codes do not share these language features.

So what does the junk say? No one is certain. "We can't prove it's a language," stresses Stanley, "but it passes the tests for language."

Once you find a gene for a disease, you can work to develop predictive tests. Richard Myers founded and heads Huntington's testing and counseling at the University. Boston University and Johns Hopkins University, which set up programs simultaneously in 1986, were the first institutions to offer such testing. Today more people have undergone testing for Huntington's than for any other disease that appears in adulthood.

While locating a gene doesn't guarantee a cure, it may point the way. Researchers hope to design drugs that can target the cause of an ailment rather than the symptoms. In collaboration with colleagues from other universities and biotechnology companies, Charles Cantor of the Biotechnology Center is working to take advantage of the natural lock-and-key mechanism of a type of protein–a string of amino acids–called streptavidin. One example of a natural lock and key is how antibodies fight infection in your body; the antibody chemically matches the infecting virus and adheres to it–rendering the virus harmless. Streptavidin's lock-and-key binding, however, is a million times stronger than that of antibodies. "You could use this natural mechanism to bring radiation right to the site of a cancerous tumor in a precise way," says Cantor.

Another possible way to treat genetic disease is to correct or replace the altered gene through gene therapy. This involves inserting corrective DNA into human cells to replace flawed genes or to produce proteins that stimulate the body's natural immune system. Such experimental gene therapy to treat Parkinson's disease is just one example of the more than 100 gene-therapy procedures now undergoing testing.

In some cases, too, finding out you are predisposed to a genetic ailment could help you take preventive actions or enable you to get treatment earlier, when it is more likely to be effective. Clinical research will also provide a piece of the genetic puzzle.

A leader in this area is Aubrey Milunsky, M.D., a professor of human genetics, pediatrics, pathology, and obstetrics at BU's School of Medicine and director of the Center for Human Genetics. As head of the human genetics program, Milunsky's landmark work has supported the development of national guidelines for folic acid supplementation to prevent neural tube defects and has focused on prenatal diagnosis and early pregnancy screening for birth defects.

"The power of genetics is that if you have the time and money, you are almost guaranteed to find the gene," says Cassandra Smith. Speaking for many researchers, she adds, "It's just a matter of perseverance."

The New Social Darwinists

John Horgan, *senior writer*

The headless woman in black leather panties has got to be the last straw. Devendra Singh, a psychologist at the University of Texas at Austin, flashes the photograph of the curvaceous torso on a giant screen during his talk on "men's preference for romantic relationships." For years Singh has been circling the globe, showing "sexy" pictures like this to men in an effort to determine whether certain female attributes are universally attractive. Although male tastes in facial structure, breast size and other features vary, Singh reports, men everywhere find women with a waist-to-hip ratio of 0.7 sexually alluring. Natural selection embedded this preference in the male psyche, Singh contends, because that ratio correlates so well with a woman's "reproductive potential."

Surely one of Singh's several hundred listeners—many of whom are female—will object that his research is offensive, silly or, at any rate, unscientific. Men's tastes are obviously dictated by culture, someone will argue, rather than by "instinct." But this is no ordinary social science meeting. It is the annual conference of the Human Behavior and Evolution Society. Attendees are trying to fulfill Charles Darwin's prophecy (reprinted on the cover of the meeting's program, along with a photograph of a barebreasted Amazonian maiden) that "in the distant future ... [p]sychology will be based on a new foundation"—that is, Darwin's own theory of evolution by natural selection.

Darwin, as usual, was right—about Darwinian psychology being in the distant future, that is. But over the past decade evolutionary theory has been racing, like a mutant virus, through the social sciences. In the seven years since the HBES was founded, it has attracted a growing number of psychologists, anthropologists, economists, historians and others seeking to understand human affairs (in all senses of the word). Publishers have released a swarm of books by scientists and journalists propounding the "new" paradigm. A highly regarded PBS series, *The Human Quest*, highlighted what it dubbed the "second Darwinian revolution" this past spring.

Watching HBES participants bonding, bickering, preening, flirting and engaging in mutual rhetorical grooming, one must concur with their basic premise. Yes, we are all animals, descendants of a vast lineage of replicators sprung from primordial pond scum. Our big, wrinkled brains were fashioned not in the last split second of civilization but during the hundreds of thousands of years preceding it. We are "Stone Agers in the fast lane," as S. Boyd Eaton, a physician at Emory University, puts it.

But just how much can the new social Darwinism tell us about our modern, culture-steeped selves? Even enthusiasts admit that the field has much to prove before it can shake the old complaint that it traffics in untestable "just-so stories" or truisms. Singh's work in "Darwinian aesthetics" is a case in point. His finding, once unpacked, hardly seems profound. Men desire young, healthy women—neither starving nor obese—who are not already pregnant and whose hips are wide enough to deliver a child. Do we really need Darwinian theory to tell us that?

Actually, we do, replies Randolph M. Nesse, a psychiatrist at the University of Michigan who helped to organize the first HBES meeting and one of the society's most respected members. Most social scientists, Nesse points out, still assert that our concepts of beauty are culturally determined; only Darwinists attempt to explain why certain aspects of beauty are universal. Nesse adds that just as it does for biology, Darwinian theory can also provide a much needed framework for the social sciences, which are now in disarray.

Yet Nesse admits that he often becomes frustrated by his field's inability to predict counterintuitive phenomena rather than to offer retroactive explanations of all too familiar ones. He would like to see researchers construct the rigorous "ladders of inference" that have made fields such as, say, molecular genetics so successful. "We're just getting started," Nesse says. "To see this as a mature field would be a mistake."

The Modular Mind

The HBES conference demonstrates, if nothing else, the astonishing ambition of the new social Darwinists. Topics range from the evolution of religious symbology to the resurgence of spouse swapping among middle-class Americans. The meeting sounds at times like a pep rally. There is much gleeful bashing of those deluded souls who think culture—whatever that is—determines human behavior. When anthropologist Lee Cronk of Texas A&M University derides cultural determinism as a "religion" rather than a rational stance, his audience roars with laughter.

But serious disagreements lurk beneath the seeming unity of the gathering. Just how malleable are our minds? To what extent are we creatures of instinct, as opposed to reason? Just how consciously do we pursue our genetic interests? To what degree do the differ-

2. DETERMINANTS OF BEHAVIOR: MOTIVATION, ENVIRONMENT, AND PHYSIOLOGY

Psychologists and others try to sidestep old pitfalls—both political and scientific—as they apply evolutionary theory to the clothed ape

ences between individuals and ethnic groups reflect genetic rather than cultural influences?

Moreover, some of the new social Darwinists, in their effort to avoid the political pitfalls into which their predecessors stumbled, have become hard to distinguish from culturalists. Most shun the naturalistic fallacy, the conflation of what is with what should and must be. This view was typified by the original social Darwinists of a century ago, who argued that those at the top of the Victorian heap deserved to be there.

Nesse and other HBES founders also deliberately chose not to include the controversial term "sociobiology" in the society's name. Sociobiology is closely associated with Edward O. Wilson of Harvard University, who was tarred as a genetic determinist for arguing in his 1975 classic *Sociobiology* and later works that evolutionary theory can illuminate the social behavior not only of termites and baboons but also of humans.

To be sure, the society's official journal is called *Ethology and Sociobiology,* and some of the veterans here still defiantly call themselves sociobiologists, out of loyalty to Wilson or sheer stubbornness. Others, while acknowledging their debt to sociobiology, contend that sociobiologists often ignored the mind's role in mediating the links between genes and human behavior. To reflect this emphasis on the mind, they call themselves evolutionary psychologists.

Leda Cosmides and John Tooby, a wife-and-husband team at the University of California at Santa Barbara, are leaders of evolutionary psychology. Some sociobiologists, they note, have implied that the human brain is a calculating machine dedicated to "maximizing fitness" in all environments. If that were true, they say, no one would forgo having children; in fact, men would all be lining up at sperm banks so that they might have as many offspring as possible.

In the (dare one say it) seminal 1992 book *The Adapted Mind,* which they coedited with Jerome H. Barkow of Dalhousie University, Cosmides and Tooby assert that the mind consists of a motley collection of specialized mechanisms, or modules, designed by natural selection to solve problems that faced our hunter-gatherer forebears, such as acquiring a mate, raising children and dealing with rivals. The solutions often involve such emotions as lust, fear, affection, jealousy and anger.

Cosmides and Tooby also emphasize, as sociobiologists often did not, that Darwinian theory need not conflict with the liberal principle that all humans are created equal (more or less). "Evolutionary psychology is, in general, about universal features of the mind," they have written. "Insofar as individual differences exist, the default assumption is that they are expressions of the same universal human nature as it encounters different environments."

Gender is the crucial exception to this rule. Evolutionary psychologists insist that natural selection has constructed the mental modules of men and women in very different ways as a result of their divergent reproductive roles. David M. Buss, an evolutionary psychologist at the University of Michigan, says his research on sexual attraction and "mate choice" reveals a distinct gender gap.

Buss has surveyed men and women worldwide about their sexual attitudes. He has concluded that men, because they can in principle father a virtually infinite number of children, are much more inclined toward promiscuity than are women. Women, because they can have on average only one child per year, are choosier in selecting a mate. Men in all cultures place a greater premium on youth and physical attractiveness—which Buss calls cues to fertility—than do women, to whom male "resources" are more important. Similarly, because men can never be sure that a child is theirs, their jealousy tends to be triggered by fears of a mate's sexual infidelity. Women, on the other hand, be-

---

Can Darwin Explain Everything?

At the annual meeting of the Human Behavior and Evolution Society, speakers invoked evolutionary theory to explain a broad range of phenomena.

Sex, Politics and Religion. Secular and religious laws in societies such as imperial Rome and medieval England, asserts Laura Betzig of the University of Michigan, represented strategies of male rulers to accumulate and retain wealth and power, which led in turn to greater sexual opportunities.

Male Dominance of Culture. The fact that art, music and literature are produced largely by men between the ages of 20 and 40 suggests that culture "is primarily sexual display by young males," says Geoffrey Miller of the University of Nottingham.

The Amorous Female Tourist. The tendency of certain affluent women to pursue sexual liaisons with low-status men while on vacation, in seeming violation of Darwinian tenets, may actually be motivated by the women's innate desire for "social connectedness," according to April Gorry of the University of California at Santa Barbara.

Female Beauty. Men desire women with full lips and small chins, says Victor S. Johnston of New Mexico State University, because these attributes correlate with high estrogen levels and thus high fertility.

Problems during Pregnancy. The hypertension afflicting some pregnant women, suggests David Haig of Harvard University, may result from a "selfish gene" strategy of the fetus; the strategy causes the fetus to draw too heavily on the mother's resources—that is, the nutrients in her blood.

come more upset at the thought of losing a mate's emotional commitment and thus his resources.

Buss realizes that these conclusions, which he spells out in his 1994 book *The Evolution of Desire*, might seem obvious to the "man in the street." But some influential social scientists, he notes, have held that the man in the street is wrong, that culture rather than nature determines sexual attitudes. This view was typified by Margaret Mead, who in her famous book *Coming of Age in Samoa* depicted a society in which men and women pursue sexual pleasure with equal abandon, and jealousy is unknown. Buss says work by him and others has shown that Mead's vision was a fantasy.

The persistence of male jealousy, Buss adds, also contradicts the suggestion of some sociobiologists that our minds rationally calculate how to maximize our reproductive prospects under any and all circumstances. Male jealousy made sense in a hunter-gatherer environment, Buss explains, because when acted on, it could improve the chances that a male's genes were propagated rather than a competitor's. But modern males, Buss says, will become enraged by a mate's unfaithfulness even if she is using birth control.

Our Cheating Hearts

One of the few HBES members who still calls herself a sociobiologist, Sarah Blaffer Hrdy of the University of California at Davis, accuses Buss of caricaturing the views of sociobiologists and even cultural determinists. If Mead saw the world through the filter of her own fantasies, Hrdy comments, so have many male investigators of sexual behavior—such as those who study the evolutionary significance of female breast symmetry.

"Men just love coming up with scenarios for female breasts because they love looking at them," Hrdy snaps. She complains that far too much time has been expended on "preference" studies like Buss's; sexual behavior is often more complex, and calculated, than such surveys suggest. For example, male jealousy may often be irrational, but the female preference for mates with money makes perfect sense today, given that women's economic opportunities are still limited in most societies. Hrdy concurs with the statement of one HBES speaker that evolutionary psychologists must move beyond their "discovery" that "men like pretty girls and women like wealthy men."

Some researchers think Cosmides has done just that. One of the mind's most useful modules, she proposes, is dedicated to detecting "cheating" by others. Her hypothesis is a corollary of a bracingly cynical concept called reciprocal altruism, first advanced in 1971 by Robert L. Trivers of Rutgers University. Trivers proposed that altruism could have arisen among our forebears only if it led to some "tit for tat" benefit.

Building on this insight, Cosmides argues that in a society bound by reciprocal altruism, natural selection would have favored both those who could cheat successfully and those who could spot cheaters. In tests with volunteers, Cosmides showed that humans are much more adept at solving problems if the solution requires the detection of cheating rather than some purely logical, abstract chain of reasoning.

At the meeting, economist Vernon Smith of the University of Arizona says his research supports the hypothesis of Cosmides. In Smith's experiments, volunteers have the opportunity to earn hundreds of dollars by successfully negotiating various complex transactions with others. (Needless to say, Smith has no trouble recruiting volunteers for his research.) The transactions are all variations of the famous Prisoner's Dilemma: each participant must decide whether to betray his or her counterparts and earn a guaranteed sum or trust them and possibly earn more—or even less—than the original amount.

Smith expected his subjects to calculate their selfish interests with cold rationality; that is the prediction of rational-choice theory, which is gospel among most economists. But the volunteers tended to be more trusting initially and, if their trust was betrayed, more unforgiving than they would be if behaving rationally. Smith was puzzled by his results until he discovered the writings of Cosmides and Tooby, who have emphasized the role of emotion in social transactions.

The modularity model has attracted mental health researchers as well. Alan M. Leslie, a psychologist at Rutgers, presents evidence that autism stems from a disorder of what he calls the theory-of-mind mechanism. According to this hypothesis, normal children have an innate ability to create internal representations, or "theories," of others' mental states. This ability has obvious adaptive value, Leslie explains, because it allows us more effectively to predict and manipulate the behavior of others. Autistic children often score well on intelligence tests—unless those tests require them to empathize with or predict the behavior of others.

10. New Social Darwinists

Is Language an Instinct?

Another convert to evolutionary psychology is Steven Pinker, a linguist at the Massachusetts Institute of Technology. In a lecture at the HBES meeting, Pinker, who plans to spend the next year working with Cosmides and Tooby in Santa Barbara, delivers a Cliff Notes version of his well-received 1994 book *The Language Instinct*. Language is far too complex, Pinker contends, to be entirely learned; it must stem from an innate program hardwired into our brains. Moreover, language is common to all cultures (unlike reading and writing), and all physiologically normal children learn to speak fluently with little or no effort. Research has also shown that all languages share common features, suggesting that natural selection favored certain syntactic structures.

"I'm going to make some extremely banal points," Pinker adds. Language, he asserts, almost certainly arose because it was adaptive—that is, it conferred benefits on our hunter-gatherer ancestors. Language would allow early hominids to share learned skills related to toolmaking, hunting and other activities. Those especially adept at language would be able to manipulate others, form alliances and enjoy other advantages that would translate into more offspring. "I don't intend these points to be taken as revolutionary," Pinker says, "but they are generally denied when they are brought up at all."

In fact, these "banal" points are denied by none other than Pinker's legendary M.I.T. colleague and fellow linguist Noam A. Chomsky. Evolutionary psychologists are all, in a sense, heirs of Chomsky's. Almost 40 years ago Chomsky routed the behaviorists' tabula-rasa view of the mind by arguing convincingly that language is innate. But since then, Chomsky has cast doubt on the assumption that language is an adaptive trait, favored by natural selection.

Some Darwinists hint that Chomsky's position must be linked somehow to his leftist politics. Chomsky retorts that he simply recognizes, as Pinker and others do not, the limits of Darwinian explanations. He accepts that natural selection may have played *some* role in the evolution of language and other human attributes. But given the enormous gap between human language and the relatively simple communication systems of other animals, Chomsky says, and given our fragmentary knowledge of the past, science can tell us little about how language evolved.

Just because language is adaptive now, Chomsky elaborates, does not

53

2. DETERMINANTS OF BEHAVIOR: MOTIVATION, ENVIRONMENT, AND PHYSIOLOGY

mean that it arose in response to selection pressures. Language may have been an incidental by-product of a spurt in intelligence that only later was coopted for various uses. The same may be true of other properties of the human mind. Evolutionary psychology, Chomsky complains, is not a real science but "a philosophy of mind with a little bit of science thrown in." The problem, he adds, is that "Darwinian theory is so loose it can incorporate anything."

Even at the meeting, some investigators find fault with the emphasis of evolutionary psychology on specialized rather than general-purpose abilities. James H. Fetzer, a philosopher at the University of Minnesota, argues that the subjects in the cheating experiments of Cosmides could have been displaying not some innate talent but a learned ability; after all, situations involving potential deception are common in the modern era, too. Fetzer contends that evolutionary psychologists too quickly dismiss the possibility that humans may possess an all-purpose "heuristics" program; modern civilization and science itself testify to the power of our ability to learn through simple trial and error.

Steven J. Mithen, an archaeologist at the University of Reading, agrees. He faults evolutionary psychologists for implying that the "ancestral environment" was uniform and static rather than highly variable in space and time. The fluidity of the conditions under which our ancestors evolved, Mithen argues, might have favored those whose problem-solving skills, too, were adaptable rather than compartmentalized.

The Docile Yanomamö

But just how adaptable are we? In attempting to explain behavior that does not accord with Darwinian tenets, some theorists have postulated that conformity—or "docility"—is an adaptive trait. Those who go along, get along. In an article in *Science* in 1990 the economist and Nobel laureate Herbert A. Simon of Carnegie Mellon University conjectured that docility could explain why, for example, people obey religious tenets that curb their sexuality and why men fight in wars when as individuals they have little to gain and much to lose.

Although this hypothesis cleverly coopts the culturalists' position, it could also undermine the status of evolutionary psychology as a legitimate science. If a given behavior accords with Darwinian tenets, fine; if it does not, it merely demonstrates our docility. The theory becomes falsification-proof (thus demonstrating Chomsky's point that Darwin can account for anything). Acknowledging the tendency of humans to conform to their culture poses another problem for Darwinian theorists. Given the interconnectedness of all modern cultures, some of the universal, seemingly adaptive attitudes and actions documented by researchers such as Buss might actually result from docility. That is what the culturalists have said all along.

Indeed, Napoleon A. Chagnon, a prominent "Darwinian anthropologist" at Santa Barbara, sounds like a culturalist when he interprets his own work. For more than 20 years Chagnon has studied the behavior of the Yanomamö, one of the few Amazonian tribes still clinging to its primordial way of life. In this polygynous society, men in one village often raid other villages, killing men they encounter there and kidnapping women. Chagnon has found a correlation between the number of homicides that men commit and the number of offspring that they have. On the other hand, those who shrink from violent encounters—Chagnon calls them wimps—are usually "wiped out."

Chagnon has been accused of implying that male violence and even warfare are instinctual and therefore inevitable. He insists that is not his position. The Yanomamö men, Chagnon says, engage in aggressive behavior because it is esteemed by their culture. If they were raised in a society that revered not violence but, say, farming skills, they would quickly conform to that system. Chagnon acknowledges that his view is not so different from that of Stephen Jay Gould of Harvard University, who also emphasizes the malleability of human nature—and is considered by many HBES members to be an archenemy of their enterprise. "Steve Gould and I probably agree on a lot of things," Chagnon says.

The Wicked Stepfather Syndrome

Two other Darwinian researchers who warn against overinterpreting their findings are Margo Wilson and Martin

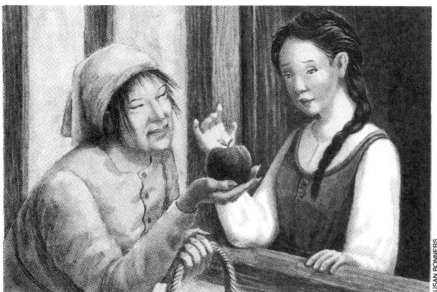
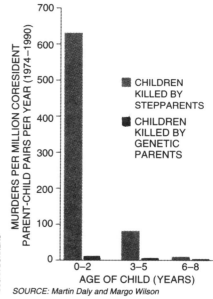

EVIL STEPPARENTS, notorious from fairy tales such as the Grimm brothers' *Snow-White*, may have a basis in fact. Children age two or younger in Canada were some 60 times more likely to be killed by a stepparent than by a genetic parent.

Daly of McMaster University. This married couple has examined what Darwinists consider to be the most perverse of human acts, a parent's murder of his or her own child. Evolutionary theory predicts that we should be particularly solicitous toward those to whom we are most closely related. After analyzing murder records from the U.S. and Canada, Wilson and Daly determined that children younger than two were at least 60 times more likely to be killed by a stepparent—and almost always a stepfather—than by a natural parent. The results agreed with evolutionary theory after all.

Wilson and Daly, like David Buss, are sensitive to charges that they have "discovered" the obvious: people like their own children more than the children of others; this message, after all, is embodied in such fairy tales as *Cinderella* and *Snow-White*. Wilson contends that most social scientists have dismissed this "folk wisdom" about evil stepparents rather than trying to determine whether it has any basis.

Wilson and Daly's research is often cited as a model of Darwinian social science, because it addresses an important issue and rests on a large empirical foundation. But even they concede that their work raises some obvious questions. Families with a stepparent might be less stable financially and emotionally than families that have remained intact. Moreover, many stepfathers might have assumed the burden of stepchildren reluctantly when they married. Controlling for such factors is next to impossible, Wilson says.

Some critics have suggested that Wilson and Daly should compare the homicide rates for adopted children with that for natural children. Wilson responds that performing such a study would be extremely difficult, in part because many adoptive parents want to conceal their relationship to their children. If such data were available, she predicts, they would show little or no effect, because couples who adopt are carefully screened for financial security, emotional stability and other factors. They may also be more motivated to have children than many natural parents are.

Wilson and Daly have been contacted by both prosecutors and defense lawyers involved in cases in which a stepparent has killed a child. The defense lawyers are seeking to exonerate their clients on the grounds that "it was in their genes." Applying the same logic, prosecutors have asked whether Wilson and Daly would support stiff sentences to deter other stepparents inclined to commit such a crime. Wilson and Daly have declined to support either position. They emphasize that no one should infer from their results that stepparents are fated to abuse their children; after all, most stepparents treat their children benignly.

The Guy in the Black Hat

The work of Wilson and Daly—and of Chagnon—raises what is, for those who pursue genetic explanations of human behavior, another divisive issue. Why do some men resort to violence when others, faced with similar situations, refrain from doing so? Wilson, Daly and Chagnon all downplay the possibility that some men are more genetically inclined toward violence than others; the researchers cite environmental factors, such as differences in upbringing, as more likely causes of behavioral differences. This view conforms to the party line of evolutionary psychology, which holds that with the important exception of sex, all humans are born with essentially the same psychological endowment. Cosmides and Tooby have speculated that genetic variation among individuals may protect our species from disease or parasites but should have few significant behavioral consequences.

In fact, the surest way to annoy evolutionary psychologists is to lump them together with behavioral geneticists, who tend to ascribe differences among individuals and even ethnic groups to genetic variation. "I'm the guy in the black hat here," says David C. Rowe of the University of Arizona, one of the few behavioral geneticists invited to give a talk at the conference. (His talk is scheduled for the final session of the final day, after many attendees have left.)

Rowe understands why evolutionary psychologists disavow behavioral genetics: this position makes their work easier both politically and scientifically. If all commonalities can be ascribed to genes and all disparities to the environment, the task of constructing models is enormously simplified; evolutionary psychologists can also distance themselves from the race-obsessed science exemplified by last year's notorious best-seller *The Bell Curve*.

But Rowe still finds the position of Cosmides and Tooby a bit disingenuous. If genes can account for our commonalities, he points out, they can also account for our differences; moreover, evolution would not occur without individual variation. A growing body of evidence, Rowe notes, shows a correlation between genetic variation and such significant behavioral traits as aggression, extroversion, intelligence, homosexuality and depression.

These findings—when combined with the obvious fact that humans conform to their culture—raise what for evolutionary psychologists must be a disturbing possibility. They assume that genes underlie our commonalities and environment our differences. But the reverse may also be true. Culture may account for many of our commonalities, and our differences may reflect genetic variation.

Given their aversion to behavioral genetics, it is no wonder that many evolutionary psychologists are enamored of the work of Frank J. Sulloway. He offers a more palatable explanation for individual variation: birth order. For almost 25 years Sulloway, a historian at M.I.T., has compiled data on links between birth order and personality. Firstborn children, he has concluded, are much more likely than their younger siblings to be conservative, to support the status quo and to reject new scientific or political ideas. Later-born children, in contrast, tend to be more adventurous, radical, open-minded, willing to take risks.

Sulloway acknowledges that in 1983 two Swiss psychiatrists surveyed all the previous literature on birth-order effects and concluded that they were illusory. Sulloway says his meta-analysis of their data turned up a "huge" effect that they missed. He contends that most of the great revolutions in modern history—scientific and political—have been led and supported by later-borns and opposed by "stubborn" firstborns. Darwin, for example, was the fifth of six children, and those who supported his theory also tended to be later-borns.

Evolutionary psychology, Sulloway says, accounts for these findings. The longer children survive beyond the perils of infancy, the more likely it is that they will reproduce and thus propagate their parents' genes (other factors being equal). Parents thus tend to invest more "resources" in older children. Firstborns seek to exploit this situation by maintaining a close relationship with their parents and other authorities. Later-borns, with less to lose, have more incentive to embrace change and disorder. "From a Darwinian point of view, it is just impossible that birth-order effects don't exist," declares Sulloway (who, needless to say, is a later-born).

Sulloway's theory, although acclaimed on the front page of the *Wall Street Journal*, has not undergone peer review yet. Sulloway has packed his analysis of history into an 800-page book, entitled *Born to Rebel*, scheduled to be published next year. Like many other listeners,

2. DETERMINANTS OF BEHAVIOR: MOTIVATION, ENVIRONMENT, AND PHYSIOLOGY

George C. Williams of the State University of New York at Stony Brook is both fascinated by and skeptical of Sulloway's results. "I keep thinking of counterexamples," Williams says. Isaac Newton, for example, was a firstborn.

The Darwinian Society

Williams is one of the most venerated elders of the HBES and of evolutionary biology in general. In his classic work *Adaptation and Natural Selection*, published in 1966, he posed a question that still inspires his younger colleagues: "Is it not reasonable to anticipate that our understanding of the human mind would be aided greatly by knowing the purpose for which it was designed?"

Williams remains active in the field he helped to create. In *Why We Get Sick: The New Science of Darwinian Medicine*, published this year, he and Nesse argue that evolutionary theory can help physicians understand and treat physical and mental disorders. Williams also has high hopes for what he calls Darwinian epistemology. Is there some adaptive reason, he asks, why we organize reality into space and time? After all, one profound lesson of modern physics is that our "commonsense" views of space and time are highly arbitrary. But Williams, noting how easy it is to misunderstand and misapply evolutionary theories of human nature, admits he has "some nervous hesitation about the whole business."

Lionel Tiger, an anthropologist at Rutgers, contends that Darwinian science inevitably will, and should, have legal, political and moral consequences; some of the most pressing issues of the 1990s —abortion, birth control, sexual discrimination, homosexuality—are "in Darwin's beat." Tiger says he knows of at least one Supreme Court justice and several high-ranking Pentagon officials who have taken an interest in evolutionary psychology and are considering applying it in their realms. Ready or not, here comes the Darwinian society.

Further Reading

THE RED QUEEN: SEX AND THE EVOLUTION OF HUMAN NATURE. Matt Ridley. Penguin Books, 1993.

THE MORAL ANIMAL: THE NEW SCIENCE OF EVOLUTIONARY PSYCHOLOGY. Robert Wright. Pantheon Books (Random House), 1994.

EVOLUTIONARY PSYCHOLOGY: A NEW PARADIGM FOR PSYCHOLOGICAL SCIENCE. David M. Buss in *Psychological Inquiry*, Vol. 6, No. 1, pages 1-30; 1995.

Revealing the Brain's Secrets

Is space truly the final frontier? Not according to scientists who are probing what they call the most complex and challenging structure ever studied: the human brain. "It is the great unexplored frontier of the medical sciences," said neurobiologist John E. Dowling, professor of natural science at Harvard University. Just as space exploration dominated science in the 1960s and 1970s, the human brain is taking center stage in the 1990s.

It may seem odd to compare an organ that weighs only about three pounds to the immensity of the universe. Yet the human brain is as awe-inspiring as the night sky. Its complex array of interconnecting nerve cells chatter incessantly among themselves in languages both chemical and electrical. None of the organ's magical mysteries has been easy to unravel. Until recently, the brain was regarded as a black box whose secrets were frustratingly secure from reach.

Now, an explosion of discoveries in genetics and molecular biology, combined with dramatic new imaging technologies, have pried open the lid and allowed scientists to peek inside. The result is a growing understanding of what can go wrong in the brain, which raises new possibilities for identifying, treating, and perhaps ultimately preventing devastating conditions such as Alzheimer's disease or stroke.

"The laboratory bench is closer to the hospital bed than it has ever been," said neurobiologist Gerald Fischbach, chairman of neurobiology at Harvard Medical School, where the brain and its molecular makeup are a primary focus of research.

One important challenge is to understand the healthy brain. By studying brain cells and the genetic material inside them, scientists are discovering how groups of specialized cells interact to produce memory, language, sensory perception, emotion, and other complex phenomena. Figuring out how the healthy brain goes about its business is an essential platform that researchers need in order to comprehend what goes wrong when a neurological disease strikes.

There have also been great strides toward elucidating some of the common brain disorders that rob people of memory, mobility, and the ability to enjoy life. The most promising of these fall into several broad categories.

- The discovery of disease-producing genetic mutations has made it possible not only to diagnose inherited disorders, but in cases such as Huntington's disease, to predict who will develop them. These findings have also pointed the way toward new therapies.
- Insights into the programmed death of nerve cells may lead to drugs that can halt the progression of degenerative diseases or contain stroke damage.
- Naturally occurring chemicals that protect nerve cells from environmental assaults may hold clues about preventing disease or reversing neurologic injury.
- Information about brain chemistry's role in mood and mental health has already helped people burdened by depression, for example, and is expected to benefit others as well.

Genetics opens a new door

Discovering a gene associated with a disease is like unlocking a storehouse of knowledge. Once researchers have such a gene, they may be able to insert it into experimental systems such as cell cultures or laboratory animals. This makes it easier to discern the basic mechanisms of the disorder, which in turn helps scientists figure out what diagnostic tests or therapies might be best. When a new treatment is proposed, genetically engineered models of human diseases make testing quicker and more efficient.

2. DETERMINANTS OF BEHAVIOR: MOTIVATION, ENVIRONMENT, AND PHYSIOLOGY

In recent years, scientists have found abnormal genes associated with Huntington's disease (HD), Alzheimer's disease (AD), amyotrophic lateral sclerosis (ALS or Lou Gehrig's disease), one form of epilepsy, Tay-Sachs disease, two types of muscular dystrophy, and several lesser-known neurological conditions.

A decade-long search for the HD gene ended in 1993, when Harvard researchers Marcy MacDonald and James Gusella, working with scientists at other institutions, identified a sequence of DNA that produces symptoms of the disease if it is repeated enough times. Huntington's is a progressive and ultimately fatal hereditary disorder that affects about 25,000 people in the United States. It typically strikes at midlife, and the researchers discovered that the more copies of the sequence a person inherited, the earlier symptoms show up.

Scientists quickly developed a highly reliable assay that enables people with a family history of HD to find out if they or their unborn fetus harbors the dangerous mutation. But because no cure for the disease exists, few people have rushed to have themselves tested.

Demand might increase, however, if scientists can use the HD gene to design effective treatments. Genes contain the assembly instructions for proteins, the molecules that carry out the day-to-day operations of the body. Scientists strive to identify the protein made by a disease-producing gene and to figure out what it does, which in turn helps them understand the event that initiates the disease process.

The HD gene codes for a protein that appears to contribute to the premature death of certain neurons. It is the loss of these cells that results in the involuntary movements and mental deterioration typical of Huntington's. When researchers know more about this protein, they may be able to develop drugs or other therapies that could slow the onset of symptoms or even block them entirely.

A downward spiral
The gradual extinction of certain brain cells is also the underlying cause of Alzheimer's disease. In this case, the impact is progressive loss of memory, changes in personality, loss of impulse control, and deterioration in reasoning power. Under the microscope, the brains of people who died with AD are studded with abnormalities called amyloid plaques and neurofibrillary tangles. About 20% of all AD cases are inherited, and these people develop symptoms earlier in life than those with the more common form, which typically appears well after age 65.

In recent years, scientists have discovered several different genetic mutations that can

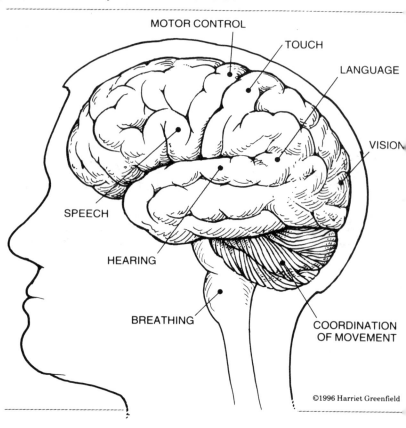
©1996 Harriet Greenfield

cause the unusual, inherited form of AD. One of these abnormal genes has successfully been introduced into mice by researchers at several pharmaceutical companies, and experts believe that this animal model will help them understand how all forms of the disease progress at the cellular and molecular level.

So far, it looks as though some of the animals' brains develop amyloid plaques like the ones that build up in humans. Long-standing doubt about whether plaques cause symptoms may be resolved by future observations of whether these genetically engineered mice show signs of memory loss. If there is a strong correlation between amyloid accumulation and symptom severity, these mice will be used to test drugs that might keep plaques from forming.

The cell death story
Unlike other types of cells, nerve cells (neurons) are meant to last a lifetime because they can't reproduce themselves. Struck by the realization that abnormal cell death is the key factor in neurologic problems ranging from Alzheimer's to stroke, scientists have embarked on a crusade aimed at understanding why nerve cells die and how this might be prevented.

It's normal to lose some brain cells gradually. Trouble arises when a large population of cells dies all of a sudden, as in a stroke, or when too many of a certain type die over time, such as in Alzheimer's or Parkinson's (PD) disease. While some scientists remain skeptical that inquiries into cell death will ever lead to effective means for preventing or treating neurodegenerative diseases, many others are enthusiastically pursuing this line of research.

Some scientists are racing to develop *neuroprotective* drugs that could guard brain cells against damage and death or even help them regenerate. There are many different ideas about how to do this.

For example, although Harvard scientists have identified the gene for HD and the protein it makes, they don't understand the mechanisms that lead to symptoms. One theory is that a phenomenon called *excitotoxicity* is responsible, and that Huntington's is only one of many diseases in which this process plays a role.

The idea behind excitotoxicity is that too much of a good thing is bad for cells. Glutamate, for example, is an ordinarily benign chemical messenger that stimulates certain routine cellular activities. Under extraordinary circumstances, however, "cells can be so excited by glutamate that they wear themselves out and die," said John Penney Jr., a neurologist at Massachusetts General Hospital and a Harvard professor of neurology.

Sending a signal
One of the many types of doorways built into the walls of nerve cells is a structure called an NMDA receptor. One of its functions is to allow small amounts of calcium (a substance usually shut out of the cell) to enter it. This happens when the NMDA receptor is stimulated by glutamate. If excess glutamate is present, too much calcium rushes in — an influx that is lethal to the cell.

Someday it may be possible to halt the advance of Huntington's by injecting drugs which block the NMDA receptor so that calcium can't get in. In animal experiments, scientists have demonstrated that such receptor-blocking agents can keep brain cells from dying. Harvard researchers are seeking approval for a clinical trial that will test such neuroprotective drugs in patients with symptomatic disease. If participants obtain any relief from this treatment, the next step will be to determine whether this approach can prevent symptoms in patients who have the gene but do not have symptoms.

Scientists also hope that neuroprotection can be used to limit brain damage due to stroke. When a stroke shuts down the supply of blood to part of the brain, neurons in the immediate area die within minutes. Over the next several hours, more distant cells in the region are killed as excitotoxic signals spread. In an effort to limit the extent of brain damage, researchers are currently treating small numbers of patients with intravenous doses of experimental agents such as NMDA receptor blockers and free radical scavengers. Other neuroprotective agents under development, include protease inhibitors, nitric oxide inhibitors, and nerve growth factors.

"Our dream is a safe and effective neuroprotectant that can be given to the stroke patient in the ambulance or shortly after arrival in the emergency room," said neurologist Seth Finkelstein, an associate professor at Harvard Medical School who conducts basic research at Massachusetts General Hospital. "That's the holy grail of neuroprotective treatment."

Applications for Alzheimer's
Neuroprotection is also making waves in Alzheimer's research, as scientists strive to inhibit the type of cell death that typifies this disease. One group of investigators has identified several *peptides* (small protein molecules) that block the formation of amyloid plaque in the test tube, said neurobiologist Huntington Potter, an associate professor at Harvard Medical School. The researchers hope to test these peptides in humans.

Brain cells manufacture several neuroprotective chemicals on their own, which scientists call *neurotrophic* or nerve growth factors. These small proteins may hold the key to keeping cells alive even in the face of stroke, degenerative diseases, or even spinal cord injury.

Relieving Depression

People who are depressed have less of the neurotransmitter serotonin than those who aren't. In the picture on the left, the axon terminal of one nerve cell releases serotonin, which travels across the synapse and activates the cell body (receiving cell). Serotonin is then reabsorbed by the sending cell. On the right, a selective serotonin reuptake inhibitor (SSRI), such as the antidepressant Prozac, slows the reabsorption of serotonin, keeping it in the synapse longer and boosting its effect on the receiving cell.

2. DETERMINANTS OF BEHAVIOR: MOTIVATION, ENVIRONMENT, AND PHYSIOLOGY

For example, several different neurotrophic factors are being tested in the laboratory to determine if they could protect the dopamine-producing cells that die prematurely in people with Parkinson's disease. Other uses are being studied as well, and some researchers anticipate that these chemicals will be tested in humans before the decade draws to a close.

Mood, mind, and brain chemistry

Scientists have discovered that a surprising number of mental disorders, from depression to schizophrenia, are the result of brain chemistry gone awry. And this understanding has led them to design new medications for treating specific mental disorders and behavior problems.

The best known of this new breed of drugs is fluoxetine (Prozac), one of several selective serotonin reuptake inhibitors (SSRIs). It was possible to design these agents, which are widely prescribed to alleviate depression and related disorders, only after scientists came to understand how nerve cells communicate at the molecular level.

Each nerve cell has an *axon*, a long branch that reaches out and touches other nerve cells. A tiny space called a *synapse* separates the axon terminal (which sends a message) and the cell body (that receives it), and this is where the action is. The sending cell releases *neurotransmitters* (chemical messengers) into the synapse which either excite or inhibit a receiving cell that is equipped with the proper receptors. Messages pass from cell to cell in this manner, eventually leading to a physiologic action. In each synapse, the cell that sent the message sops up leftover neurotransmitters and stores them for future use. People who are depressed have less serotonin than those who aren't, and the SSRIs block the reuptake of this chemical, thereby boosting the effect of a small amount on the receiving cell. *(See illustration* **"Relieving Depression."**)

But Prozac and its relatives are only the tip of the iceberg. As researchers work to understand the roles of different chemical messengers and the highly specific receptors that bind them, a whole new approach to the treatment of mental disorders is evolving. The identification of highly specialized receptors is already paving the way for ever more specific drugs to treat these conditions.

Schizophrenia therapy is a case in point. As devastating as this form of mental illness is, treatments have sometimes appeared worse than the disease. Until very recently, the only drugs that relieved symptoms could also lead to spasmodic, uncontrollable movements known as *tardive dyskinesia*. This is because these agents block all types of receptors for dopamine, a neurotransmitter that is a key player in normal movement as well as in this mental disorder. Now there is a new drug for schizophrenia, clozapine, that blocks only a small subclass of dopamine receptors. It relieves symptoms of the illness in some people without leading to abnormal movements. Still, it can have other serious side effects.

Tailored to fit

The bottom line for the treatment of behavior and emotional disorders may be that drugs will become ever more specialized. Just as computers now help salespeople fit blue jeans to the individual purchasers, it is not inconceivable that psychopharmacologists may someday tailor drugs to the needs of each patient.

What does the future of brain research hold? Dr. Dowling anticipates that medications that can slow the process of degenerative disease, correct the chemical imbalances that cause mental disorders, prevent stroke damage, and repair spinal cord injuries may all be on the horizon. "We have learned so much about the cellular and molecular aspects of the brain," Dr. Dowling said. "We stand at a time of great opportunity, when we can take tremendous advantage of these things and turn them into practical clinical therapies."

— KATHLEEN CAHILL ALLISON

Man's World, Woman's World? Brain Studies Point to Differences

Gina Kolata

Dr. Ronald Munson, a philosopher of science at the University of Missouri, was elated when Good Housekeeping magazine considered publishing an excerpt from the latest of the novels he writes on the side. The magazine eventually decided not to publish the piece, but Dr. Munson was much consoled by a letter from an editor telling him that she liked the book, which is written from a woman's point of view, and could hardly believe a man had written it.

New scanner finds more evidence of how the sexes differ in brain functions.

It is a popular notion: that men and women are so intrinsically different that they literally live in different worlds, unable to understand each other's perspectives fully. There is a male brain and a female brain, a male way of thinking and a female way. But only now are scientists in a position to address whether the notion is true.

The question of brain differences between the sexes is a sensitive and controversial field of inquiry. It has been smirched by unjustifiable interpretations of data, including claims that women are less intelligent because their brains are smaller than those of men. It has been sullied by overinterpretations of data, like the claims that women are genetically less able to do everyday mathematics because men, on average, are slightly better at mentally rotating three dimensional objects in space.

But over the years, with a large body of animal studies and studies of humans that include psychological tests, anatomical studies, and increasingly, brain scans, researchers are consistently finding that the brains of the two sexes are subtly but significantly different.

Now, researchers have a new noninvasive method, functional magnetic resonance imaging, for studying the live human brain at work. With it, one group recently detected certain apparent differences in the way men's and women's brains function while they are thinking. While stressing extreme caution in drawing conclusions from the data, scientists say nonetheless that the groundwork was being laid for determining what the differences really mean.

"What it means is that we finally have the tools at hand to begin answering these questions," said Dr. Sally Shaywitz, a behavioral scientist at the Yale University School of Medicine. But she cautioned: "We have to be very, very careful. It behooves us to understand that we've just begun."

The most striking evidence that the brains of men and women function differently came from a recent study by Dr. Shaywitz and her husband, Dr. Bennett A. Shaywitz, a neurologist, who is also at the Yale medical school. The Shaywitzes and their colleagues used functional magnetic resonance imaging to watch brains in action as 19 men and 19 women read nonsense words and determined whether they rhymed.

In a paper, published in the Feb. 16 issue of Nature, the Shaywitzes reported that the subjects did equally well at the task, but the men and women used different areas of their brains. The men used just a small area on the left side of the brain, next to Broca's area, which is near the temple. Broca's area has long been thought to be associated with speech. The women used this area as well as an area on the right side of the brain. This was the first clear evidence that men and women can use their brains differently while they are thinking.

Another recent study, by Dr. Ruben C. Gur, the director of the brain behavior laboratory at the University of Pennsylvania School of Medicine, and his colleagues, used magnetic resonance imaging to look at the metabolic activity of the brains of 37 young men and 24 young women when they were at rest, not consciously thinking of anything.

In the study, published in the Jan. 27 issue of the journal Science, the investigators found that for the most part, the brains of men and women at rest were indistinguishable from each other. But there was one difference, found in a brain structure called the limbic system that regulates emotions. Men, on average, had higher brain activity in the more ancient and primitive regions of the limbic system, the parts that are more involved with action. Women, on average, had more activity in the newer and more complex parts of the limbic system, which are involved in symbolic actions.

Men have larger brains; women have more neurons.

Dr. Gur explained the distinction: "If a dog is angry and jumps and bites, that's an action. If he is angry and bares his fangs and growls, that's more symbolic."

Dr. Sandra Witelson, a neuroscientist at McMaster University in Hamilton, Ontario, has focused on brain anatomy, studying people with terminal cancers that do not involve the brain. The patients have agreed to participate in neurological and psychological tests and then to allow Dr. Witelson and her colleagues to examine their brains after they die, to look for relationships between brain structures and functions. So far she has studied 90 brains.

Several years ago, Dr. Witelson reported that women have a larger corpus callosum, the tangle of fibers that run down the center of the brain and enable the two hemispheres to communicate. In addition, she said, she found that a region in the right side of the brain that corresponds to the region women used in the reading study by the Shaywitzes was larger in women than in men.

Most recently, Dr. Witelson discovered, by painstakingly counting brain cells, that although men have larger brains than women, women have about 11 percent more neurons. These extra nerve cells are densely packed in two of the six layers of the cerebral cortex, the outer shell of the brain, in areas at the level of the temple, behind the eye. These are regions used for understanding language and for recognizing melodies and the tones in speech. Although the sample was small, five men and four women, "the results are very, very clear," Dr. Witelson said.

Going along with the studies of brain anatomy and activity are a large body of psychological studies showing that men and women have different mental abilities. Psychologists have consistently shown that men, on average, are slightly better than women at spatial tasks, like visualizing figures rotated in three dimensions, and women, on average, are slightly better at verbal tasks.

Dr. Gur and his colleagues recently looked at how well men and women can distinguish emotions on someone else's face. Both men and women were equally adept at noticing when someone else was happy, Dr. Gur found. And women had no trouble telling if a man or a woman was sad. But men were different. They were as sensitive as women in deciding if a man's face was sad—giving correct responses 90 percent of the time. But they were correct about 70 percent of the time in deciding if women were sad; the women were correct 90 percent of the time.

"A woman's face had to be really sad for men to see it," Dr. Gur said. "The subtle expressions went right by them."

Studies in laboratory animals also find differences between male and female brains. In rats, for example, male brains are three to seven times larger than female brains in a specific area, the preoptic nucleus, and this difference is controlled by sex hormones that bathe rats when they are fetuses.

"The potential existence of structural sex differences in human brains is almost predicted from the work in other animals," said Dr. Roger Gorski, a professor of anatomy and cell biology at the University of California in Los Angeles. "I think it's a really fundamental concept and I'm sure, without proof, that it applies to our brains."

But the question is, if there are these differences, what do they mean?

Dr. Gorski and others are wary about drawing conclusions. "What happens is that people overinterpret these things," Dr. Gorski said. "The brain is very complicated, and even in animals that we've studied for many years, we don't really know the function of many brain areas."

This is exemplified, Dr. Gorski said, in his own work on differences in rat brains. Fifteen years ago, he and his colleagues discovered that males have a comparatively huge preoptic nucleus and that the area in females is tiny. But Dr. Gorski added: "We've been studying this nucleus for 15 years, and we still don't know what it does. The most likely explanation is that it has to do with sexual behavior, but it is very, very difficult to study. These regions are very small and they are interconnected with other things." Moreover, he said, "nothing like it has been shown in humans."

And, with the exception of the work by the Shaywitzes, all other findings of differences in the brains or mental abilities of men and women have also found that there is an amazing degree of overlap. "There is so much overlap that if you take any individual man and woman, they might show differences in the opposite direction" from the statistical findings, Dr. Gorski said.

Dr. Munson, the philosopher of science, said that with the findings so far, "we still can't tell whether the experiences are different" when men and women think. "All we can tell is that the brain processes are different," he said, adding that "there is no Archimedean point on which you can stand, outside of experience, and say the two are the same. It reminds me of the people who show what the world looks like through a multiplicity of lenses and say, 'This is what the fly sees.' " But, Dr. Munson added, "We don't know what the fly sees." All we know, he explained, is what we see looking through those lenses.

Some researchers, however, say that the science is at least showing the way to answering the ancient mind-body problem, as applied to the cognitive worlds of men and women.

Dr. Norman Krasnegor, who directs the human learning and behavior branch at the National Institute of Child Health and Human Development, said the difference that science made was that when philosophers talked about mind, they "always were saying, 'We've got this black box.' " But now, he said, "we don't have a black box; now we are beginning to get to its operations."

Dr. Gur said science was the best hope for discovering whether men and women inhabited different worlds. It is not possible to answer that question simply by asking people to describe what they perceive, Dr. Gur said, because "when you talk and ask questions, you are talking to the very small portion of the brain that is capable of talking." If investigators ask people to tell them what they are thinking, "that may or may not be closely related to what was taking place" in the brain, Dr. Gur said.

On the other hand, he said, scientists have discovered that what primates perceived depends on how their brains function. Some neurons fire only in response to lines that are oriented at particular angles, while others seem to recognize faces. The world may well be what the philosopher Descartes said it was, an embodiment of the workings of the human mind, Dr. Gur said. "Descartes said that we are creating our world," he said. "But there is a world out there that we can't know."

Dr. Gur said that at this point he would hesitate to baldly proclaim that men and women inhabit different worlds. "I'd say that science might be leading us in that direction," he said, but before he commits himself he would like to see more definite differences in the way men's and women's brains function and to know more about what the differences mean.

Dr. Witelson cautioned that "at this point, it is a very big leap to go from any of the structural or organizational differences that were demonstrated to the cognitive differences that were demonstrated." She explained that "all you have is two sets of differences, and whether one is the basis of the other has not been shown." But she added, "One can speculate."

Dr. Witelson emphasized that in speculating she was "making a very big leap," but she noted that "we all live in our different worlds and our worlds depend on our brains.

"And," she said, "if these sex differences in the brain, with 'if' in big capital letters, do have cognitive consequences, and it would be hard to believe there would be none, then it is possible that there is a genuine difference in the kinds of things that men and women perceive and how these things are integrated. To that extent it may be possible that in some respects there is less of an easy cognitive or emotional communication between the sexes as a group because our brains may be wired differently."

The Shaywitzes said they were reluctant even to speculate from the data at hand. But, they said, they think that the deep philosophical questions about the perceptual worlds of men and women can eventually be resolved by science.

"It is a truism that men and women are different," Dr. Bennett Shaywitz said. "What I think we can do now is to take what is essentially folklore and place it in the context of science. There is a real scientific method available to answer some of these questions."

Dr. Sally Shaywitz added: "I think we've taken a qualitative leap forward in our ability to ask questions." But, she said, "the field is simply too young to have provided more than a very intriguing appetizer."

Approaches to Understanding Male-Female Brain Differences

Studies of differences in perception or behavior can suggest how male and female thinking may diverge; studies of structural or metabolic differences can suggest why. But only now are differences in brain organization being studied.

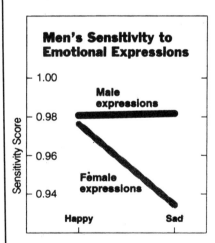

A study compared how well men and women recognized emotions in photos of actors portraying happiness and sadness. Men were equally sensitive to a range of happy and sad faces in men but far less sensitive to sadness in women's faces.

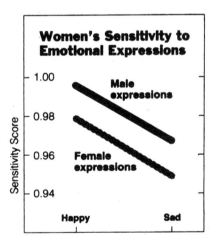

The women in the study were generally more sensitive to happy faces than to sad ones. They were also better able to recognize sadness in a man's face. For both sexes, sensitivity scores reflected the percent of the time the emotion was correctly identified.

KERNEL OF FEAR

How can just the smell of smoke make a veteran relive all the horrors of combat in hallucinatory detail? The answer lies in the amygdala, a tiny brain structure in which nerve pathways shackle innocent stimuli to memories of unbearable terror.

Mark Caldwell

Mark Caldwell is a professor of English at Fordham University and author of The Last Crusade: The War on Consumption 1862–1954. *For the January* Discover, *Caldwell wrote about the discoveries of new cellular organelles and the first successful repair of a defective gene.*

Fear may not be one of the more pleasurable emotions, but it is an effective survival tool. Sheer terror efficiently propels you away from the predator that wants to eat you; anxiety, fear's milder (if more gnawing), civilized form, chivies you into meeting the deadline set by a scary superior. In either case, the reward you get for enduring the cold sweat and the pounding heartbeat is that you live on to gather up another lunch or meet another deadline.

Unfortunately, fear sometimes floods out beyond the channels where it's useful. Take the experience of the "Gunny," as he asked to be identified: the Gunny was stationed with the Marines in Vietnam from 1969 to 1971. He is a compact, powerfully built man with a threateningly shaved head but a disconcertingly kind gaze and a gentle voice. "I go into deep flashbacks," he says. "It's like I'm right there again—the sounds, the smells, the screaming. It's almost like a blackout; the present doesn't exist. It can be snowing and I sweat like I'm in the jungle." So debilitating did these attacks become that one day in 1987 the Gunny walked away from his Pittsburgh post office job and spent the next three years in the backcountry of Pennsylvania—emerging only when he found himself stalking hunters in the woods. Scared by this silently rising pressure of violence, he forced himself back into civilization and began treatment.

The Gunny suffers from post-traumatic stress disorder, a pathological form of anxiety. The syndrome typically begins with a trauma beyond the range of normal human experience—combat, say, or a disaster like the Kobe earthquake or the World Trade Center bombing. Some people emerge unscarred by such experiences, but PTSD patients are uncontrollably and often permanently affected. Small irritants like a thunderclap can set in motion tidal waves of panic, even full-color flashbacks, during which sufferers relive horrors that may have vanished from their conscious memories.

The war in Vietnam spawned a near epidemic of PTSD. In fact, U.S. soldiers' experiences there gave rise to what's now regarded as the classic form of the disorder. Vets like the Gunny, who is undergoing treatment at the National Center for PTSD (a unit of the Veterans Affairs Medical Center), in West Haven, Connecticut, are far from unusual. "I can numb out for hours, not thinking of anything," echoes George K., another patient at the center. "But then something will remind me and take me back—the odor of a certain kind of wood burning, or even of a plant, since I live in Florida and the vegetation is a lot like Vietnam's."

Traditional psychotherapy has had at best mixed success in treating PTSD—its tools, as many therapists will admit, are blunt and imprecise, not finely matched to the physiological mechanism of the disease. George K. and the Gunny are part of a therapy program with confessedly modest goals: getting the patients to accept their disorder as chronic and their progress as a matter of halting, reversible steps. But bizarre though the experiences of PTSD sufferers may be, and frustrating as the condition is to treat, it's no longer as mysterious as its quasi-hallucinatory manifestations might suggest. Neurobiologists have now identified and begun to disentangle the cranial wiring that gives rise to it—opening up the possibility, they believe, of treatment based on the anatomy of the syndrome. The more visionary researchers in the field dream

13. Kernel of Fear

of drugs engineered to zero in on the cerebral mechanisms that go haywire during a PTSD attack.

The key to their hopes is an unprepossessing piece of the brain, a chickpea-size tangle of neurons called the amygdala. The term, Latin for "almond," describes the structure's shape. As with most brain structures, you've got two more or less symmetrical amygdalae—one on the right, another on the left, just behind your ears. "Just above the ear is the temporal lobe of your brain," explains Joseph LeDoux of New York University's Center for Neural Science. "The amygdala's on the interior underside of it."

Anatomists first encountered the amygdala centuries ago, though they hadn't a clue as to what it did. Recently, however, amygdala research has flourished as several radically different approaches to studying the brain have come together, giving neuroscientists a sharper picture of the biology of terror. The work is in three parts. First researchers like LeDoux perform behavioral experiments: they subject test animals to fear-causing stimuli, such as a mildly unpleasant pulse of electricity, then measure the animals' responses. Next they track those responses to particular parts of the brain. Finally they peer deep into the microscopic reaches of those structures, tracing the intricate nerve-to-nerve signaling that accompanies the reaction.

The behavioral experiments at the base of this work wouldn't, in principle, surprise a tyro in sophomore biology. It's been nearly a century, after all, since Ivan Petrovich Pavlov stumbled on the discovery that the brain changes itself in response to a consistently administered stimulus. When Pavlov's assistant brought his lab dogs meat regularly, they soon began salivating every time they saw him. Somewhere in the dogs' brains, Pavlov's lab assistant and yumminess, however improbably, had been joined by a firm physiological bond.

As one vet was leaving the church on his wedding day, a car backfired. The war was 25 years and a world away, but he still ran for cover.

Pavlov's salivating dogs bear some relevance to human fear in general, and PTSD patients in particular, in that the reactions are a response to specific stimuli. But PTSD sufferers bolt into panic at stimuli most of us would find at most mildly startling. Psychologist Michael Davis of the Yale School of Medicine recalls one Vietnam veteran who, years into therapy for PTSD, had gotten well enough to marry: "But as he was leaving the church with his new bride, a car backfired. He dove into the bushes. Now, there should have been all kinds of signals in the environment that told him everything was okay. It was 25 years later; he was in the United States, not Vietnam; he was at a church; he was wearing a white tuxedo, not battle fatigues. But when that primordial stimulus came through, he ran for cover. People with anxiety problems just don't respond adequately to safety signals."

Approximating an experience like this with lab animals is tricky. If you give a rat a mild shock and accompany the experience with a flash of light, the rat will soon exhibit a startle response—usually by freezing in place—when it sees the light alone. But suppose you want to equate the rat's learned behavior with a human's experience of acquired fear. How do you know that a rat is feeling fear just because you see it freeze?

Davis, among others, has addressed this difficulty by devising some ingenious experimental techniques. One is called, unmellifluously, the fear-potentiated startle paradigm. First you give the rat a series of shocks to the foot, each accompanied by a flash of light; the rat learns to freeze when it sees the light. Next you expose it to a burst of white noise, which predictably makes it jump. Then you accompany the white noise with the light flash, and now the rat jumps higher than it does when it hears the noise alone. Which proves two things. First, the light in itself is a neutral stimulus (because it doesn't make the rat leap). Second, the light—through its association with the shocks—has acquired the ability to intensify the rat's fear reaction to other startling events, such as a sharp noise. The light triggers a learned fear rather than causing the fear directly.

It works in humans too—only with us you assess startle by measuring how strongly we blink our eyes. In one experiment, Davis and his colleagues found that eye-blink reflexes intensify if subjects are warned to expect a shock from an electrode fastened to their wrists—demonstrating that a piece of information not painful in itself can tap a reservoir of learned fear in the brain.

Where in the brain is this linkage between stimuli forged? By the 1950s and 1960s the amygdala had already started to emerge as a suspiciously significant site. Researchers found that when a monkey's amygdala was damaged, the animal became tamer, less responsive to threats, and generally less fearful. A bit later, using electrical probes in living animals, they showed that in experiences of remembered fear the amygdala, figuratively, lights up like a Christmas display. "If we stimulate the amygdala electrically with a very low current," Davis says, "we can facilitate startle: it's just like a natural fear situation." Conversely, Davis and others had learned by the mid-1980s that fear-potentiated startle disappears if you remove a key part of an animal's amygdala. Show a lab rat its inaugural cat and its blood pressure and heart rate shoot up, apparently by instinct. But take out its amygdala and the rat blithely ignores predators.

For obvious reasons, this kind of experiment can't be done on humans, and suggestive as the animal work is, neurologists have been hesitant to make the leap. But late last year a group of researchers from the University of Iowa College of Medicine offered persuasive evidence that the phenomenon does indeed extend to people. Their patient, S. M., suffers from a disease that destroyed her right and left amygdalae—a rare phenomenon. Her condition hasn't damaged her memory or emotions, except in the case of fear. She can't recognize—can't even imitate—a fearful human facial expression.

Recent technological advances have allowed neuroscientists to begin more detailed brain mapping. Researchers are delving into minute nerve circuits that course through the amygdala and link it with other parts of the brain. "When I started working in this field, it was very, very difficult to figure out how certain areas of the brain connect to other areas," Davis remarks. "But one of the wonderful things that have happened in the last 15 years is that we've begun to be able to track the connections." Such work became possible thanks to advances in microbiology, the field that in the last decade or so has uncovered so much about the innards of living cells, including nerves.

2. DETERMINANTS OF BEHAVIOR: MOTIVATION, ENVIRONMENT, AND PHYSIOLOGY

The mapping began with axons—the long, snaky parts of nerve cells, which connect the cells to one another. Axons, Davis explains, are full of distinctive proteins that shuttle up and down their length, bearing biochemical messages. "People found you could inject a fluorescent dye that these proteins would take up, then transport all the way back along the axon to the cell body." Davis and his colleagues introduced just such a dye into the relay of nerves that produce a startle response in rats. "It led straight back to the amygdala," he says.

Show a lab rat a cat and its blood pressure and heart rate shoot up. But take out its amygdala and the rat blithely ignores predators.

By patiently applying such techniques, Davis and others have begun to assemble a vividly colored road map of neurons to and from the amygdala, and they've found that the tentacles reach in some surprising directions. A tangle of input nerves enters the amygdala in two regions called the basal and lateral nuclei. Another important knot of nerves courses outward from an area called the central nucleus and leads ultimately to all the end points that administer the visible business of fear—the nerves and muscles that make you jump out of your chair when a car backfires, raise your blood pressure, and speed your heartbeat.

The researchers have also found that although information can flow into the amygdala from the cortex—the section of the brain traditionally associated with higher mental functions like reasoning—it can arrive there from more primitive regions as well, areas that in humans, at least, seem independent of consciousness. You can seriously damage the part of an animal's cortex that interprets auditory signals, yet the amygdala, receiving and processing signals that bypass the cortex, will still teach the animal fear.

This connection begins to hint at how, if you're pathologically anxious, you can undergo fission at the sound of a thunderclap, even though your conscious mind tells you you're safe at home in Des Moines by your VCR. A trauma sensitizes the amygdala, imprinting it with a potent yet unconscious memory of fear, training it to jerk all the neural cords of terror every time your five senses transmit a stimulus that, no matter how innocently, echoes the primal episode. The thunderclap, let us say, is like a gunshot. The gunshot was experienced a quarter century ago in a field in Southeast Asia and is entwined with images of death. "Once these pathways are glued together," LeDoux says, "the link is there. A stimulus, like the sound of guns, gets tied up with the horror of seeing the bodies."

Now, unfortunately, when the innocent sound of thunder reaches your ear, a signal bypasses the cortex, traveling from your ear into the amygdala, where the traumatic combat experience has permanently linked it to an outbound circuit that activates all the dolor of panic. Any deliberate, reasoned attempts to deal with the remembered trauma are subverted by neural circuits completely beyond your conscious control.

But how is it that other, associated stimuli also get tied up with the same irrational response? "Say you saw your buddy blown up in front of you in the desert in Kuwait," Davis explains, "and say you were in deep sand at the time. Now every time you see sand on the beach, it re-creates this fear. That's the conditioning process—sand paired with an awful event."

We can guess what's happening on the cell-to-cell level. The key players here are neurotransmitters—chemicals that relay information by squirting out from the axon of one cell, crossing the synapse (the minute gap between nerves), and activating a chemical receptor on the next cell in line. Perhaps the most widely known neurotransmitter is serotonin, and it owes its current celebrity to its tendency to be affected by Prozac, the supercelebrity of antidepressants. But in the amygdala another neurotransmitter, called glutamate, appears to dominate.

When you zoom down to the microscopic world of the nerve cells, the operation of glutamate becomes very complicated indeed. But while neurobiologists are quick to point out that they can't yet show in minute detail what goes on during a PTSD flashback, they can speculate plausibly about how glutamate transmission might lay down a permanent trace through the brain that—in PTSD—would repeatedly allow an inherently innocuous noise like a car backfiring to provoke an uncontrollable onslaught of panic.

Glutamate transmission can work in two ways, each involving a different receptor on the tail end of the nerve cell that receives a signal. When activated, one of these—called the AMPA receptor—allows a transient impulse to speed through the system from point A to point B. Like the wake of a rowboat, all vestiges of the signal vanish almost as soon as the impulse has passed. For PTSD, though, you need permanent learning. The glutamate system might manage that too, by means of another receptor, this one called NMDA. When activated, the NMDA initiates a series of complicated biochemical changes inside the cell that allow learning to take place, laying down a permanent trace, like the imprint of a mountain bike's tire along a dirt trail. Activating the NMDA receptor makes it permanently easier for signals to leap across the synapse, just as the bike's tire track smooths the route for later cyclists, as if inviting more and more of them to follow it.

Now, normally the NMDA receptor is blocked; it won't engage unless one of several things happens first. But, fascinatingly, one of the things that can liberate it is an activated AMPA receptor. That offers an intriguing (though admittedly speculative) model of how PTSD conditioning might take place. Suppose a transient stimulus—let's say it's the crash of a howitzer firing in battle—activates an AMPA receptor in the amygdala. That would unblock the cell's NMDA receptor, allowing a second stimulus—say, body parts flying—to imprint an essentially indelible trajectory from the senses into the amygdala and out again.

LeDoux cautions that research hasn't yet reached the point at which we can make a complete voyage from this microscopic nerve world to a full-fledged human memory, which involves thousands of neurons signaling in complex patterns in many parts of the brain. Still, the glutamate system can give us a tantalizing glimpse.

What's important here is that it may not be just the sound of the explosion that gets linked to the fearful response. Thanks to the first signal's success in unlocking the NMDA receptor, other signals arriving at the same time, carrying information about the look of the sand, say, or the heat of the desert wind, are joined by glutamate to the same fearful response. Decades after the initial event, a neutral stimulus like the sight of a sandy beach may follow a glutamate-lit path that leads to terror.

13. Kernel of Fear

The message, then, for some researchers is clear: alter the biochemistry of the amygdala and you change, maybe drastically, the experience of fear.

Sadly, that step won't be easy. For one thing, a drug that safely affects glutamate transmission has yet to be found. For another, the amygdala itself is far from well understood. "The brain is fantastically complicated," Davis concedes, "just like the immune system." The amygdala sends a tangle of pathways in and out of the brain's other parts, and there's strong evidence that it's involved in many phenomena beyond fear and other emotions. It's been convincingly identified as a modulator of social behavior, and it may also be implicated in schizophrenia, epilepsy, and Alzheimer's disease. Nevertheless, despite such daunting complexity, the progress researchers have made so far has emboldened many to hope for designer drugs to block the episodes of uncontrollable stress that mark conditions like PTSD.

Of course, tempting though the prospect might be, nobody wants to get rid of fear altogether. "You have to be anxious enough to meet your deadline," Davis notes. "So you don't want to turn off your amygdala totally." Still, patients like the vets at West Haven's National Center for PTSD, who suffer surges of unendurable stress, need and deserve something to keep their terror at bay. No such drug has yet appeared: that's the disappointing news. But as the amygdala gives up more and more of its secrets, it may ultimately grant inventive pharmacologists an opening to block fear in its most nightmarish—and least useful—forms.

The Brain Manages Happiness And Sadness in Different Centers

Daniel Goleman

The essence of emotion—the rapture of happiness, the numbness of depression, the angst of anxiety—is as evanescent as a spring rainbow. It is hard enough for a poet to capture, let alone a neuroscientist.

Now brain researchers, in their own fashion, have begun to do so. A major result emerging from the new research is that the brain does not have just a single emotional center, as has long been believed, but that different emotions involve different structures. Another is that the brains of men and women seem to generate certain emotions with different patterns of activity.

The new advances are made possible by fast imaging methods that allow researchers to take snapshots of the brain in action. The snapshots are short enough that they roughly parallel the duration of an emotion, however fleeting. They have already resulted in a radical redrawing of the neurological map for emotion, showing regions of emotional activity both in and beyond the limbic system, a ring of structures around the brain stem, which for 50 years was considered the brain's emotional center.

One surprising result of the remapping is that emotional opposites, like happiness and sadness, are not registered that way in the brain, but rather entail quite independent patterns of activity, according to a report this month in The American Journal of Psychiatry.

"It's because happiness and sadness involve separate brain areas that we can have bittersweet moments, like when a child is leaving home for college and you're sad, but happy, too," said Dr. Mark George, a psychiatrist and neurologist at the National Institute of Mental Health in Bethesda, Md., and the lead author of the report.

When a woman feels sad, Dr. George discovered with a brain imaging method known as positron emission tomography, her brain shows increased activity in the structures of the limbic system near the face, and more activity in the left prefrontal cortex than in the right. His studies were conducted in women to avoid the confounding difficulty of possible differences between the sexes.

When his 11 subjects felt happy, the characteristic pattern was a decrease of activity in the regions of the cerebral cortex that are committed to forethought and planning. These regions are in the temporal-parietal area of the cortex, located just over and a bit behind the ears, and the right prefrontal lobe, just behind the forehead. "Those neocortical region are used in complex planning—it's interesting these shut down in happiness," Dr. George said.

The cue for sadness was to ask the subjects to recall personal events in their lives such as deaths and funerals, or to look at a picture of a sad face. For happiness, the cue was to remember joyous times such as births and weddings, or to look at happy faces.

In earlier research, Dr. George found that the neocortical areas become even less active when volunteers received injections of morphine or cocaine. "There seems to be a continuum in brain activity in the same regions from transient happiness to ecstasy," he said.

Another key change was in the amygdala, a pair of almond-shaped structures in the limbic system. The amygdala area "activates during sadness," Dr. George said. But the structures change only slightly when a person is happy. "The left amygdala seems to shut down a bit, while the right goes up," he said.

Such findings are mapping out a new neuroanatomical atlas for the emotions, one that eventually may give psychiatrists new guides to treating mental illness. "The brain mechanisms of emotional change are perhaps the most central question in psychiatry," said Dr. Robert Robinson, chief of psychiatry at the University of Iowa Hospitals and Clinics in Iowa City.

Many serious psychiatric disorders such as depression and panic attacks, are extremes of ordinary emotion. Studies of anxiety, for instance show that the brain regions that are most active while people are

14. Brain Manages Happiness and Sadness

How the Brain Computes Tears and Laughter

The brain handles happiness and sadness in different areas, not in a single emotional center as was thought. New fast scanning methods show that happiness is marked by a decrease in activity in the cortex, in areas responsible for forethought and planning. Sadness is associated with enhanced activity in regions of the limbic system. PET scans below show changes in activity of subjects experiencing the two emotional states.

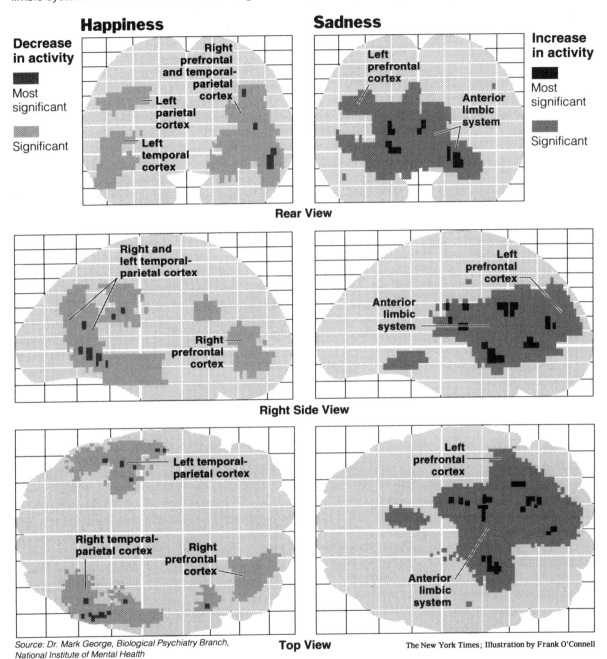

Source: Dr. Mark George, Biological Psychiatry Branch, National Institute of Mental Health

The New York Times; Illustration by Frank O'Connell

anxious are even more active during panic attacks. Locating the primary sites of various emotions represents a major step toward understanding what is going wrong when these sites become overactive.

The recent findings on sadness offer a new twist: brain areas involved in ordinary sadness almost completely shut down when a person is clinically depressed. "Sadness and depression seem to involve the same brain region, the left prefrontal cortex, in different ways," said Dr. George. "It gets more active during ordinary sadness, but shuts down in people with clinical depression. Perhaps the left prefrontal cortex somehow burns itself out when sadness persists for several months."

Many people with severe depression no longer feel sadness or any other emotion. "They're emotionally numb," said Dr. George.

He has also studied the locations of happiness and sadness in men, though these studies have not been published. He has found that the processing of emotion is yet another aspect in which the brains of men and women apparently differ. "When they are sad, women activate the anterior limbic system much more than do men," said Dr. George. "At the same time, women seem to experience a more profound sadness than do men. It makes me wonder if this might be related to why women have twice the risk of depression as do men."

In a study still in progress, Dr. George is mapping anger and anxiety. "Other work on anxiety implicates the right temporal area of the cerebral cortex, and our findings seem to support that," Dr. George said.

For anger, a main area of increased activity appears to be the anterior septum, which is in the center of the brain. "In cats, if you stimulate this area with an electrode the cat lashes out in rage at anything nearby," said Dr. George.

Before imaging, neuroscientists' principal method of mapping the sites of emotions in the brain rested on analyzing what was missing in patients who had had brain injuries or strokes. The technique is like drawing a diagram of a house's electrical wiring by pulling out the fuses one by one.

But the brain imaging techniques are still far from perfect. PET scans require subjects to be injected with a mildly radioactive chemical and make images that are averaged from multiple readings instead of from a single scan. And a serious problem with the magnetic resonance imaging technique is that a patient must lie in a metal cylinder, an experience that has been likened to being trapped in a coffin. "While you're in those machines it's very difficult to have reactions other than those to the machine itself," said Dr. Paul Ekman, director of the Human Interaction Laboratory at the University of California at San Francisco, who recently spent three hours in such a machine.

To overcome the problem, researchers have gotten their subjects into the desired emotional states with such prods as a scene from the film "The Godfather" in which a decapitated horse's head is found in a bed, a joyous scene from "On Golden Pond" in which Jane Fonda dances with her father, Henry Fonda, and even—to elicit fear in people with a snake phobia—a live (but friendly) python perched atop the doughnutlike PET scan equipment that surrounds the head. Patients having magnetic resonance imaging can watch films through a kind of periscope.

Dr. Ekman and colleagues plan to study how emotions are evoked by seeing which brain areas light up in response to stimuli like remembering an upsetting event, seeing an image of a sad face or putting one's facial muscles in the configuration typical of various emotions.

The investigation is of crucial importance for researchers, since the means they employ to evoke an emotion while capturing brain images may itself affect the image they get.

A team led by Dr. Richard Lane at the University of Arizona in Tucson compared the brain areas involved when people either watched film clips that evoked happiness or sadness, or called to mind happy or sad moments. In all cases there was heightened activity in the thalamus and the prefrontal cortex, suggesting a role for these regions in each of these emotions, no matter how it was evoked.

"The prefrontal cortex monitors a person's emotional state, no matter what it is, to generate an appropriate response," said Dr. Lane, "while the thalamus participates in how that response is executed."

During the film—not during emotional memories—two key areas of the limbic system were active: the amygdala and the hippocampus, suggesting that these structures are involved in evaluating whether a situation is of emotional import, Dr. Lane said.

On the other hand, during the recall of sad or happy events there was more activity in the anterior insular region, an area of the cortex with strong connections to the limbic system, implying a special role for this area in emotional memories. "The anterior insular region seems to be involved in investing thoughts or memories with emotional significance," said Dr. Lane.

That same region is also active during anticipatory anxiety, such as when someone is waiting to receive a mild electric shock, according to new findings by Dr. Eric Reiman, a psychologist at the University of Arizona in Phoenix, and a colleague of Dr. Lane's.

"The vast majority of findings until now about the brain's emotional regions has been based on emotions in laboratory animals, all of which are induced by external means, such as shocks," said Dr. Reiman. "But the results with people who are evoking emotions through memories are showing that a very different set of brain areas are active than had been thought from the animal research."

The exploration of the brain's topography for emotions through imaging is its earliest stages and, like any forays into new terrain, may produce distorted maps, researchers warn.

"We need to be cautious about interpreting these findings on the regions involved in emotions," said Dr. Richard Davidson, a psychologist at the University of Wisconsin and a participant in some of the research. "We're just beginning to work out the technical difficulties in capturing neuroanatomical images from people during something so private and fleeting as an emotion."

FAITH & HEALING

Can prayer, faith and spirituality really improve your physical health? A growing and surprising body of scientific evidence says they can.

Claudia Wallis

Draped in embroidered cloth, laden with candles, redolent with roses and incense, the altar at the Santa Fe, New Mexico, home of Eetla Soracco seems an unlikely site for cutting-edge medical research. Yet every day for 10 weeks, ending last October, Soracco spent an hour or more there as part of a controlled study in the treatment of AIDS. Her assignment: to pray for five seriously ill patients in San Francisco.

Soracco, an Estonian-born "healer" who draws on Christian, Buddhist and Native American traditions, did not know the people for whom she was praying. All she had were their photographs, first names and, in some cases, T-cell counts. Picturing a patient in her mind, she would ask for "permission to heal" and then start to explore his body in her mind: "I looked at all the organs as though it is an anatomy book. I could see where things were distressed. These areas are usually dark and murky. I go in there like a white shower and wash it all out." Soracco was instructed to spend one hour a day in prayer, but the sessions often lasted twice as long. "For that time," she says, "it's as if I know the person."

Soracco is one of 20 faith healers recruited for the study by Dr. Elisabeth Targ, clinical director of psychosocial oncology research at California Pacific Medical Center in San Francisco. In the experiment, 20 severely ill AIDS patients were randomly selected; half were prayed for, half were not. None were told to which group they had been assigned. Though Targ has not yet published her results, she describes them as sufficiently "encouraging" to warrant a larger, follow-up study with 100 AIDS patients.

Twenty years ago, no self-respecting M.D. would have dared to propose a double-blind, controlled study of something as intangible as prayer. Western medicine has spent the past 100 years trying to rid itself of remnants of mysticism. Targ's own field, psychiatry, couldn't be more hostile to spirituality: Sigmund Freud dismissed religious mysticism as "infantile helplessness" and "regression to primary narcissism." Today, while Targ's experiment is not exactly mainstream, it does exemplify a shift among doctors toward the view that there may be more to health than blood-cell counts and EKGs and more to healing than pills and scalpels.

"People, a growing number of them, want to examine the connection between healing and spirituality," says Jeffrey Levin, a gerontologist and epidemiologist at Eastern Virginia Medical School in Norfolk. To do such research, he adds, "is no longer professional death." Indeed, more and more medical schools are adding courses on holistic and alternative medicine with titles like Caring for the Soul. "The majority, 10 to 1, present the material uncritically," reports Dr. Wallace Sampson of Stanford University, who recently surveyed the offerings of every U.S. medical school.

This change in doctors' attitudes reflects a broader yearning among their patients for a more personal, more spiritual approach to health and healing. As the 20th century draws to an end, there is growing disenchantment with one of its greatest achievements: modern, high-tech medicine. Western medicine is at its best in a crisis—battling acute infection, repairing the wounds of war, replacing a broken-down kidney or heart. But increasingly, what ails America and other prosperous societies are chronic illnesses, such as high blood pressure, backaches, cardiovascular disease, arthritis, depression and acute illnesses that become chronic, such as cancer and AIDS. In most of these, stress and life-style play a part.

"Anywhere from 60% to 90% of visits to doctors are in the mind-body, stress-related realm," asserts Dr. Herbert Benson, president of the Mind/Body Medical Institute of Boston's Deaconess Hospital and Harvard Medical School. It is a triumph of medicine that so many of us live long enough to develop these chronic woes, but, notes Benson, "traditional modes of therapy—pharmaceutical and surgical—don't work well against them."

Not only do patients with chronic health problems fail to find relief in a doctor's office, but the endless high-tech scans and tests of modern medicine also often leave them feeling alienated and uncared for. Many seek solace in the offices of alternative therapists and faith healers—to the tune of $30 billion a year, by some estimates. Millions more is spent on best-selling books and tapes by New Age doctors such as Deepak Chopra, Andrew Weil and Larry Dossey, who offer an appealing blend of medicine and Eastern-flavored spirituality.

Some scientists are beginning to look seriously at just what benefits patients may derive from spirituality. To their surprise, they are finding plenty of relevant data buried in the medical literature. More than 200 studies that touch directly or indirectly on the role of religion have been ferreted out by Levin of Eastern

2. DETERMINANTS OF BEHAVIOR: MOTIVATION, ENVIRONMENT, AND PHYSIOLOGY

Virginia and Dr. David Larson, a research psychiatrist formerly at the National Institutes of Health and now at the privately funded National Institute for Healthcare Research. Most of these studies offer evidence that religion is good for one's health. Some highlights:

▶ A 1995 study at Dartmouth-Hitchcock Medical Center found that one of the best predictors of survival among 232 heart-surgery patients was the degree to which the patients said they drew comfort and strength from religious faith. Those who did not had more than three times the death rate of those who did.

▶ A survey of 30 years of research on blood pressure showed that churchgoers have lower blood pressure than non-churchgoers—5 mm lower, according to Larson, even when adjusted to account for smoking and other risk factors.

▶ Other studies have shown that men and women who attend church regularly have half the risk of dying from coronary-artery disease as those who rarely go to church. Again, smoking and socioeconomic factors were taken into account.

▶ A 1996 National Institute on Aging study of 4,000 elderly living at home in North Carolina found that those who attend religious services are less depressed and physically healthier than those who don't attend or who worship at home.

▶ In a study of 30 female patients recovering from hip fractures, those who regarded God as a source of strength and comfort and who attended religious services were able to walk farther upon discharge and had lower rates of depression than those who had little faith.

▶ Numerous studies have found lower rates of depression and anxiety-related illness among the religiously committed. Nonchurchgoers have been found to have a suicide rate four times higher than church regulars.

There are many possible explanations for such findings. Since churchgoers are more apt than nonattendees to respect religious injunctions against drinking, drug abuse, smoking and other excesses, it's possible that their better health merely reflects these healthier habits.

Some of the studies, however, took pains to correct for this possibility by making statistical adjustments for lifestyle differences. Larson likes to point out that in his own study the benefits of religion hold up strongly, even for those who indulge in cigarette smoking. Smokers who rated religion as being very important to them were one-seventh as likely to have an abnormal blood-pressure reading as smokers who did not value religion.

Churchgoing also offers social support—which numerous studies have shown to have a salutary effect on well-being. (Even owning a pet has been shown to improve the health of the lonesome.) The Dartmouth heart-surgery study is one of the few that attempts to tease apart the effects of social support and religious conviction. Patients were asked separate sets of questions about their participation in social groups and the comfort they drew from faith. The two factors appeared to have distinct benefits that made for a powerful combination. Those who were *both* religious and socially involved had a 14-fold advantage over those who were isolated or lacked faith.

Could it be that religious faith has some direct influence on physiology and health? Harvard's Herbert Benson is probably the most persuasive proponent of this view. Benson won international fame in 1975 with his best-selling book, *The Relaxation Response*. In it he showed that patients can successfully battle a number of stress-related ills by practicing a simple form of meditation. The act of focusing the mind on a single sound or image brings about a set of physiological changes that are the opposite of the "fight-or-flight response." With meditation, heart rate, respiration and brain waves slow down, muscles relax and the effects of epinephrine and other stress-related hormones diminish. Studies have shown that by routinely eliciting this "relaxation response," 75% of insomniacs begin to sleep normally, 35% of infertile women become pregnant and 34% of chronic-pain sufferers reduce their use of painkilling drugs.

In his latest book, *Timeless Healing* (Scribner; $24), Benson moves beyond the purely pragmatic use of meditation into the realm of spirituality. He ventures to say humans are actually engineered for religious faith. Benson bases this contention on his work with a subgroup of patients who report that they sense a closeness to God while meditating. In a five-year study of patients using meditation to battle chronic illnesses, Benson found that those who claim to feel the intimate presence of a higher power had better health and more rapid recoveries.

"Our genetic blueprint has made believing in an Infinite Absolute part of our nature," writes Benson. Evolution has so equipped us, he believes, in order to offset our uniquely human ability to ponder our own mortality: "To counter this fundamental angst, humans are also wired for God."

In Benson's view, prayer operates along the same biochemical pathways as the relaxation response. In other words, praying affects epinephrine and other corticosteroid messengers or "stress hormones," leading to lower blood pressure, more relaxed heart rate and respiration and other benefits.

Recent research demonstrates that these stress hormones also have a direct impact on the body's immunological defenses against disease. "Anything involved with meditation and controlling the state of mind that alters hormone activity has the potential to have an impact on the immune system," says David Felten, chairman of the Department of Neurobiology at the University of Rochester.

It is probably no coincidence that the relaxation response and religious experience share headquarters in the brain. Studies show that the relaxation response is controlled by the amygdala, a small, almond-shaped structure in the brain that together with the hippocampus and hypothalamus makes up the limbic system. The limbic system, which is found in all primates, plays a key role in emotions, sexual pleasure, deep-felt memories and, it seems, spirituality. When either the amygdala or the hippocampus is electrically stimulated during surgery, some patients have visions of angels and devils. Patients whose limbic systems are chronically stimulated by drug abuse or a tumor often become religious fanatics. "The ability to have religious experiences has a neuro-anatomical basis," concludes Rhawn Joseph, a neuroscientist at the Palo Alto VA Medical Center in California.

Many researchers believe these same neuronal and hormonal pathways are the basis for the renowned and powerful "placebo effect." Decades of research show that if a patient truly believes a therapy is useful—even if it is a sugar pill or snake oil—that belief has the power to heal. In one classic 1950 study, for instance, pregnant women suffering from severe morning sickness were given syrup of ipecac, which induces vomiting, and told it was a powerful new cure for nausea. Amazingly, the women ceased vomiting. "Most of the history of medicine is the history of the placebo effect," observes Benson in *Timeless Healing*.

Though Benson devotes much of his book to documenting the power of the placebo effect—which he prefers to call "remembered wellness"—he has come to believe the benefits of religious faith are even greater. "Faith in the medical treatment," he writes, "[is] wonderfully therapeutic, successful in treating 60% to 90% of the most common medical problems. But if you so believe, faith in an invincible and infallible force carries even more healing power... It is a supremely potent belief."

Do the faithful actually have God on their side? Are their prayers answered? Benson doesn't say. But a true scientist, insists Jeffrey Levin, cannot dismiss this possibility: "I can't directly study that, but as an honest scholar, I can't rule it out."

A handful of scientists have attempted to study the possibility that praying works through some supernatural factor. One of the most cited examples is a 1988 study by cardiologist Randolph Byrd at San Francisco General Hospital. Byrd took 393 patients in the coronary-care unit and randomly assigned half to be prayed for by born-again Christians. To eliminate the placebo effect, the patients were not told of the experiment. Remarkably, Byrd found that the control group was five times as likely to need antibiotics and three times as likely to develop complications as those who were prayed for.

Byrd's experiment has never been replicated and has come under some criticism for design flaws. A more recent study of intercessory prayer with alcoholics found no benefit, while Elisabeth Targ's study of AIDS patients is still too small to produce significant results.

Science may never be able to pin down the benefits of spirituality. Attempts by Benson and others to do so are like "trying to nail Jell-O to the wall," complains William Jarvis, a public-health professor at California's Loma Linda University and the president of the National Council Against Health Fraud. But it may not be necessary to understand how prayer works to put it to use for patients. "We often know something works before we know why," observes Santa Fe internist Larry Dossey, the author of the 1993 best seller *Healing Words*.

A TIME/CNN poll of 1,004 Americans conducted last week by Yankelovich Partners found that 82% believed in the healing power of prayer and 64% thought doctors should pray with those patients who request it. Yet even today few doctors are comfortable with that role. "We physicians are culturally insensitive about the role of religion," says David Larson, noting that fewer than two-thirds of doctors say they believe in God. "It is very important to many of our patients and not important to lots of doctors."

Larson would like physicians to be trained to ask a few simple questions of their seriously or chronically ill patients: Is religion important to you? Is it important in how you cope with your illness? If the answers are yes, doctors might ask whether the patient would like to discuss his or her faith with the hospital chaplain or another member of the clergy. "You can be an atheist and say this," Larson insists. Not doing so, he argues, is a disservice to the patient.

Even skeptics such as Jarvis believe meditation and prayer are part of "good patient management." But he worries, as do many doctors, that patients may become "so convinced of the power of mind over body that they may decide to rely on that, instead of doing the hard things, like chemotherapy."

In the long run, it may be that most secular of forces—economics—that pushes doctors to become more sensitive to the spiritual needs of their patients. Increasingly, American medicine is a business, run by large HMOs and managed-care groups with a keen eye on the bottom line. Medical businessmen are more likely than are scientifically trained doctors to view prayer and spirituality as low-cost treatments that clients say they want. "The combination of these forces—consumer demand and the economic collapse of medicine—are very powerful influences that are making medicine suddenly open to this direction," observes Andrew Weil, a Harvard-trained doctor and author of *Spontaneous Healing*.

Cynics point out that there is an even more practical reason for doctors to embrace spirituality even if they don't believe. The high cost of malpractice insurance gives physicians an incentive to attend to their patients' spiritual needs—and, if necessary, get on their knees and pray with them. Not only might it help restore their image as infallible caregivers, but if something does go wrong, patients who associate their doctors with a higher power might be less likely to sue.

—*Reported by Jeanne McDowell/Los Angeles, Alice Park/New York and Lisa H. Towle/Raleigh*

Problems Influencing Personal Growth

At each stage of development from infancy to old age, humans are faced with new challenges. The infant has the rudimentary sensory apparati for seeing, hearing, and touching but needs to begin coordinating stimuli into meaningful information. For example, early in life the baby begins to recognize familiar and unfamiliar people and usually becomes attached to the primary caregivers. In toddlerhood, the same child must master the difficult skills of walking, talking, and toilet training. This energetic, mobile, and sociable child also needs to learn the boundaries set on his or her behavior by others. As the child matures, not only do physical changes continue to take place, but the family composition may change when siblings are added, parents divorce, or mother and father work outside the home. Playmates become more influential, and others in the community such as day-care workers and teachers have an increasing influence on the child. The child eventually may spend more time at school than at home. The demands in this new environment require that the child sit still, pay attention, learn, and cooperate with others for long periods of time, behaviors perhaps never before extensively demanded of him or her.

In adolescence the body noticeably changes. Peers may pressure the individual to indulge in new behaviors such as using illegal drugs or engaging in premarital sex. Some older teenagers are said to be faced with an identity crisis when they must choose among career, education, and marriage. The pressures of work and family life exact a toll on less mature youths, while others are satisfied with the workplace and home.

Adulthood and middle age may bring contentment or turmoil as individuals face career peaks, empty nests, advancing age, and perhaps the death of loved ones such as parents. Again, some individuals cope more effectively with these events than do others.

At any step in the developmental sequence, unexpected stressors challenge individuals. These stressors include major illnesses, accidents, natural disasters, economic recessions, and family or personal crises. It is important to remember, however, that an event need not be negative to be stressful. Any major life change may cause stress. As welcome as weddings, new babies, and job promotions may be, they, too, can be stressful because of the changes in daily life they require. Each challenge and each change must be met and adjusted to if the individual is going to move successfully to the next stage of development. Some individuals continue along their paths unscathed; others do not fare so well.

This unit of the book examines major problems in various stages of life from childhood to old age. The first article commences our chronological look at problems of development. In "Clipped Wings," the results of a report on the deleterious effects of drugs, alcohol, and other substances on the fetus are shared with the reader. As the article suggests, even before birth problems for our development exist.

Toddlerhood is the next stage of development. Many American parents need to decide whether both parents will work, and, if so, whether the child will be placed in child care. In "How Kids Benefit from Child Care," Vivian Cadden reveals the results of a survey of working mothers whose children were in day care. The mothers nearly unanimously agreed that this early experience provided advantages for their children.

We next examine the influence of mothers and fathers on the child. In "Fathers' Time," Paul Roberts investigates the roles of mothers and fathers in their child's development. Roberts reveals that each parent seems to serve a distinct role. In fact, though the father's role has often been ignored by psychological researchers, they report that fathers are more important to development than we ever thought.

The fourth essay in this unit examines a fascinating topic, memories of childhood abuse. A controversy exists in society as well as in the psychological literature about whether some people's memories are real or fictitious. In "Lies of the Mind," Leon Jaroff discusses these memories and describes how false memories rip families apart. Jaroff also shares with the reader some methods for coping with abuse, real or not.

Child abuse is not our society's only childhood problem, however. Myra and David Sadker's research clearly demonstrates that American schools are unfair to girls. Compared to boys, who are more actively engaged in the learning process by their teachers, girls have become spectators in educational settings. The Sadkers' point is made in "Why Schools Must Tell Girls: 'You're Smart, You Can Do It.'"

In a second article on schools, Margot Hornblower suggests that schools need to expand their roles, given all the changes in our society. She recommends that schools become holistic communities that educate not just children but parents and that schools should act as sur-

UNIT 3

rogate parents to those children whose parents are unavailable or unwilling to care for and love them. She suggests that better schools will decrease delinquency, enhance achievement, and invariably serve children well in other capacities.

Adolescence is the next life stage. A prevalent social problem in the United States is teen pregnancy. The United States has the highest teen pregnancy rate of any industrialized Western society. In "Helping Teens Avoid Negative Consequences of Sexual Activity," Jeannie Rosoff examines many relevant issues, all aimed at reducing the teen pregnancy rate.

Adulthood is the next growth stage. Adulthood is often ignored in favor of childhood, but author Gail Sheehy says that adulthood is important and that adults pass through several important stages. In "New Passages," Sheehy discusses her notion that there are three distinct phases of adulthood and emphasizes midlife.

Is it true that as we age our brains lose power? "Is It Normal Aging?" discusses the causes and consequences of Alzheimer's disease. This useful selection helps the reader determine whether cognitive problems are mere age-related changes or the beginning of this ravaging disease.

The ultimate developmental stage is death. Death is a topic that both fascinates and frightens most of us. There are some individuals, however, who choose to die. In "The Mystery of Suicide," David Gelman grapples with the serious topic of suicide while our society currently struggles with right-to-die and euthanasia issues.

Looking Ahead: Challenge Questions

Individuals face challenges at every phase of development. What challenges are typical of each stage, as mentioned in this unit? What are others that have not been mentioned? What stage do you believe is most demanding? Why?

If drugs and other addictive substances have detrimental effects on the fetus, should we hold addicted parents responsible for the care and treatment of their addicted and deformed infants? Why or why not? If you answered "yes," what should we do? For example, should we imprison them for neglect? What other factors besides drugs and alcohol influence prenatal life?

How can we enhance children's early development? How important is the parent-infant relationship? Is there any such thing as natural motherly love, and if so, how important is it? How does divorce affect the child-parent relationship? How does both parents' working affect their children? Should working parents place their children in day care? What are the advantages of day care? The disadvantages?

How do mothers and fathers differ in their role as parents? What purpose do the differences serve? Should psychological research attend more to the role of fathers? Why or why not?

Many issues face American children. This unit examines gender roles, child abuse, and teen pregnancy. What are their effects on American children? Describe some other problems and their effects on the child not mentioned in the readings.

What are false memories of abuse? How can we tell the difference between real or imagined abuse? What programs are available for survivors of abuse, real or imagined?

There is little discussion in these articles of children from other cultures. Some cultures rear their children quite differently from the way Americans do. What lessons can we learn from these cultures that we might incorporate into our child-rearing methods? What strategies and techniques could we teach others?

How are boys and girls treated differently in school? What are the later consequences of the differences in treatment? What can Americans do to ensure that girls are treated fairly and well in our public schools? What other roles should our schools take on? Should schools become "parents" to American children? Why or why not?

What determines adolescent pregnancy? Is this an issue just for girls? Explain. Is it primarily minority adolescents who become pregnant? What are some other social problems affecting adolescents?

Is adulthood as important to growth as childhood? How many stages do adults pass through? Discuss whether or not American adults face more crises today than did earlier generations. What could we do to change society so that adulthood provides continual positive growth experiences? What link is there, if any, between critical life events in adulthood and propensity for illness?

What myths do we hold about middle and old age? What truth is there to these myths? How can social scientists and older adults change our attitudes and correct any misinformation? What positive changes does research suggest come from aging? What negative changes occur as a result of aging? How is the brain involved in these changes?

Nearly everyone fears death. Explain whether or not this is a sign of poor coping. How might people learn to cope better with the prospect of their own or another's death? Why should we fear or not fear death? Explain whether or not you agree or disagree that death should be speeded along if the quality of life has declined.

What is suicide? Explain why you agree or disagree that people should be able to end their lives by suicide when quality declines. Why do you think most people commit suicide? How and when should we intervene with an individual if she or he decides to commit suicide?

Clipped Wings
*The Fullest Look Yet at How
Prenatal Exposure to Drugs, Alcohol, and Nicotine
Hobbles Children's Learning*

Lucile F. Newman and Stephen L. Buka

Lucile F. Newman is a professor of community health and anthropology at Brown University and the director of the Preventable Causes of Learning Impairment Project. Stephen L. Buka is an epidemiologist and instructor at the Harvard Medical School and School of Public Health.

SOME FORTY thousand children a year are born with learning impairments related to their mother's alcohol use. Drug abuse during pregnancy affects 11 percent of newborns each year—more than 425,000 infants in 1988. Some 260,000 children each year are born at below normal weights—often because they were prenatally exposed to nicotine, alcohol, or illegal drugs.

What learning problems are being visited upon these children? The existing evidence has heretofore been scattered in many different fields of research—in pediatric medicine, epidemiology, public health, child development, and drug and alcohol abuse. Neither educators, health professionals, nor policy makers could go to one single place to receive a full picture of how widespread or severe were these preventable causes of learning impairment.

In our report for the Education Commission of the States, excerpts of which follow, we combed these various fields to collect and synthesize the major studies that relate prenatal exposure to nicotine, alcohol, and illegal drugs[*] with various indexes of students' school performance.

The state of current research in this area is not always as full and satisfying as we would wish. Most of what exists is statistical and epidemiological data, which document the frequency of certain high-risk behaviors and correlate those behaviors to student performance. Such data are very interesting and useful, as they allow teachers and policy makers to calculate the probability that a student with a certain family history will experience school failure. But such data often cannot control for the effects of other risk factors, many of which tend to cluster in similar populations. In other words, the same mother who drinks during her pregnancy may also use drugs, suffer from malnutrition, be uneducated, a teenager, or poor—all factors that might ultimately affect her child's school performance. An epidemiological study generally can't tell you how much of a child's poor school performance is due exclusively to a single risk factor.

Moreover, the cumulative damage wrought by several different postnatal exposures may be greater than the damage caused by a single one operating in isolation. And many of the learning problems that are caused by prenatal exposure to drugs can be compounded by such social factors as poverty and parental disinterest and, conversely, overcome if the child lives in a high-quality postnatal environment.

All of these facts make it difficult to isolate and interpret the level and character of the damage that is caused by a single factor. Further, until recently, there was little interest among researchers in the effects of prenatal alcohol exposure because there was little awareness that it was affecting a substantial number of children. The large cohort of children affected by crack is just now entering the schools, so research on their school performance hasn't been extensive.

What does clearly emerge from the collected data is that our classrooms now include many students whose ability to pay attention, sit still, or fully develop their visual, auditory, and language skills was impaired even before they walked through our schoolhouse doors. On the

---

[*] The full report for the ECS also addressed the effect on children's learning of fetal malnutrition, pre- and postnatal exposure to lead, and child abuse and neglect.

brighter side, the evidence that many of these impairments can be overcome by improved environmental conditions suggests that postnatal treatment is possible; promising experiments in treatment are, in fact, under way and are outlined at the end of this article.

1. Low Birthweight

The collection of graphs begins with a set on low birthweight, which is strongly associated with lowered I.Q. and poor school performance. While low birthweight can be brought on by other factors, including maternal malnutrition and teenage pregnancy, significant causes are maternal smoking, drinking, and drug use.

Around 6.9 percent of babies born in the United States weigh less than 5.5 pounds (2,500 grams) at birth and are considered "low-birthweight" babies. In 1987, this accounted for some 269,100 infants. Low birthweight may result when babies are born prematurely (born too early) or from intrauterine growth retardation (born too small) as a result of maternal malnutrition or actions that restrict blood flow to the fetus, such as smoking or drug use.

In 1987, about 48,750 babies were born at very low birthweights (under 3.25 lbs. or 1,500 grams). Research estimates that 6 to 8 percent of these babies experience major handicaps such as severe mental retardation or cerebral palsy (Eilers et al., 1986; Hack and Breslau, 1986). Another 25 to 26 percent have borderline I.Q. scores, problems in understanding and expressing language, or other deficits (Hack and Breslau, 1986; Lefebvre et al., 1988; Nickel et al., 1982; Vohr et al., 1988). Although these children may enter the public school system, many of them show intellectual disabilities and require special educational assistance. Reading, spelling, handwriting, arts, crafts, and mathematics are difficult school subjects for them. Many are late in developing their speech and language. Children born at very low birthweights are more likely than those born at normal weights to be inattentive, hyperactive, depressed, socially withdrawn, or aggressive (Breslau et al., 1988).

New technologies and the spread of neonatal intensive care over the past decade have improved survival rates of babies born at weights ranging from 3.25 pounds to 5.5 pounds. But, as Figures 2 and 3 show, those born at low birthweight still are at increased risk of school failure. The increased risk, however, is very much tied to the child's postnatal environment. When the data on which Figure 2 is based are controlled to account for socioeconomic circumstances, very low-birthweight babies are approximately twice, not three times, as likely to repeat a grade.

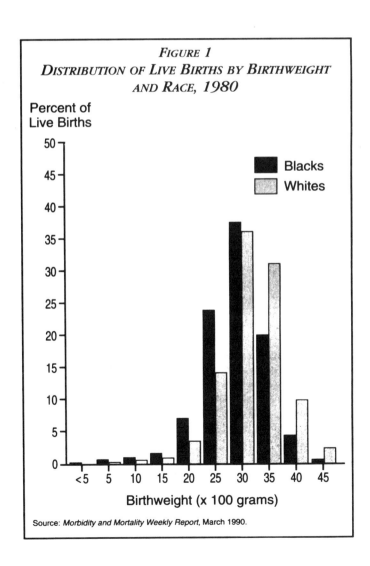

FIGURE 1
DISTRIBUTION OF LIVE BIRTHS BY BIRTHWEIGHT AND RACE, 1980

Source: *Morbidity and Mortality Weekly Report*, March 1990.

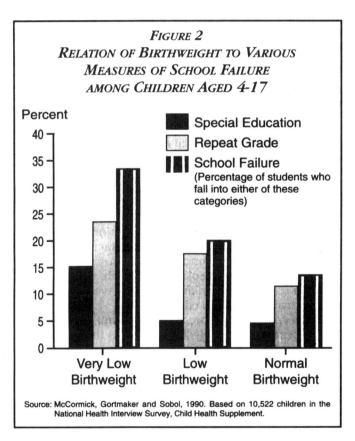

FIGURE 2
RELATION OF BIRTHWEIGHT TO VARIOUS MEASURES OF SCHOOL FAILURE AMONG CHILDREN AGED 4-17

Source: McCormick, Gortmaker and Sobol, 1990. Based on 10,522 children in the National Health Interview Survey, Child Health Supplement.

3. PROBLEMS INFLUENCING PERSONAL GROWTH

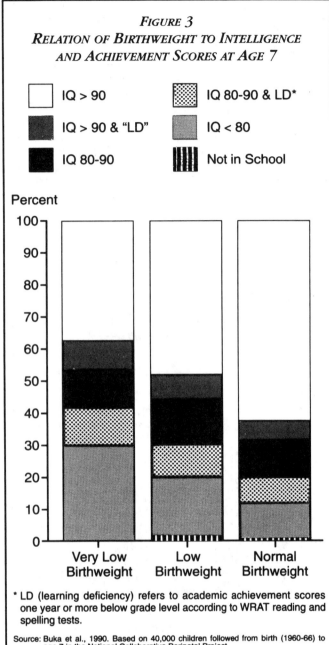

FIGURE 3
RELATION OF BIRTHWEIGHT TO INTELLIGENCE AND ACHIEVEMENT SCORES AT AGE 7

* LD (learning deficiency) refers to academic achievement scores one year or more below grade level according to WRAT reading and spelling tests.

Source: Buka et al., 1990. Based on 40,000 children followed from birth (1960-66) to age 7 in the National Collaborative Perinatal Project.

Indeed, follow-up studies of low-birthweight infants at school age have concluded that "the influence of the environment far outweighs most effects of nonoptimal prenatal or perinatal factors on outcome" (Aylward et al., 1989). This finding suggests that early assistance can improve the intellectual functioning of children at risk for learning delay or impairment (Richmond, 1990).

2. Maternal Smoking

Maternal smoking during pregnancy has long been known to be related to low birthweight (Abel, 1980), an increased risk for cancer in the offspring (Stjernfeldt et al., 1986), and early and persistent asthma, which leads to, among other problems, frequent hospitalization and school absence (Streissguth, 1986). A growing number of new studies has shown that children of smokers are smaller in stature and lag behind other children in cognitive development and educational achievement. These children are particularly subject to hyperactivity and inattention (Rush and Callahan, 1989).

Data from the National Collaborative Perinatal Project on births from 1960 to 1966 measured, among other things, the amount pregnant women smoked at each prenatal visit and how their children functioned in school at age seven. Compared to offspring of nonsmokers, children of heavy smokers (more than two packs per day) were nearly twice as likely to experience school failure by age seven (see Figure 4). The impact of heavy smoking is apparently greater the earlier it occurs during pregnancy. Children of women who smoked heavily during the first trimester of pregnancy were more than twice as likely to fail than children whose mothers did not smoke during the first trimester. During the second and third trimesters, these risks decreased. In all of these analyses, it is difficult to differentiate the effects of exposure to smoking before birth and from either parent after birth; to distinguish between learning problems caused by low birthweight and those caused by other damaging effects of smoking; or, to disentangle the effects of smoke from the socioeconomic setting of the smoker. But it is worth noting that Figure 4 is based on children born in the early sixties, an era when smoking mothers were fairly well distributed across socioeconomic groups.

One study that attempted to divorce the effects of smoking from those of poverty examined middle-class children whose mothers smoked during pregnancy (Fried and Watkinson, 1990) and found that the infants showed differences in responsiveness beginning at one week of age. Later tests at 1, 2, 3, and 4 years of age showed that on verbal tests "the children of the heavy smokers had mean test scores that were lower than those born to lighter smokers, who in turn did not perform as well as those born to nonsmokers." The study also indicated that the effects of smoke exposure, whether in the womb or after birth, may not be identifiable until later ages when a child needs to perform complex cognitive functions, such as problem solving or reading and interpretation.

3. Prenatal Alcohol Exposure

Around forty thousand babies per year are born with fetal alcohol effect resulting from alcohol abuse during pregnancy (Fitzgerald, 1988). In 1984, an estimated 7,024 of these infants were diagnosed with fetal alcohol syndrome (FAS), an incidence of 2.2 per 1,000 births (Abel and Sokol, 1987). The three main features of FAS in its extreme form are facial malformation, intrauterine growth retardation, and dysfunctions of the central nervous system, including mental retardation.

There are, in addition, about 33,000 children each year who suffer from less-severe effects of maternal alcohol use. The more prominent among these learning impairments are problems in attention (attention-deficit disorders), speech and language, and hyperactivity. General school failure also is connected to a history of fetal alcohol exposure (Abel and Sokol, 1987; Ernhart et al., 1985). Figure 5 shows the drinking habits of women of childbearing age by race and education.

When consumed in pregnancy, alcohol easily crosses the placenta, but exactly how it affects the fetus is not well known. The effects of alcohol vary according to how far along in the pregnancy the drinking occurs. The first trimester of pregnancy is a period of brain growth and organ and limb formation. The embryo is most susceptible to alcohol from week two to week eight of development, a point at which a woman may not even know she is pregnant (Hoyseth and Jones, 1989). Researchers have yet to determine how much alcohol it takes to cause problems in development and how alcohol affects each critical gestational period. It appears that the more alcohol consumed during pregnancy, the worse the effect. And many of the effects do not appear until ages four to seven, when children enter school.

Nearly one in four (23 percent) white women, eighteen to twenty-nine, reported "binge" drinking (five

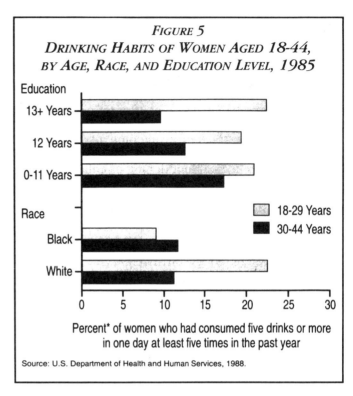

FIGURE 5
DRINKING HABITS OF WOMEN AGED 18-44, BY AGE, RACE, AND EDUCATION LEVEL, 1985

Percent* of women who had consumed five drinks or more in one day at least five times in the past year

Source: U.S. Department of Health and Human Services, 1988.

drinks or more a day at least five times in the past year). This was nearly three times the rate for black women of that age (about 8 percent). Fewer women (around 3 percent for both black and white) reported steady alcohol use (two drinks or more per day in the past two weeks).

4. Fetal Drug Exposure

The abuse of drugs of all kinds—marijuana, cocaine, crack, heroin, or amphetamines—by pregnant women affected about 11 percent of newborns in 1988—about 425,000 babies (Weston et al., 1989).

Cocaine and crack use during pregnancy are consistently associated with lower birthweight, premature birth, and smaller head circumference in comparison with babies whose mothers were free of these drugs (Chasnoff et al., 1989; Cherukuri et al., 1988; Doberczak et al., 1987; Keith et al., 1989; Zuckerman et al., 1989). In a study of 1,226 women attending a prenatal clinic, 27 percent tested positive for marijuana and 18 percent for cocaine. Infants of those who had used marijuana weighed an average of 2.8 ounces (79 grams) less at birth and were half a centimeter shorter in length. Infants of mothers who had used cocaine averaged 3.3 ounces (93 grams) less in weight and .7 of a centimeter less in length and also had a smaller head circumference than babies of nonusers (Zuckerman et al., 1989). The study concluded that "marijuana use and cocaine use during pregnancy are each independently associated with impaired fetal growth" (Zuckerman et al., 1989).

In addition, women who use these substances are like-

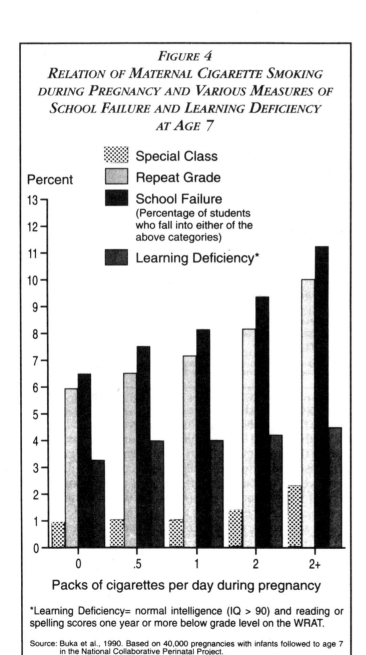

FIGURE 4
RELATION OF MATERNAL CIGARETTE SMOKING DURING PREGNANCY AND VARIOUS MEASURES OF SCHOOL FAILURE AND LEARNING DEFICIENCY AT AGE 7

*Learning Deficiency= normal intelligence (IQ > 90) and reading or spelling scores one year or more below grade level on the WRAT.

Source: Buka et al., 1990. Based on 40,000 pregnancies with infants followed to age 7 in the National Collaborative Perinatal Project.

3. PROBLEMS INFLUENCING PERSONAL GROWTH

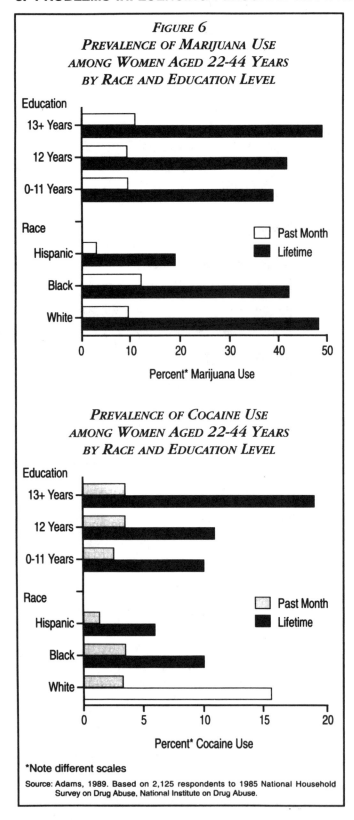

FIGURE 6
PREVALENCE OF MARIJUANA USE AMONG WOMEN AGED 22-44 YEARS BY RACE AND EDUCATION LEVEL

PREVALENCE OF COCAINE USE AMONG WOMEN AGED 22-44 YEARS BY RACE AND EDUCATION LEVEL

*Note different scales

Source: Adams, 1989. Based on 2,125 respondents to 1985 National Household Survey on Drug Abuse, National Institute on Drug Abuse.

aged nearly a pound (14.6 ounces or 416 grams) smaller than those born to women who had normal weight gain and did not use cigarettes, marijuana, and cocaine (see Table 1). The effect of these substances on size is more than the sum of the risk factors combined.

Like alcohol use, drug use has different effects at different points in fetal development. Use in very early pregnancy is more likely to cause birth defects affecting organ formation and the central nervous systems. Later use may

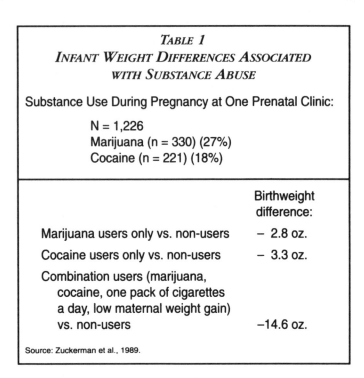

TABLE 1
INFANT WEIGHT DIFFERENCES ASSOCIATED WITH SUBSTANCE ABUSE

Substance Use During Pregnancy at One Prenatal Clinic:

N = 1,226
Marijuana (n = 330) (27%)
Cocaine (n = 221) (18%)

	Birthweight difference:
Marijuana users only vs. non-users	– 2.8 oz.
Cocaine users only vs. non-users	– 3.3 oz.
Combination users (marijuana, cocaine, one pack of cigarettes a day, low maternal weight gain) vs. non-users	–14.6 oz.

Source: Zuckerman et al., 1989.

ly to smoke and to gain less weight during pregnancy, two factors associated with low birthweight. The cumulative effect of these risk factors is demonstrated by the finding that infants born to women who gained little weight, who had smoked one pack of cigarettes a day, and who tested positive for marijuana and cocaine aver-

result in low birthweight due to either preterm birth or intrauterine growth retardation (Kaye et al., 1989; MacGregor et al., 1987; Petitti and Coleman, 1990). While some symptoms may be immediately visible, others may not be apparent until later childhood (Weston et al., 1989; Gray and Yaffe, 1986; Frank et al., 1988).

In infancy, damaged babies can experience problems in such taken-for-granted functions as sleeping and waking, resulting in exhaustion and poor development. In childhood, problems are found in vision, motor control, and in social interaction (Weston et al., 1989). Such problems may be caused not only by fetal drug exposure but also by insufficient prenatal care for the mother or by an unstimulating or difficult home environment for the infant (Lifschitz et al., 1985).

WHAT CAN be done to ameliorate the condition of children born with such damage? Quite a bit, based on the success of supportive prenatal care and the results of model projects that have provided intensive assistance to both baby and mother from the time of birth. These projects have successfully raised the I.Q. of low- and very-low birthweight babies an average of ten points or more—an increase that may lift a child with below-average intelligence into a higher I.Q. category (i.e., from retarded to low average or from low average to average). Generally known as either educational day care or infant day care, these programs provide a developmentally stimulating environment to high-risk babies and/or intensive parent support to prepare the parent to help her child.

In one such program based at the University of California/Los Angeles, weekly meetings were held among staff, parents, and infants over a period of four years. By the project's end, the low-birthweight babies had caught up in mental function to the control group of normal birthweight children (Rauh et al., 1988). The Infant Health and Development Project, which was conducted in eight cities and provided low-birthweight babies with pediatric follow-up and an educational curriculum with family support, on average increased their I.Q. scores by thirteen points and the scores of very-low birthweight children by more than six points. Another project targeted poor single teenage mothers whose infants were at high risk for intellectual impairment (Martin, Ramey and Ramey, 1990). One group of children was enrolled in educational day care from six and one-half weeks of age to four and one-half years for five days a week, fifty weeks a year. By four and one-half years, the children's I.Q. scores were in the normal range and ten points higher than a control group. In addition, by the time their children were four and one-half, mothers in the experimental group were more likely to have graduated from high school and be self-supporting than were mothers in the control group.

These studies indicate that some disadvantages of poverty and low birthweight can be mitigated and intellectual impairment avoided. The key is attention to the cognitive development of young children, in conjunction with social support of their families.

HOW KIDS BENEFIT FROM CHILD CARE

In a breakthrough study, over 1,700 readers reveal that their children learn critical academic and social skills from being in day care

Vivian Cadden

Vivian Cadden, a WORKING MOTHER contributing editor, is a member of the board of the Child Care Action Campaign.

Attitudes among working women toward child care have changed profoundly. A solid three out of four mothers of infants, toddlers and preschoolers believe that their child is learning more in day care than he or she would staying home with Mom all day. This surprisingly positive view of the advantages of child care emerges from a survey of 1,762 readers of WORKING MOTHER.

"The recognition that a quality child care arrangement can actually be *educational* for children represents an entirely new perspective; as recently as fifteen years ago, child care was seen as just an unavoidable necessity for working families," says Barbara Reisman, executive director of the Child Care Action Campaign (CCAC), which coauthored the survey. (The results of the questionnaire will be presented at the CCAC conference, "Child Care and Education: The Critical Connection," taking place in New York City March 31st through April 2nd.)

In fact, so great is the acceptance of child care now, that working mothers are almost unanimously (97 percent) convinced that their child benefits from it because it is educational, contributes to personal development and builds social skills. The women also have decided opinions on how young children learn and why certain forms of care are more conducive to learning than others:

- Eighty-five percent say that because their youngster is in child care he or she is "more independent."
- Eighty percent believe that "children who have had good child care are readier for first grade than other children."
- Three quarters say their kids gain valuable social skills in child care.
- Signaling a new trend, a majority (56 percent) prefer center-based care as a learning environment.
- Women have a new respect for teachers as professionals who are experts on child development.
- Respondents believe that one-on-one care, whether by a nanny, a relative or the mother herself, is of lesser educational value than group care.

What Children Learn

Parents put an especially high premium on the social skills their child gains from a group experience. In answer to an open-ended question, "What is the most important thing your youngster has learned from child care?", the most frequent responses were "learning to share" and "making friends." It is these perceptions that lead mothers to believe that their child is learning more from outside care than he would staying home with Mom.

"The most important thing my daughter has learned is how to interact with other children and adults. I don't think she would have received the stimulation and encouragement at home that she has received from her center's director, teachers and classmates," writes a woman from Waverly Hall, Georgia.

A San Ramon, California, mother says, "In addition to sharing and taking turns, my two-year-old has learned a wonderful quality—empathy. If Amanda sees another child cry, she asks what's wrong and tries to cheer him up."

A majority of women say that their youngster is "more outgoing" and "happier" because of being in child care; about half believe that he or she is "smarter," "less clingy" and "more cooperative."

Mothers of three- and four-year-olds are likely to talk about academic accomplishments that they believe contribute to

17. Kids Benefit from Child Care

their youngster's readiness for first grade: the growth of vocabulary and mastery of ABCs and numbers and color.

A Norfolk, Virginia, mother, for instance, is proud that her four-year-old "can count to twenty, knows her ABCs and can recognize letters."

Many mothers have such a strong belief in the benefits of group care that they would want their child to spend part of the day or several days a week in group care even if they didn't work. A Freeport, New York, woman writes, "Our center offers so much that I'm not trained to do. . . . I have often said that even if I didn't work I would want my son to attend this center a couple of days a week!"

Good Marks for Centers

One notable finding of the survey is a new enthusiasm for center-based care and a preference for it over every other type of care. This mirrors a trend in the country at large, but the preference is greater among WORKING MOTHER readers.

Overall, 57 percent of mothers in the survey have their youngster in a child care center, while 32 percent use a family day care home; 5 percent have in-home care, and 3 percent rely on a spouse or other relative. Even mothers of infants under two use center care about as often

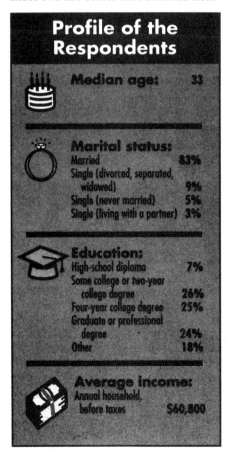

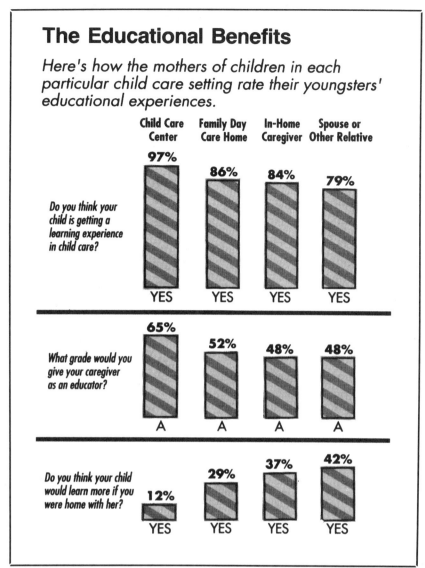

as they do family day care. And a whopping 72 percent of three- and four-year-olds are cared for in centers.

Even more striking is the degree of satisfaction mothers express with center care and their faith in its educational content. On practically every question dealing with the educational value of care, the center comes out on top. Mothers were asked, for example, "What grade would you give your caregiver for the job she is doing at providing learning experiences for your child?" Sixty-five percent of those whose child attends a center answered "A," compared to only 52 percent of those with a child in family care. And barely half—48 percent—were as pleased with the learning experience a child got from a nanny or relative. (See "The Educational Benefits.")

A Lowell, Massachusetts, respondent whose six-year-old and three-year-old have been in centers since infancy writes, "Our children have gained insight into many facets of life, which I believe they would not have experienced if they had stayed home with me: exposure to many different types of adults and children; a wide variety of toys, games, books and activities; learning about cooperation and sharing; being able to giggle and act silly with lots of friends one day and being alone in a cozy corner with a book the next day; being in a physical environment that supports children's needs instead of placing limitations on them; being in a place where children are not pushed to learn but where they learn and discover because it's fun and they want to do it."

Anne Mitchell, senior consultant to CCAC on the New York City conference, marveled at the sophistication of readers' views as expressed in their replies. "Clearly, these women know the kind of

3. PROBLEMS INFLUENCING PERSONAL GROWTH

environment in which children learn and flourish," she says.

The high regard for center care is all the more remarkable because over the years such care has so often come under attack. Mothers are aware of this, and many comment on it in their letters.

The Lowell, Massachusetts, mother says of her children's center, "This is the kind of day care center that should be featured when television journalists insist on 'exposing the care that children get in the day care centers of our nation.'"

"Many of us," a Brooklyn mother adds, "are disgusted by the negative media coverage of child care centers."

Teachers Are Pros

Readers also voice great respect for the people who care for their children. Likely to be well educated themselves (see "Profile of the Respondents"), these women value the training their children's caregivers have acquired.

A mother with a graduate degree who has a one-year-old daughter in a center says, "I don't have the experience nor do I know how and what to teach a kid!" Another writes, "I feel teachers are better geared to educate a small child. After all, that's what they went to college for."

Many women feel that if they were home all day they wouldn't be concentrating on educational activities for their child as teachers are able to do. A mother from Newnan, Georgia, puts it this way: "The day care center doesn't have to worry about washing clothes, cleaning house, running errands and getting distracted."

A Bloomington, Indiana, mother writes, "I am not as focused on creative ideas for children." As an example, she describes how her four-year-old learned to lace his shoes at his center by lacing a shoe box that had been made into a mock shoe. "I was so amazed," she says, "that I brought the teacher flowers!"

After citing some of the things her toddler has learned in child care, a Newark, Delaware, mother says, "I, too, have learned from child care, observing the teachers. I have learned how to talk to Jennifer in a positive and encouraging way. I have learned how much she is capable of doing. I have learned to give her choices whenever possible, to encourage her to make decisions."

Readers also understand that teaching young children is not a matter of formal indoctrination. "Learning is not shoved down my son's throat. He learns by playing and the thoughtful direction of his teachers" is how one mother puts it.

In fact, her enlightened view that "children learn through playing" is shared almost unanimously by the respondents: Ninety-eight percent agree.

One-on-One Care

The respondents' enthusiasm about the educational value of day care does not carry over to their assessment of one-on-one care provided by nannies or relatives.

Only 12 percent of mothers who use center care believe their child would learn more if they stayed home. But a hefty 42 percent of those who rely on a spouse or other relative think so. And 37 percent of moms with a nanny feel they could give their child a better learning experience if they stayed home.

The marked confidence in group care and more tepid enthusiasm for individual care represents a real turnabout in women's opinion. An affluent Arlington, Virginia, mother with an infant in center care says, "I am particularly interested in your

---

What Government Should Do

One of the most remarkable findings of the survey is how strongly women feel about the need for public schools to accommodate the changing needs of society. The vast majority, for instance, want before- and after-school care for elementary-age children. In fact, at a time when most people feel enormously burdened by taxes, 85 percent of the respondents not only think public schools should provide such care, but an amazing 74 percent would be willing to pay higher taxes for it.

There is less enthusiasm for schools getting involved in child care for the very young, however. Only 29 percent of the women support public-school programs for three-to-five-year-olds and a meager 18 percent want such programs for children from birth through three.

What should public schools provide?

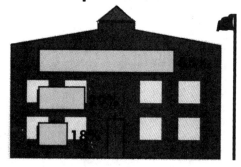

- Before- and after-school programs
- Child care for kids three and up
- Child care for kids from birth onward

What would you pay more taxes for?

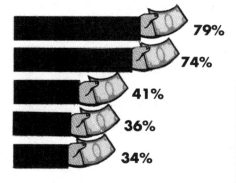

- Better public schools — 79%
- Before- and after-school programs — 74%
- Child care for four-year-olds — 41%
- Child care for three-year-olds and up — 36%
- Child care for infants and toddlers — 34%

17. Kids Benefit from Child Care

survey because I have begun to believe that as social creatures, babies and children are meant to be around many more familiar people than is the norm in our culture. Many societies have a much broader, extended family network in which children are with many older children and adults throughout the day. It strikes me as odd that we see mother and child cloistered at home as the ideal."

The Income Factor

Across the board, no matter what their income, mothers believe almost unanimously that their child benefits from child care. But their answers to other questions suggest that income (with the consequent ability or inability to afford high-quality care) plays an important part in determining the learning experience the youngster receives.

- Asked "Would you change your child's arrangement if another affordable option were available?", about 32 percent of mothers with household incomes under $20,000 replied "yes." Only 17 percent with household incomes of $100,000 and over would make a change.
- Twenty-eight percent of those in the lowest income group believe their child would learn more if Mom stayed home; only 18 percent of those with household incomes of $100,000 and over think so.

These findings are consistent with other studies, in which respondents with family incomes above $60,000 express high levels of general satisfaction with their child care arrangement, while respondents with incomes below $20,000 are less satisfied.

The outstanding impression that has emerged from the survey results and the readers' letters is that working mothers with children in quality child care believe their youngsters are getting the best of two worlds. As an Aurora, Colorado, woman with a two-year-old and a six-year-old puts it: "My children are growing up seeing Mom and Dad as their base, but also having the ability to branch out in relationships and experiences they would not have readily received staying at home with me all day."

Editor's note: Readers who need assistance finding child care in their area can call the National Association of Child Care Resource and Referral Agencies at this number: 1-800-424-2246.

Fathers' Time

Their style is vastly different, but dads can no longer be looked on as second bananas in the parenting biz. New studies show fathers are crucial for the emotional and intellectual growth of their kids, influencing how they ultimately turn out. Writer/father PAUL ROBERTS reports on the importance of being a papa. Actor/father BILL MOSELEY's dispatches reveal what it's like on the front lines.

Paul Roberts

PAUL ROBERTS is a Seattle-based freelance writer. Actor BILL MOSELEY interviewed Timothy Leary for *PT* in 1995.

This was supposed to be the Golden Era of Paternity. After decades of domestic aloofness, men came charging into parenthood with an almost religious enthusiasm. We attended Lamaze classes and crowded into birthing rooms. We mastered diapering, spent more time at home with the kids, and wallowed in the flood of "papa" literature unleashed by Bill Cosby's 1986 best-seller *Fatherhood*.

Yet for all our fervor, the paternal revolution has had a slightly hollow ring. It's not simply the relentless accounts of fatherhood's dark side—the abuse, the neglect, the abandonment—that make us so self-conscious. Rather, it's the fact that for all our earnest sensitivity, we can't escape questions of our psychological necessity: What is it, precisely, that fathers do? What critical difference do we make in the lives of our children?

Think about it. The modern mother, no matter how many nontraditional duties she assumes, is still seen as the family's primary nurturer and emotional guardian. It's in her genes. It's in her soul. But mainstream Western society accords no corresponding position to the modern father. Aside from chromosomes and feeling somewhat responsible for household income, there's no similarly celebrated deep link between father and child, no widely recognized "paternal instinct." Margaret Mead's quip that fathers are "a biological necessity but a social accident" may be a little harsh. But it does capture the second-banana status that many fathers have when it comes to taking their measure as parents.

Happily, a new wave of research is likely to substantially boost that standing. Over the last decade, researchers like Jay Belsky, Ph.D., at Pennsylvania State University, and Ross Parke, Ph.D., of the University of California/Riverside Center for Family Studies, have been mapping out the psychology of the father-child bond, detailing how it functions and how it differs—sometimes substantially—from the bond between mother and child. What emerges from their work is the beginning of a truly modern concept of paternity, one in which old assumptions are overturned or, at the very least, cast in a radically different light. Far from Mead's "social accident," fatherhood turns out to be a complex and unique phenomenon with huge consequences for the emotional and intellectual growth of children.

Key to this new idea of fatherhood is a premise so mundane that most of us take it for granted: fathers parent differently than mothers do. They play with their children more. Their interactions tend to be more physical and less intimate, with more of a reliance on humor and excitement. While such distinctions may hardly seem revelatory, they can mean a world of difference to kids. A father's more playful interactive style, for example, turns out to be critical in teaching a child emotional self-control. Likewise, father-child interactions appear to be central to the development of a child's ability to maintain strong, fulfilling social relationships later in life.

But it's not simply a matter of paternal be-

Diary of a Dad

I love this time. Jane Moseley puts her hunter mare through its paces. Time slows to a trot, works up to a canter, drops to a lazy walk.

She announces she won't wear her riding hat. I insist she must. She refuses, would rather not ride. I can't believe she'd give up The Most Important Thing in her Life over this. Fine, don't ride. This triggers an outpouring of vitriol. I pay attention, but don't take it personally. Thirty minutes later she's holding my hand as we walk down Melrose.

havior differing from maternal methods. The fabric of the father-child bond is also different. Studies show that fathers with low self-esteem have a greater negative impact in their children than do mothers who don't like themselves. In addition, the father-child bond seems to be more fragile—and therefore more easily severed—during periods of strife between parents.

Amid this welter of findings two things are clear. First, given our rapidly evolving conceptions of "father" and "family," fatherhood in the 1990s is probably tougher, psychologically, than at any other time in recent history. Plainly put, there are precious few positive role models to guide today's papas. Yet at the same time, the absence of any guidance holds hidden promise. Given the new information on fatherhood, the potential for a rich and deeply rewarding paternal experience is significantly greater today than even a generation ago. "The possibilities for fathering have never been better," Belsky says. "Culturally speaking, there is so much more that fathers are 'allowed' to do."

Our Forefathers

The surge of interest in fatherhood has a distinctly modern feel, as if after thousands of years of unquestioned maternal preeminence, men are just now discovering and asserting their parental prerogatives. But in fact, this unquestioned maternal dominance is itself a relatively recent development. Up until the mid-1700s, when most fathers worked in or near the home and took a much greater hand in child rearing, Western culture regarded them and not mothers as the more competent parent—and ultimately held them more responsible for how their children turned out. Not only were books and manuals on parenting written chiefly for men, according to R. L. Griswold, author of *Fatherhood in America*, men were routinely awarded custody of their kids in cases of divorce.

With the Industrial Revolution, however, more fathers began working outside their homes and thus were effectively removed from domestic life. As Vicky Phares, Ph.D., assistant professor of psychology at the University of South Florida, wrote in *Fathers and Developmental Psychopathology*, industrialization ushered in the "feminization of the domestic sphere and the marginalization of fathers' involvement with their children." By the mid-1800s, Phares notes, "child-rearing manuals were geared toward mothers, and this trend continued for the most part until the mid-1970s."

The implication here—that parental roles have largely been defined by economics—is still a subject of cultural debate. Less arguable, however, is the fact that by the turn of the twentieth century, both science and society saw the psychology of parenting largely as the psychology of motherhood. Not only were mothers somehow more "naturally" inclined to parent, they were also genetically better prepared for the task. Indeed, in 1916, Phares notes, one prominent investigator went so far as to "prove" the existence of the maternal instinct—and the lack of paternal equivalent—largely based on the notion that "few fathers were naturally skilled at taking care of infants."

Granted, bogus scientific claims were plentiful in those times. But even Freud, who believed fathers figured heavily in children's development of conscience and sexual identity, dismissed the idea that they had any impact until well past a child's third year. And even then, many psychologists argued, these paternal contributions consisted primarily of providing income, discipline, and a masculine role model, along with periodic injections of what might be called "real world" experience—that is, things that took place outside the home. "The classical psychological view held that a father's 'job' was to expand his children's horizon beyond the bosom of the family and the mother-child relationship," Belsky observes. "Mothers preserved and protected children from discomfort. But fathers imposed a realistic, the world-is-tough perspective."

By the 1920s, the classic "mother-centric" view was showing its cracks. Not only did subsequent empirical studies find little hard evidence of any unique maternal instinct but, as Phares points out, the phenomenon of "mother-blaming"—that is, blaming mothers for all the emotional and behavioral problems of their children—prodded some researchers (and, no doubt, a good many mothers) to ask whether fathers might share some of the responsibility.

By the 1950s, science began to recognize that there was some paternal impact on early childhood—even if it was only in the negative context of divorce or the extended absence of a father. Psychologist Michael Lamb, Ph.D., research director at the National Institute for Child Health and Human Development in Bethesda, Maryland, explains: "The assumption was that by comparing the behavior and per-

---

After Jane and I had a snack, she wanted to box. So we waltzed around for 20 minutes, floating like a butterfly (me), stinging like a bee (Jane). I've taught her the rudiments of pugilism: how to make a fist (don't wrap your fingers around your thumb); how she should always stand sideways to her opponent, watching the hands not the eyes, etc. After a few fun-filled injury-free rounds, I came to my senses and ended our play.

Jane is an only child, so I figure it's my job to play with her as a brother or provide her with a sibling—playing with her is easier!

3. PROBLEMS INFLUENCING PERSONAL GROWTH

sonalities of children raised with and without fathers, one could—essentially by a process of subtraction—estimate what sort of influence fathers typically had."

What Dads Do

It wasn't until the feminist movement of the 1970s that researchers thought to ask whether dads could be as nurturing as moms. To everyone's astonishment, the answer was yes.

Actually, that was half the answer. Subsequent inquiries showed that while fathers could be as nurturing as mothers, they tended to leave such duties to moms. Hardly news to millions of overworked women, this finding was crucial. For the first time, researchers began systematically studying how and why male and female parenting strategies diverged, and more to the point, what those differences meant for children.

Although the total fatherhood experience runs from conception on, research has focused most keenly on the first few years of the parent-child relationship. It's here that children are most open to parental influence; they function primarily as receivers, consuming not only huge quantities of nourishment and comfort but stimuli as well. For decades, investigators have understood that infants not only enjoy taking in such rudimentary knowledge but absolutely require it for intellectual, physical, and especially emotional growth.

Without such constant interaction, argues W. Andrew Collins, Ph.D., of the University of Minnesota's Institute for Child Development, infants might never fully develop a sense of comfort and security. As important, they might not develop a sense of being connected to—and thus having some degree of control over—the world around them. "The key ingredient is a 'contingent responsiveness,'" says Collins, "where infants learn their actions will elicit certain reliable responses from others."

It's also during this crucial period that one of the most fundamental differences between male and female parenting styles takes place. Work by several psychiatrists, including San Diego's Martin Greenberg, M.D., and Kyle Pruett, M.D., a professor of psychiatry at the Yale Child Study Center, suggests that while new mothers are inclined to relate to their infants in a more soothing, loving, and serious way, new fathers "hold their children differently and have a different kind of patience and frustration cycle than mothers," Pruett observes.

I crave adult company, but I don't have a baby-sitter for tonight. So I'm trying to lug Jane all the way to Santa Monica to see Wing Chun, a kung-fu movie she says she doesn't want to see. Oh, no you don't, kid, it's my time now, and we're going to Santa Monica. Of course, Jane winds up loving the movie. Later that night we watch a video of Captains Courageous. I am reminded of all the songs that the two of us have made up over the past several years: "Feed Lot," "Ain't No Bridge," "Don't Drink the Water," "When the Vulture Swoops," etc. (Lyrics upon request).

Why it is fathers behave this way isn't entirely clear. (And when fathers are primary caregivers, they are likely to display many of the so-called maternal traits.) Some studies suggest these gender differences are part of a larger male preference for stimulating, novel activities that arises from neurobiological differences in the way stimuli and pleasure are linked in male and female brains, and likely a result of genetics. Individuals high in the sensation-seeking trait are far more likely to engage in new and exciting pastimes. Though not all guys qualify as sensation seekers, the trait is far more common in men—particularly young ones—than it is in women, and might help explain why any young fathers start off having a parenting style that's stimulating for them as well as their child.

The Daddy Dynamic

Whatever its origins, this more playful, jocular approach carries major consequences for developing children. Where the "average" mother cushions her baby against irritating stimulation, the "average" father heaps it on, consistently producing a broader range of arousal. The resulting ups and downs force children to "stretch," emotionally and physically.

This emotion-stretching dynamic becomes more pronounced as father-child relationships enter into their second and third years. When playing, fathers tend to be more physical with their toddlers—wrestling, playing tag, and so on—while mothers emphasize verbal exchanges and interacting with objects, like toys. In nearly all instances, says Lamb, fathers are much more likely "to get children worked up, negatively or positively, with fear as well as delight, forcing them to learn to regulate their feelings."

In a sense, then, fathers push children to cope with the world outside the mother-child bond, as classical theory argued. But more than this, fathering behavior also seems to make children develop a more complex set of interactive skills, what Parke calls "emotional communication" skills.

First, children learn how to "read" their father's emotions via his facial expressions, tone of voice, and other nonverbal cues, and respond accordingly. Is Daddy really going to chase me down and gobble me up, or is he joking? Did I really hurt Daddy by poking him in the eye? Is Daddy in the mood to play, or is he tired?

Second, children learn how to clearly communicate their own emotions to others. One common example is the child who by crying lets her daddy know that he's playing too roughly or is scaring her. Kids also learn to indicate when interactions aren't stimulating enough; they'll show they've lost interest by not responding or wandering off.

Finally, children learn how to "listen" to their own emotional state. For instance, a child soon learns that if he becomes too "worked up" and begins to cry, he may in effect drive his play partner away.

The consequences of such emotional mastery are far-reaching. By successfully coping with stimulating, emotionally stretching interactions, children learn that they can indeed ef-

Made Jane cry—down on her for not helping me put away the groceries, make dinner. She wanted to play Super Mario Bros. (So did I.) She called me an idiot. I yelled at her about not pulling her oar—sounded just like my dad—and sent her to her room. I kept her in there for a few minutes, felt bad, knocked on the door, and sat on her bed and apologized for losing my temper. "You hurt my feelings," she sniffed.

CREATING A NEW PATRIARCHY

Even the most dedicated dads quickly discover that the road to modern fatherhood is strewn with obstacles. Positive role models are in short supply and personal experiences are usually no help. Jerrold Lee Shapiro, Ph.D., professor of psychology at Santa Clara University, says understanding your relationship with your own father is the first step. If not, you're bound to automatically and unconciously replicate things from your childhood.

Here are several strategies both parents can use to strengthen the father-child bond.

◆ Start early. While involvement doesn't always equal intimacy, fathers who immerse themselves in all aspects of parenting from birth on are more likely to be closer to their children. Take part in as many prenatal activities as possible and schedule at least a week away from work after the baby is born to practice parenting skills and overcome anxieties about handling the baby.

◆ Create "fathering space": Schedule times and activities in which you take care of your newborn entirely on your own. The traditional practice of deferring to mothers as "experts" gives new fathers few chances to hone their parenting skills, bolster their confidence, and build solid bonds with baby.

Sue Dickinson, M.S.W., a marriage and family therapist in Cle Elum, Washington, suggests persuading mom to go out of the house so you can have the experience of being *the* parent. Martin Greenberg, M.D., recommends bundling your baby in a chest pack and going for walks. The feeling of a baby's body—together with his or her warmth and smell—is captivating.

◆ Articulate feelings. Although fatherhood is routinely described as "the most wonderful experience" a man can have, new fathers may feel anxious, fearful, and frustrated. They may also be jealous of the time their wives spend with the baby and of their wives' "natural" parenting skills. These feelings may only make it harder for you to wholeheartedly participate in parenting and create distance between you and your child. New fathers need to identify such feelings and discuss them with their wives.

◆ Mind the details. Tune in to your children and avoid relying on mom to "read" what your baby wants.

◆ Respect diversity. Accept your partner's parenting style without criticizing. Mothers often regard fathers' more boisterous style as too harsh or insensitive. But such criticism can derail a dad's desire for involvement. "Just because he's doing something you wouldn't do doesn't make it wrong," says Jay Belsky, Ph.D. Mothers have to temper their need to protect and remember dads offer things moms don't.

◆ Be realistic. Fathers who want to adopt a more hands-on approach than they themselves experienced are often frustrated when kids don't immediately respond. But children accustomed to having mom as the primary caregiver simply cannot adapt to "sudden" paternal involvement overnight. Above all, parenting requires patience.

3. PROBLEMS INFLUENCING PERSONAL GROWTH

fect change both on internal matters (their feelings) and in the outside world (their father's actions). In that regard, links have been found between the quality of father-child interactions and a child's later development of certain life skills, including an ability to manage frustration, a willingness to explore new things and activities, and persistence in problem solving.

As important as learning to regulate the emotional intensity of their interactions is children's ability to master the larger interactive process, the give and take that makes up social communication. "Kids who learn how to decode and encode emotions early on will be better off later when it comes to any social encounter," Parke says.

Such benefits have been intensely studied in the area of sibling relationships. Work by Belsky and Brenda Volling, Ph.D., an assistant professor of psychology at the University of Michigan, suggests that the emotion-management "lessons" learned by children from their fathers during play are applied later in interactions with siblings—and ultimately with people outside the family—and lead to more cooperation and less fighting. The press release announcing Belsky and Volling's research quipped, "If Adam had been a better father, things might have turned out differently for Cain and Abel."

Such findings come with plenty of caveats. A mother's more comforting manner is just as crucial to her children, helping them foster, among other things, a critical sense of security and self-confidence. Indeed, a mere preference for stimulating activities does not a good father make; obviously, the quality of father-child interactions is important. Successful fathers both monitor and modulate their play, maintaining a level of stimulation that keeps children engaged without making them feel like they've been pushed too far. This requires complete engagement—something many of today's busy fathers find difficult to manage. "What often happens is fathers don't pay attention to the cues their kids are sending," Belsky says. "A kid is crying 'uncle' and his father doesn't hear it."

Of course, fathers aren't the only parent who can teach these coping skills. Mothers physically play with their kids and, depending on the dynamics and history of the family, may also be the ones providing more of a "paternal" influence—teaching coping skills through play. Yet this "stretching" role typically falls to fathers because men gravitate toward less intimate, more physical interactions. And, as Reed Larson, Ph.D., a psychologist at the University of Illinois-Champagne, observes, "when dads stop having fun interacting with their kids, they're more likely than mothers to exit."

Whether these differences are genetic, cultural, or, more likely, a combination of the two, is still hotly debated. But the fact remains that in terms of time spent with children, fathers typically spend more of it playing with their kids than mothers do—a difference that from very early on, children pick up on. Studies show that during stressful situations, one-year-old and 18-month-old babies more often turn to their primary caretaker—in most families, mom—for help. By contrast, when researchers measured so-called affiliative behaviors like smelling and vocalizing, during their first two years, babies showed a preference for their fathers. Just as dramatic, almost as soon as a child can crawl or walk, he or she will typically seek out dad for play and mom for comfort and other needs.

DOWNSIDE OF THE DADDY TRACK

On the face of it, fathers would seem to enjoy considerable advantages over mothers during their children's first years. Not only do they do less of the dirty work, but it's almost as if they've been anointed to handle the fun art of parenting. Yet as time goes on this situation changes dramatically. While a mother's more intimate, need-related approach to parenting generally continues to cement her bond with her children, a father's more playful and stimulating style steadily loses its appeal. By the age of eight or nine, a child may already be angry at his father's teasing, or bored or annoyed by his I'm-gonna-gitcha style.

This discrepancy often becomes quite pronounced as children reach adolescence. Research suggests that preteens and teens of both sexes continue to rely on their mothers for intimacy and needs, and increasingly view her as the favored parent for topics requiring sensitivity and trust. By contrast, Parke says, the joking, playful style that serves fathers so well during children's first years may begin to alienate teens, giving them the impression that their father doesn't take their thoughts and needs seriously.

Adding to this tension is the father's traditional role as the dispenser of discipline and firmness. It's hypothesized that fathers' less intimate interactive style may make it easier—although not more pleasant—for them to play the "heavy." In any case, adolescents come to see

---

Anna's sleeping over. Earlier in the evening, Jane was on the floor of her bedroom looking up my shorts, laughing, saying she saw my penis. Later, I spy Jane and Anna holding up our cat Jackson. Must be a penis hunt, little-girl style. It's already in full swing and they're seven and eight!

In addition to being cook, chauffeur, maid, and spiritual protector, I am also Sex Authority! Two years ago, I explained, in a general way, the birds and the bees to Jane, correcting the misinformation she'd been given by her good friend Olivia.

their fathers as the harsher, more distant parent. This feeling may increase teenagers' tendency to interact more often and intimately with their mothers, which in turn only heightens the sense of estrangement and tension between fathers and their kids.

As to whether fathers' possibly not being at home as much as mothers makes it easier or more difficult for them to be the disciplinarian, Parke says there are too many other factors involved to make such a determination. He does note, however, that many mothers faced with unruly kids still employ the threat, "Wait 'til your father gets home."

Clearly, the distance between fathers and adolescent children is not solely as result of fathers' playfulness earlier on. A central function of adolescence is a child's gradual movement toward emotional and physical autonomy from both parents. But studies suggest this movement is most directly and forcefully spurred by fathers' less intimate ways.

Does a father's parenting style during adolescence produce more closeness between father and child? The answer is probably no, says Parke. But if the question is, does a father's style serve a launching, independence-gaining function, the answer is probably yes. "Mothers' continued nurturance maintains a child's connectedness to the family, while fathers encourage differentiation," Parke says. In fact, according to a recent survey of adolescents by Israeli researchers Shmuel Shulman, Ph.D., and Moshe Klein, Ph.D., most perceived their fathers as being the primary source of support for their teenage autonomy.

Such notions will undoubtedly strike some as disturbingly regressive, as if researchers have simply found new, complex ways to justify outdated stereotypes of paternal behavior. For as any sensitive observer knows, the totality of fatherhood goes well beyond a tendency toward stimulating interactions and away from intimacy. Nonetheless, this does appear to be a central component of fathering behavior and may help explain why some seemingly antiquated modes of fathering persist. Despite evolution in gender roles, Belsky says, fathers are still more likely to provide less sensitivity, require kids to adjust to 'tough' realities, and perhaps be less understanding and empathetic.

Yet if the father-child bond truly serves as a mechanism for preparing children for the external world, the bond itself seems remarkably sensitive, even vulnerable, to that world. External variables, such as a father's relationships beyond his family—and in particular his experience in the workplace—appear to be linked to both the kinds of fathering behavior he exhibits and the success he achieves with it. Some of these links are obvious. Few would be surprised to learn that fathers with high-stress jobs are apt to be more distant from their kids or use harsher, physical discipline when dealing with youthful infractions.

Other links between a man's external world and the way he fathers are more subtle. According to Parke, there are significant and intriguing fathering differences between men whose jobs involve a great degree of independence and those who are heavily managed. Fathers with workplace autonomy tend to expect and encourage more independence in their children. Moreover, they generally place grater emphasis on a child's intent when assessing misbehavior, and aren't inclined toward physical discipline. By contrast, men in highly supervised jobs with little autonomy are more likely to value and expect conformity from their kids. They're also more likely to consider the consequences of their children's misbehavior when meting out punishment, and discipline them physically.

This so-called spillover effect is hardly mysterious. We would expect parents whose jobs reward them for creativity, independence, and intent to value those qualities, and to emphasize them in their interactions with their children. Not that men have a monopoly on job spillover. A mother whose job is stressful probably isn't able to parent at one hundred percent either.

D_{ADS} W_{HO} D_{ISCONNECT}

Other factors may also have a greater impact on the father-child bond than on the bond between mother and child. "If things aren't going well in a marriage," says Lamb, "it's more likely to have a negative impact on a father's relationship with his child. " This is surely due in part to a child's history of intimacy with his or her mother. But Lamb also speculates that fathers simply find it easier to "disconnect" from their kids during times of conflict.

Speculations like these raise the specter of some genetic explanation. If fathers are inclined to relate to their children in a less intimate way, they may naturally be less capable of building and maintaining strong parent-child bonds. Yet while Lamb and Parke acknowledge some degree of innate, gender-related parenting differences, they place far more emphasis on cultural or learned factors.

Jane's legs hurt tonight; she calls them growing pains. I got mad, then simmered down (when my fear subsided), gave her Tylenol after she brushed her teeth. Read her a chapter from Great Expectations.

When Jane's sick, her mother takes such good care of her with medicines, doctors. I was raised Christian Scientist, taught that sickness and injury are illusions that should be healed with prayer and proper thinking. I'm just getting over my anger, my fear of disease, doctors, medicine.

3. PROBLEMS INFLUENCING PERSONAL GROWTH

Lately, I've felt a little more thin-skinned with Jane. I think it dates back to around the time of her Christmas break. Jane's not as cuddly, pliable, obedient as she was before. Rather, she's more headstrong, defiant, sometimes openly mocking of me, my authority.

I guess she's becoming independent, setting her own boundaries. Yipes! Thankfully, Lucinda explained this. I figured Jane was going through a bad patch, or maybe her friends or mother were encouraging her to resist my fine parenting! Instead, it's my parenting that's helped foster her confidence.

Bill Moseley

Of these, the most important may be the parenting models today's men and women have from their own childhoods—models that very likely ran along traditional lines, and most significantly indicated mothering was mandatory and fathering far more discretionary. A mother may be angry and depressed. Lamb says, "but parenting has to be done and the buck stops with her, whereas dads have traditionally been given leeway."

It's changing, of course. New legal sanctions, such as those against deadbeat dads, coupled with a rising sense—not just among conservatives—of fathers' familial obligations, are making it tougher for men to simply walk away physically or emotionally. Today men getting divorced are likely to fight for primary or joint custody of their kids. We may even reach a point where one parent isn't deemed mandatory and the other "allowed" to drop back.

BRINGING THE REVOLUTION HOME

Researchers say the more compelling changes in fathering are, or ought to be, taking place not just on a social level but on a personal one. One of the simplest steps is refiguring the division of parental duties: mom takes on some of the play master role, while dad does more of the need-based parenting—everything from changing diapers to ferrying the kids to dance lessons. By doing more of the "mandatory" parenting, Parke says, fathers will encourage their kids to see them not simply as a playmate, but as a comfort provider too.

No one's advocating a complete role reversal, or suggesting a complete shift is possible. Parke says men have difficulty "giving up their robust interactive styles, even when they are the parent staying at home." Instead, families should take advantage of the difference between men's and women's parenting approaches. Since fathers' boisterous antics seem to help prepare children for life outside the family, mothers shouldn't cancel this out by intervening or being overly protective.

At the same time, a more androgynous approach has its advantages. Children will be less inclined to mark one parent for fun and the other for comfort. For fathers this might mean more opportunities to deal with emotional ups and downs and develop the empathy and emotional depth.

Of course, fathers will experience difficulties making this shift. Yet the potential rewards are huge. Not only will we give our children more progressive examples of parenting—examples that will be crucial when they raise their own children—but we'll greatly enhance our own parenting experiences.

Fatherhood may be more confusing and open-ended than ever before, but the possibilities—for those willing to take the risks—are endless. "In the theater of modern family life," says Belsky, "there are just many more parts that fathers can play."

LIES OF THE MIND

Repressed-memory therapy is harming patients, devastating families and intensifying a backlash against mental-health practitioners

LEON JAROFF

SUFFERING FROM A PROLONGED BOUT OF DEPRESSION AND desperate for help, Melody Gavigan, 39, a computer specialist from Long Beach, California, checked herself into a local psychiatric hospital. As Gavigan recalls the experience, her problems were just beginning. During five weeks of treatment there, a family and marriage counselor repeatedly suggested that her depression stemmed from incest during her childhood. While at first Gavigan had no recollection of any abuse, the therapist kept prodding. "I was so distressed and needed help so desperately, I latched on to what he was offering me," she says. "I accepted his answers."

When asked for details, she wrote page after page of what she believed were emerging repressed memories. She told about running into the yard after being raped in the bathroom. She incorporated into another lurid rape scene an actual girlhood incident, in which she had dislocated a shoulder. She went on to recall being molested by her father when she was only a year old—as her diapers were being changed—and sodomized by him at five. Following what she says was the therapist's advice, Gavigan confronted her father with her accusations, severed her relationship with him, moved away and formed an incest survivors' group.

But she remained uneasy. Signing up for a college psychology course, she examined her newfound memories more carefully and concluded that they were false. Now Gavigan has begged her father's forgiveness and filed a lawsuit against the psychiatric hospital for the pain that she and her family suffered.

Gavigan is just one victim of a troubling psychological phenomenon that is harming patients, devastating families, influencing new legislation, taking up courtroom time, stirring fierce controversy among experts and intensifying a backlash against all mental-health practitioners: the "recovery"—usually while in therapy—of repressed memories of childhood sexual abuse, satanic rituals and other bizarre incidents (*see box*).

"If penis envy made us look dumb, this will make us look totally gullible," says psychiatrist Paul McHugh, chairman of the psychiatry department at Johns Hopkins University. "This is the biggest story in psychiatry in a decade. It is a disaster for orthodox psychotherapists who are doing good work."

No one questions that childhood sexual abuse is widespread and underreported. The subject, rarely mentioned and then only in hushed tones until the 1980s, has become the stuff of talk shows, movies and feature articles. Indeed, many, perhaps millions of Americans have jarring and humiliating memories of abuse, recollections that, painful as they are, have stayed with them through the years.

But can memories of repeated incest and other bizarre incidents be so repressed that the victim is totally unaware of them until they emerge during therapy or as the result of a triggering sight, smell or sound?

Across the U.S. in the past several years, literally thousands of people—mostly women in their 20s, 30s and 40s—have been coming forward with accusations that they were sexually abused as children, usually by members of their own family, at home or, in many cases, at hidden sites where weird rituals were practiced. Says McHugh, "It's reached epidemic proportions."

Unlike the countless adults who have lived for years with painful memories of actual childhood sexual abuse, most individuals with "recovered memory" initially have no specific recollection of incest or molestation. At worst, they have only a vague feeling that something may have happened. Others, simply seeking help to alleviate depression, eating disorders, marital difficulties or other common problems, are informed by unsophisticated therapists or pop-psychology books that their symptoms suggest childhood sexual abuse, all memories of which have been repressed.

In the course of the therapy, many of these troubled souls conjure up exquisitely detailed recollections of sexual abuse by family members. Encouraged by their therapists to reach deeper into the recesses of their memories—often using techniques such as visualization and hypnosis—some go on to describe events that sorely strain credulity, particularly tales of their forced childhood participation in satanic rituals involving animal and infant sacrifices, as well as sexual acts.

In many cases the therapists conclude, and eventually convince the patients through suggestion, that the repressed memories of childhood abuse have caused them to "dissociate." As a result, they appear to develop multiple-personality disorder, the strange and, until recently, rare condition brought to wide public attention by

3. PROBLEMS INFLUENCING PERSONAL GROWTH

the 1973 book, *Sybil*, which describes the condition of a woman who develops several strikingly different but interchangeable personas.

Legislatures in nearly half the states have responded to the widespread public acceptance of recovered memories by applying a strange twist to venerable statute-of-limitations laws. In general, the new legislation allows alleged victims of child abuse to sue the accused perpetrators within three to six years after the repressed memories emerge. This means that with little more than the recollection of the accuser, a parent or other relative can be hauled into court decades after the supposed crime.

Taking advantage of the newly enacted legislation, some of the supposed victims have successfully brought civil and even criminal actions against members of their own families. Juries have awarded them damages, and in a few cases the accused parent has been sentenced to jail—based entirely on the recovered memory of his adult offspring.

To many critics of the recovered-memory movement, the accusations and convictions are reminiscent of the 17th century Salem witchcraft trials, in which elderly women and an occasional man were condemned to death, often on the basis of a single unsubstantiated charge that they had demonstrated witchlike behavior.

"Recovered-memory therapy will come to be recognized as the quackery of the 20th century," predicts Richard Ofshe, a social psychologist at the University of California, Berkeley. And in the process, Emory University psychiatry professor George Ganaway fears, it may "trigger a backlash against [legitimate charges of] child abuse. As these stories are discredited, society may end up throwing the baby out with the bath water—and the hard-earned credibility of the child-abuse-survivor movement will go down the drain."

The backlash has already begun. In Texas this summer, a woman patient won a settlement from two therapists and a psychiatric hospital after suing them for therapeutic negligence and fraud. She claimed that four years of recovered false memories had made her a "walking zombie." It was the first of what some reputable therapists fear will be many such rulings that will ultimately give their profession a black eye.

An increasing number of recovered-memory accusers have recanted, and some have reunited with their families and joined them in suing the therapists and clinics they claim led them astray. Many of them are among the more than 7,000 individuals and families who have sought assistance from the False Memory Syndrome Foundation, a Philadelphia-based organization that has taken the lead in publicizing the wrongdoings and in helping the victims of recovered-memory therapy. Pamela Freyd, who co-founded FMSF in 1992, has yet to be reconciled with her accuser daughter.

Growing controversy and concern in the mental-health community has led the American Psychological Association to appoint a false-memory working group to investigate the phenomenon. At a meeting of the American Psychiatric Association last May, the issue of false memories was addressed in three sessions and heatedly debated by experts on both sides. The American Medical Association's house of delegates also indicated its discomfort with such memory-enhancement techniques as guided imagery, hypnosis and body massage, all of which heighten suggestibility and are widely employed by recovered-memory therapists. Use of these practices in eliciting accounts of childhood sexual abuse, the AMA delegates concluded, was "fraught with problems of potential misapplication."

> I wish I could say the debate just involves a few kooks. It's much broader, happening among the cream of the crop of psychiatrists.

"I wish I could say the debate just involves a few kooks," says Stephen Ceci, a Cornell University developmental psychologist who is a member of the American Psychological Association's work group. "It's much broader than that, happening among the cream of the crop of psychiatrists and clinical psychologists." The battle could not have come at a worse time, says Ceci; some professionals are currently pushing for increased coverage of mental health in the President's proposed national health plan. "It's not a good time for us to be airing our dirty laundry."

Still, the opposing camps are doing just that, arguing bitterly about repressed memories. Critics of recovered-memory therapy insist that there is no scientific evidence for the reality of repression and that many, if not most, of the recovered-memory claims are false. Advocates have no doubts, citing studies on amnesia and clinical experience showing that repression is commonplace. Given that psychology is an inexact science, any resolution of the issue seems distant, at best.

Judie Alpert, a professor of applied psychology at New York University, refutes the critics of recovered-memory therapy. "There is absolutely no question that some people have repressed some memories of early abuse that are just too painful to remember," she says. "In their 20s and 30s some event triggers early memories, and slowly they return. The event has been so overwhelming that the little girl who is being abused can't tolerate to be there in the moment, so she leaves her body, dissociates, as if she is up on a bookshelf looking down on the little girl who is being abused. Over time, she pushes it deep down because she can't integrate the experience."

Christine Courtois, also in the APA work group and a clinical director at the Psychiatric Institute in Washington, charges that criticism of the recovered-memory phenomenon is part of a backlash against society's tardy recognition of widespread sexual abuse. The "wholesale degradation of psychotherapy by some critics," she says, represents "displaced rage" at therapists for bringing the issue to public attention.

That kind of reasoning does not sit well with Margaret Singer, a retired professor from the University of California, Berkeley, and an expert on cults and influence techniques. She has interviewed 50 people who once believed they had recovered repressed memories of incest or ritual abuse but now think they were mistaken. All 50, Singer emphasizes, were in therapy when they "recovered" terrifying memories of abuse. "These people are reporting to me that their therapists were far more sure than they were that their parents had molested them."

Singer insists that trauma does not cause people to repress memories, although bits and pieces of experience can be lost through amnesia. In fact, she says, trauma has just the opposite effect: people can't forget it. As an example, she cites the cases of Vietnam veterans who suffer flashbacks and posttraumatic stress disorder.

Psychologist Ofshe is particularly disdainful of the concept of what he calls "robust" repression: the instantaneous submergence of any memory of sexual abuse. Recovered-memory therapists, he says, "have invented a mechanism that supposedly causes a child's awareness of sexual assault to be driven entirely from consciousness." According to these therapists, Ofshe explains, "there is no limit to the number of traumatic events that can be repressed, and no limit to the length of time over which the series of events can occur." Belief in robust repression, he concludes, "can be found only on the lunatic fringes of science and the mental-health professions."

"Repression definitions are so loose

and varied, so abundant, so shifting that it is like trying to shoot a moving target," says Elizabeth Loftus, professor of psychology and law at the University of Washington and an authority on cognitive processes, long-term memory and eyewitness testimony. "If repression is the avoidance in your conscious awareness of unpleasant experiences that come back to you, yes, I believe in repression. But if it is a blocking out of an endless stream of traumas that occur over and over that leave a person with absolutely no awareness that these things happen, that make them behave in destructive ways and re-emerge decades later in some reliable form, I don't see any evidence for it. It flies in the face of everything we know about memory."

If such recovered memories are indeed false, where do they originate? From two sources, critics say: the popular culture and misguided or inept therapy. Sensational tales about recovered memories of incest have been grist for celebrity-magazine cover stories. And repressed-memory incest and satanic-ritual-abuse victims have been featured prominently on Geraldo, Oprah, Sally Jessy Raphaël and other daytime TV talk shows.

In bookstores, pop-psychology sections are filled with dozens of self-help survivor titles. By far the most controversial and best selling (more than 700,000 copies) of these books is *The Courage to Heal* by Ellen Bass and Laura Davis. In their 1988 publication, considered the bible of the recovered-memory movement, they include such dogma as "If you think you were abused and your life shows the symptoms, then you were," and "If you don't remember your abuse, you are not alone. Many women don't have memories ... this doesn't mean they weren't abused." Like many of the authors of these self-help books, neither Davis nor Bass has any academic training in psychology, although Davis claims to be an incest survivor. Yet many therapists urge their patients to read *Courage* and other similar volumes.

Many of these books contain laundry lists of symptoms of repressed-memory victims. They inform their readers that even though they have no memory of the acts, they may have been victims of childhood sexual or ritual abuse if they experience some of the following conditions: depression, anxiety, loss of appetite or eating disorders, sexual problems and difficulty with intimacy. The all-inclusive nature of that list, critics say, suggests that among the entire U.S. population, only the rare individual has managed to escape childhood sexual abuse. That doesn't seem to surprise therapist E. Sue Blume. In her book *Secret Survivors*, she writes, "It is not unlikely that *more than half of all women* are survivors of childhood sexual trauma."

ALMOST ANY NIGHT, IN ANY major American city, adult incest and ritual-abuse survivor meetings are held in church basements and community rooms. Churches and other institutions also offer counseling for dissociative disorders and satanic-ritual-abuse victims.

Private psychiatric hospitals, which advertise in medical journals and airline magazines, are profiting as well. "We can help you remember and heal," promises one ad

It Came From Outer Space

Nancy, a West Coast attorney, remembered details of the incident only four months ago, after she began hypnotherapy sessions. Now, she recalls how one spring night in 1989 she awoke in a stupor to see a strange craft outside her window. She was taken into the vehicle and examined by a team of strange beings. A silver tube was inserted into her to extract an ovum. She breaks down as she describes the abduction. "People say 'How do you know?' You don't know. You're never sure what happened."

As thousands of therapy patients are "discovering" repressed memories of childhood sexual abuse, a smaller number are adding a new twist: they are recalling abductions by aliens. Under hypnosis, Los Angeles film producer Michael Bershad recalled his car being pulled to the side of the road by a bright object. "I got out of the car and saw five guys under 4 ft. tall. They led me inside the craft." A leader examined him, opening up his back to poke around his vertebra. The extraterrestrials also extracted sperm. "I had a lot of shame," says Bershad. "It was humiliating and degrading."

A painful sincerity unites those who have dredged up memories of UFO abductions. Many suffer from insomnia and shy away from telling anyone what they believe may have happened for fear of being perceived as crazy. "Virtually all abductees are opposed to the idea that these things really happen," explains Budd Hopkins, author of two books about contact with aliens. "They don't want these things to be real. There is no pleasure in this experience."

Harvard psychiatrist John Mack, who won a Pulitzer in 1977 for his psychological study of Lawrence of Arabia, takes the stories literally. "I encountered something here very early on, which I saw did not fit anything I had ever come across in 40 years of psychiatry." He has treated more than 70 abductees, whom he calls "experiencers."

A few researchers argue that alien abductions may be disguised memories of sexual abuse. Others assert that abduction memories may also be unwittingly planted by over-zealous therapists. "I believe these victims believe it," says Ray Hyman, professor of psychology at the University of Oregon. "People are trying to please the hypnotist. The therapist and patient collaborate with each other to produce the story." Hypnosis can be extremely effective in eliciting fantasies that therapists can use in treating patients. The technique, however, can also create false memories. Says Ray William London, president of the American Boards of Clinical Hypnosis: "It isn't a way of validating an abduction or anything else."

William Cone, a psychologist in Newport Beach, California, who specializes in treating alleged abductees, finds similarities between some of his patients and people who recover memories of satanic-ritual abuse. Both have "organizing personalities"—a loose sense of self given to paranormal experiences like seeing ghosts. Many are also highly suggestible. "They are highly functioning, intelligent people and truly believe that this happened," says Cone. "I try not to believe or disbelieve. I just sit and listen and try to help."

—*By Jeanne McDowell/Los Angeles*

3. PROBLEMS INFLUENCING PERSONAL GROWTH

for ASCA Treatment Centers in Compton, California. "Remembering incest and childhood abuse is the first step to healing."

The thriving recovered-memory industry dismays psychiatrist Ganaway. "In some cases," he says, the hospitals and clinics "are memory mills with an almost assembly-line mentality," he says. "A patient comes in with no memories but leaves with memories of childhood incest or ritual abuse." Yet even some well-trained family and marriage counselors, psychologists and psychiatrists seem too quick to tie their patients' problems to repressed memories of incest and ritual abuse. "That makes psychotherapy very easy at first," explains Johns Hopkins' McHugh. "Therapists and patients can say, 'We found the secret.' The fact that the patients and families steadily become more confused, incoherent and chaotic is then believed to be an expression of the original incest." What is really happening, he says, is that "conflicts are being generated by false memories. We have found something to make therapy easy."

Some patients now leave their therapist's office convinced that they suffer from multiple-personality disorder, which is said to stem from repressed memories of early childhood trauma, including physical and sexual abuse. Until the publication of *Sybil*, MPD was apparently rare; around the world, only a few hundred cases had been documented over the previous three centuries. Since then, however, many thousands of supposed cases of MPD have been identified in the U.S. alone—most of them incorrectly, say critics, by therapists who are looking for an easy solution in their search for evidence of childhood sexual abuse or who too easily accept the likelihood of the disorder. One problem, says Ganaway, is that once these patients have been diagnosed with MPD, they are convinced that they have it, tend to exhibit what they think are the symptoms and often reinterpret their entire life histories accordingly.

Those charges infuriate Dr. Richard Kluft, a Philadelphia psychiatrist, who works extensively with MPD patients. "It's an absolute lie that MPD is a rare psychiatric disorder," he says. He attributes the sharp rise in reported MPD cases to the rise of feminism and the resulting willingness of people "to speak out more openly on issues of exploitation and abuse."

Another doctor who believes that MPD is fairly common is Bennett Braun, medical director of the dissociative-disorders program at Rush-Presbyterian-St. Luke's Medical Center in Chicago. Braun says the number of cases of MPD has risen not for faddish reasons but because therapists have become better at recognizing the symptoms.

In his 12-bed unit at Rush North Shore Medical Center in Skokie, a branch of Rush-Presbyterian-St. Luke's Medical Center, Braun treats MPD cases, some of whom think that they are victims of satanic-ritual abuse. When he first began to hear the satanic stories in 1985, Braun says, he was incredulous. Now, having heard similar tales from many people from different states and countries and having treated more than 200 of them, he declares, "Yes, there is satanic-ritual abuse."

If some of the recovered memories of familial childhood abuse sound fanciful, the recollections of satanic-ritual abuse are downright bizarre. These tales have proliferated since the publication in 1980 of *Michelle Remembers*, a book about a belatedly aware satanic-ritual victim. They describe a massive secret conspiracy to abuse children sexually in order to brainwash them into worshipping Satan. Victims recall being raped by their parents and then by members of a cult who drink blood and sacrifice fetuses. More often than not the abusers are pillars of their communities—the mayor, police chief or school superintendent—who come out at night and join their parents in terrifying ceremonies.

> In some cases, [they] are memory mills ... A patient comes in with no memories but leaves with memories of incest or ritual abuse.

But could such satanic rituals be that commonplace, let alone exist at all? In 1990, a group of researchers at the State University of New York at Buffalo conducted a nationwide sample of clinical psychologists, asking them if they had encountered claims of ritual abuse. Some 800 of the psychologists, about a third of the sample, had treated at least one case.

Yet, law-enforcement authorities report that not one shred of reliable evidence has turned up to support these claims—no documented marks of torture, no bones of sacrificed adults, infants or fetuses and no reputable eyewitnesses. Lorraine Stanek, a Connecticut rehabilitation counselor for trauma survivors, also stresses the lack of evidence. "If you look at the alleged number of deaths that would be accounted for," she says, "there should be bodies in all our backyards." Still, incest-survivor groups are inundated with these claims. Monarch Resources, a California referral service for survivors, is said to receive more than 5,000 calls annually from people who believe they have been victims of satanic abuse. Alleged ritual abuse is also involved in about 16% of the calls to Philadelphia's False Memory Syndrome Foundation.

Braun demonstrated his belief in satanic rituals during a 1991 trial, when he testified in behalf of two daughters seeking damages from their 76-year-old mother. Recovering childhood memories, they had accused her of abusing them in bloody and murderous ceremonies. Both claimed that they had developed MPD as a result. After Braun told of treating similar cases, the jury found in favor of the two daughters.

Now, however, the tables have turned. Braun and the Chicago medical center are being sued for negligence by a female patient who in two years of in-patient treatment for supposed MPD "recovered" memories of involvement in satanic rituals with her father, mother and relatives. The rituals supposedly included torture, murder and cannibalism of large groups of people—as many as 50 on an average weekend. In addition, before growing doubts led the woman to terminate Braun's treatment in 1992, she had been made to believe she had 300 "alters" or personas, possibly setting a new MPD record. According to her lawyer, she is not currently undergoing any treatment and is doing well.

The ultimate victim of repressed memory may be the psychotherapeutic profession itself. "Therapists are terrified," says MPD specialist Kluft. "Many are feeling very hamstrung because they fear any time they ask a question, it can result in a lawsuit." Instead of seeing a patient "as a person in pain and in need of help," Kluft complains, "the therapist is looking at a potential litigant. Some people have discontinued treating trauma patients."

S. Scott Mayers, a psychotherapist in Venice, California, is hardly terrified. But he is cautious. "What I do to ensure that I don't inflict my agenda or opinion," he says, "is go with the patients' presentation and stay with it, using their own words, their own scenarios. I'm so cautious because we are all very suggestive."

Recovered-memory therapists might do well to heed those guidelines before they cause irreparable damage to their profession. For, as the public begins to recognize that people have been falsely accused by recovered-memory patients, says psychiatrist McHugh, it "opens us up to skepticism and dismay about our capacity to do things. This is a bubble that is going to burst. We will end up having to recreate the trust this country puts in psychotherapy."

—*Reported by* **Jeanne McDowell/Los Angeles**

Why schools must tell girls: 'YOU'RE SMART, YOU CAN DO IT'

Myra and David Sadker

Bias in education *is an issue that has stirred debate since 1954's Brown vs. Board of Education, the Supreme Court decision integrating public schools. In a new book,* Failing at Fairness: How America's Schools Cheat Girls *(Charles Scribner's Sons, $22), the focus is on girls. Authors Myra and David Sadker document how teachers and schools unwittingly shortchange girls up and down the educational ladder, from kindergarten through graduate school. Here the Sadkers, professors of education at The American University in Washington, D.C., and among the nation's leading experts in sex discrimination, describe the problem—and what educators and students are doing to combat it.*

Rachel Churner, 15, remembers seventh grade at her McKinney, Texas, middle school as the year she was scared silent. "You couldn't be too dumb because then you would be laughed at," she says. "But if you were too smart, you would be called a brain."

Rachel decided it was best for girls to be completely average. She stopped answering questions in class and tried to hide her intelligence. "If I got an A and people asked me how I did, I would say, 'I just got a B minus.' There were even times I wrote down the wrong answer to make a lower grade."

Reading from the same textbook, listening to the same teacher, sitting in the same classroom, girls and boys are getting very different educations. For 20 years, we've been watching girls in the classroom and studying their interactions with teachers. After thousands of hours of classroom observation, we remain amazed at the scope and stubborn persistence of gender bias.

These studies show that from grade school to grad school boys capture the lion's share of teachers' time and attention. Whether the class is science or social studies, English or math—and whether the teacher is female or male—girls are more likely to be invisible students, spectators to the educational process.

One reason that boys receive more teacher attention: They demand it. Boys call out eight times more often than girls—and get real feedback. But when girls call out, they're more likely to be reprimanded or to get the brushoff with responses like "OK."

'If you were too smart, you'd be called a brain.' —Rachel Churner

Girls not only are less visible in classrooms; they're missing from textbooks, too. Brand-new history textbooks still devote only 2 percent of their space to women. A simple test demonstrates the impact of this male curriculum. We've walked into classrooms—elementary, secondary, even college—and asked students to name 20 famous American women from history. We've given only one restriction: no athletes or entertainers. Few have met the challenge. Many couldn't name 10, or even five. One class of Maryland fifth-graders, embarrassed at coming up with so few, put "Mrs." in front of presidents' names, creating an instant list of famous-sounding women they knew nothing about. Other students wrote down names like Mrs. Fields, Betty Crocker and Aunt Jemima in a desperate attempt to find famous females.

Education is not a spectator sport. Over time, the lack of attention by teachers and the omission of women in textbooks takes its toll in lowered achievement, damaged self-esteem and limited career options. The proof:

• In the early grades, girls are equal to or even ahead of boys on almost every standardized test. By the time they leave high school or college, they have fallen behind.

3. PROBLEMS INFLUENCING PERSONAL GROWTH

- By high school, girls score lower on the SAT and ACT exams, crucial for college admission. The gender gap is greatest in math and science.
- On the College Board achievement exams, required by the most selective colleges, boys outscore girls on 11 of 14 tests by an average 30 points.

Girls are the only group who begin school scoring ahead and leave behind, a theft occurring so quietly that most people are unaware of its impact

---

Today, in small towns and large cities across the nation, parents and teachers, concerned about the future of America's daughters, have begun to take action. From college professors in Urbana, Ill., to elementary school teachers in Portland, Maine, educators are asking for help, signing up for workshops that we conduct on fighting gender bias in the classroom. Women's colleges such as Smith and Mount Holyoke have started sponsoring special summer sessions to help elementary and secondary school teachers battle bias against girls, especially in math and science.

And high on the agenda for change is renewed interest in girls-only education, until recently an endangered species.

Although not everyone agrees, most studies show that girls in single-sex schools achieve more, have higher self-esteem and are more interested in subjects like math and science.

Says Rachel Churner, now at Hockaday, a private all-girls school in Dallas: "Now I put my education first. I don't think that would have happened if I had stayed in my coed school."

Even coed schools are experimenting with single-sex classes. This includes some public schools, in one of the most surprising developments of the 1990s. After nine years of teaching coed high school math, Chris Mikles now teaches an all-girls Algebra II class at public Ventura (Calif.) High School. "The girls come in with such low self-esteem," she says. "I keep trying to get through to them: 'You're smart. You can do it.'"

This year, the Illinois Math and Science Academy in Aurora, a public coed residential school for 620 gifted students, is trying for the first time an experiment that tests a girls-only class. In the first part of the year, the school separated 13 girls for an all-girls calculus-based physics class. For the second half of the school year, the girls have rejoined coed classes. School officials will compare their performance with and without the boys, as well as against the girls and boys in coed classes.

Girls in the experimental class are feeling the results. In the girls-only class, Denab Bates, 17, says she was "more enthusiastic, more there than in my other classes"—asking and answering more questions, jumping "out of my seat to put a problem on the board. In my other classes, I sink back—'Oh, please, don't call on me.'" Kara Yokley, 15, also says she participated more, but she is not sure what will happen this semester as the class goes coed. "We need to make sure we don't lose our newfound physics freedom," she says.

Not every girl is as positive. "We took the same exams as the coed class, but the guys thought that girls weren't learning on the same level," worries 16-year-old Masum Momaya.

Legally, single-sex education in public schools is a sticky business. Laws like Title IX prohibit sex discrimination in public schools, including teaching girls and boys separately in most cases. In Illinois, educators say it works because IMSA is a laboratory school set up by the state to try innovations. In Ventura, Mikles says all-girls classes are permissible because they are open to male students, although not a single boy has yet enrolled.

Many educators have reservations that go beyond legal problems. They view single-sex education as a defeatist approach, one that gives up on girls and boys learning equally, side by side. Other critics say that the model focuses on "fixing up the girls" but leaves boys in the dust.

Where the Boys Are

It was not long ago that the focus was on boys—specifically, black boys, who some educators believed would benefit from separate schools. That movement has since lost steam. "Without a body of research to prove their effectiveness," Myra Sadker explains, boys-only schools "ran into legal problems."

AN UPDATE:

- **In Detroit,** the Malcom X Academy, an elementary and middle school with 500 students, and two other public schools were established in 1990 as all-boys schools. They were forced to admit girls after a judge ruled the same year that single-sex schools violated Title IX. Today, Malcolm X is 92 percent male.

- **The Milwaukee** school board wanted to create three boys-only schools in 1990, after evaluating the poor performance of many black males in public schools. School officials halted the project after the Detroit decision; instead, schools changed their curricula.

- **New York City's** Ujamaa Institute, intended for black and Hispanic boys, has yet to open since the proposal was challenged in court by the New York Civil Rights Coalition.

—*Myron B. Pitts*

Diane Ravitch of the Brookings Institution in Washington, D.C., is outspoken in her view that girls already are treated fairly in the educational system. Ravitch, assistant secretary of Education under President Bush, points to the fact that more women than men are enrolled in college, more women than men earn master's degrees, and the number of women graduating with law and medical degrees has increased dramatically since 1970. "The success of women in education has soared in the last 20 years," Ravitch says.

Despite such progress, women still tend to major in lower-paying fields, such as education and literature. Today, a woman with a college degree earns little more than a man with a high school diploma.

The remedy? Realistically, most schools remain committed to coeducation for philosophic, legal and economic reasons. Increasingly, though, educators are becoming convinced that changes need to be made. And when teachers change, so do their students. Our research suggests these key ways to make girls more active and assertive:

- Teachers and parents must encourage girls to speak up—both at home and in school.
- Textbooks need to be monitored to make sure that enough women are included.
- Seating arrangements in class need to be flexible, because students in the front or middle of the class get more attention.
- Comments to girls should encourage their academic progress. "You look so pretty today" and "Your handwriting is so neat"—standard comments to girls—are less helpful than "What a great test score" or "That was an insightful comment."

Parents, girls and even traditional women's organizations are beginning to join educators in making such simple but important changes. And groups nationwide are providing support and service. The National Women's History Project in California, for example, develops books and posters on multicultural women's history. The Girl Scouts has featured images of active girls in printed materials and highlighted badges in math and science. The Women's Educational Equity Act Publishing Center in Massachusetts says requests for materials have surged recently, especially in science and math. The American Association of University Women has sponsored research projects and roundtables. The Gender Equity in Education Act, currently before Congress, proposes programs to help pregnant teenagers, combat sexual harassment and provide gender-equity training for teachers.

Throughout the history of education in America, the angle of the school door has determined the direction girls travel to various adult destinies. Sometimes the door was locked and barred; at other times it was slightly ajar. Today girls face subtle inequities that have a powerful cumulative impact, chipping away at their achievement and self-esteem. But as a new generation of teachers and parents enters the school system, and an existing generation becomes increasingly open to reform, schools and educators appear ready to adapt—and girls will be the winners.

IT TAKES A SCHOOL

A new approach to elementary education starts at birth and doesn't stop when the bell rings

MARGOT HORNBLOWER NORFOLK

THE SIGN ON THE SQUAT BRICK schoolhouse in the midst of crime-ridden public-housing projects in Norfolk, Virginia, reads BOWLING PARK ELEMENTARY: A CARING COMMUNITY. Principal Herman Clark is one of those who does the caring, which is why every year he takes the parents of his pupils on a field trip to local attractions. One year it was to Greensville Correctional Center in Jarratt. "We got the chance to see the electric chair," he says. There have been visits to a prison in Chesapeake and a women's penal institution in Goochland. Two months ago, it was a walk through Death Row at Mecklenburg Correctional Center.

"The parents are subjected to a shakedown body search" for weapons or drugs, Clark says. "They hear the door slam. They look at the inmates and see the way the inmates look back at them. We ask the prisoners, 'Was there something that led you to this life?' They say, 'Yes, my parents were not there when I was a kid. There was nothing to do, so I did this or that [crime].' It is frightening. It makes our parents realize: this is where their child is heading." Every three years, Clark puts his pupils through a similar ordeal. "We target students who have the potential to get in trouble," he says. When a group of 26 returned from Deerfield Correctional Center, Clark says, "I was glad to see the bullies crying."

The shock treatment of the field trips is just one of many innovative therapies that Clark, a Ph.D. in education, has brought to

> **"Schools are being called on to be those 'surrogate parents' that can increase 'teachability.'"**

his school. Bowling Park is where the rhetoric of "standing for children" moves beyond talk. If children are to be rescued, the reasoning goes, who is better equipped to do so than the elementary school, a solid institution already in the business? Yet to rescue children, one must start early—even before birth. And to rescue children, whole families must be rescued along with them—hence the transformation of the neighborhood school into a "caring community." It may sound like a platitude, but it is in fact a revolution, one that is spreading through the country, from inner-city ghettos to prosperous suburbs and rural enclaves, as fast as you can say *ABC*.

One of the most far-reaching programs, which began in Missouri and has spread to 47 states, hires "parent educators" who offer parenting skills and developmental screening to families with young children, beginning in the third trimester of pregnancy. Bowling Park's Michael Bailey, a soft-spoken Mister Rogers type, hands out flyers in food-stamp lines to encourage new mothers to sign up. Each day he drives out to visit one of the 35 families who have joined the program. "Hello, teacher!" shrieks Tonesha Sims, 2½, running out of her house to hug him on a recent morning. Bailey spends an hour reviewing colors and numbers with the pigtailed toddler. As Bailey leaves, Tonesha begs, "Teacher, can I play with you next week?" Lottie Holloman, 68, her great-grandmother—and her guardian since Tonesha's mother, a drug addict, abandoned the girl to foster care—credits Bailey with inspiring her to buy books and read to the child. Children in the program get priority for slots in Bowling Park's preschool.

By delving into the critical first three years of life, schools such as Bowling Park are expanding far beyond traditional academics. But to many educators it is a logical evolution. Moving away from a narrow focus on curriculum reform, some schools are assuming responsibility for the foundations of learning—the emotional and social well-being of the child from birth to age 12. Thus anything that affects a child is the school's business—from nutrition to drug-abuse prevention to health care and psychological counseling. "Schools are being called on to be those 'surrogate parents' that can increase the 'teachability' of children who arrive on their doorsteps in poor shape," according to Joy G.

21. It Takes a School

Dryfoos, author of the 1994 book *Full-Service Schools*.

Bowling Park was chosen in 1992 as the site of the first CoZi school, a model that combines the education programs of two Yale professors, James P. Comer and Edward Zigler. Over the past three decades, Comer, a psychiatrist, has helped convert 600 mostly inner-city schools to a cooperative management in which parents, teachers and mental-health counselors jointly decide policy and focus on building close-knit relationships with children. Zigler, one of the founders of Head Start, designed "The School of the 21st Century," a program operating on 400 campuses, offering year-round, all-day preschool beginning at three, as well as before- and after-school and vacation programs. Bowling Park combines both approaches in what may be the nation's most comprehensive effort, as Zigler puts it, "[to] make the success of the child in every aspect of development our constant focus." Other CoZi schools are operating in Bridgeport, Connecticut, and in Mehlville, Missouri.

At Bowling Park staff members "adopt" a child; many take on several at a time. Often the child is one whose parent has died or gone to prison, or whose siblings are dealing drugs, or whose single mother neglects him. "We take these kids home with us for the weekend or out to eat or to get a haircut," says principal Clark. "School has to be about more than reading, writing and arithmetic. These kids need so much—and sometimes what they really need is a good hug."

In Clark's office the other day, Rashid Holbrook, 11, fidgeted with his wraparound shades and sought to explain why he had gone after a boy with an ax and spray painted a family's front steps. "I got a bad temper," he says. "When I get home at night, I pile up feelings." Rashid lives with an aunt who, Clark says, takes little interest in him. "My daddy's in prison," the boy says, showing little emotion. "He hit my momma. He went for breaking and entering and a hundred other charges." Interjects Clark: "But you're going in a different direction."

Rashid volunteers that he might be an engineer or a policeman. Why a policeman? "I don't like people doing things to other people," he says. And then after a long pause, "But I do it."

Rashid has been "adopted" by Clayton Singleton, 25, an art teacher. "We've been to art museums and shopping at the mall," says Singleton, pausing during a drawing class that sprawls over the floor of a corridor. "He was getting curious about the man-woman thing, so we had The Talk. Whatever questions he asked, he got the real answer." The talk was timely: only a few weeks before, Rashid had asked the daughter of another teacher if she wanted "to make a baby."

> "We have fine buildings. Why let them sit vacant 14 hours a day and three months of the year?"

The key to Bowling Park's success, which has shown up in higher test scores and a 97% attendance rate, is getting parents into the school. Many of them had never bothered even to walk their first-graders to class. CoZi offers "parent technicians"—two in Bowling Park's case—to visit parents at home, ask them what they need and spur them to form committees and organize projects. Responding to parent feedback, Bowling Park now offers adult-education courses, adult-exercise classes, a once-a-month Family Breakfast Club at which parents talk about children's books, a singing group and a "room moms" program that puts parents into the classroom to help teachers. Parents also pressed the principal for school uniforms—and now help launder them. Bowling Park's programs are funded through a combination of federal funds set aside for inner-city schools, parent fees, private grants and school-district money.

"This is a holistic approach," says CoZi coordinator Lorraine Flood. "If parents are not sitting at the table, we don't find out the underlying reasons for children's academic or behavioral problems." When a mother of children at the school lost her husband to cancer recently, leaving her with six sons, parent technicians set up a workshop on grief. A welfare mother, who had put her child in foster care, found her self-confidence so built up by parenting and adult-education classes and her service in the PTA that she recovered her daughter and got a secretarial job. Recently parent techs held a wedding reception at the school for a mother who finally got married. A grandfather, inspired by a writing workshop, reads his poems at school functions.

But the lessons of Bowling Park, where the student body is overwhelmingly black and low income, are not just for schools that serve the poor. In fact, Zigler's concept of expanding school into a full-day, year-round enterprise is equally crucial to middle-class parents at Sycamore Hills Elementary School in Independence, Missouri, where students are mostly white.

In Independence all 13 elementary schools work on the 21st Century model. Thirty-five percent of new parents take advantage of the state-funded home-visit program for children younger than age three. "We have fine buildings. Why let them sit vacant 14 hours a day and three months of the year?" says superintendent Robert Watkins. "Now we can see a child with a speech impediment at age three and get started on remediation."

Once start-up costs were absorbed for remodeling school basements or buying modular units, the preschool and after-school day care became mostly self-supporting: 85% of the $2 million program comes from parents' fees. "Schools should be a community hub," says fourth-grade teacher Darlene Shaw. In three decades at Sycamore Hills, she has witnessed profound change. "Out of my 23 students today, only one has a stay-at-home mom," she said. "Without consistent, quality day care, kids flounder. And for kids dealing with divorce and single-parent families, school is their stability when things are going crazy at home."

Nicole Argo, one of Shaw's fourth-graders, has tried riding the bus home after school at 3:15 p.m. But she found she would rather stay in Sycamore's after-school program. "It's boring to watch TV at home," she says. "At 21st Century you do projects and go places." So Nicole's parents—an engineer and a human-resources officer—pick her up after work at 4:30—along with her five-year-old sister Amanda—and drop them both off each morning at 6:30, more than an hour before school begins. Nearly a third of Independence's students have a similar 10-hour day on campus. "It's Bobby's second home," says Laurie French, the divorced mother of a nine-year-old with muscular dystrophy. "The staff is like family, and since Bobby was three, we've done a pretty good job raising him together." Although he walks with difficulty, Bobby takes karate lessons in the program. And lately his favorite activity has been crochet, taught at the day-care center by a volunteer grandmother.

Independence and Norfolk have not experienced opposition to their reforms, but that does not mean every school district is ready for change. Overcrowded classrooms, pinched budgets and teachers set in their ways are only a few of the obstacles. Julia Denes, assistant director of Yale's Bush Center of Child Development and Social Policy, warns, however, that not adopting CoZi-like programs will ultimately cost more. "We must invest in children at an early age to prevent special needs and delinquency," she says. That's the message too of principal Clark's field trips.

Helping Teenagers Avoid Negative Consequences of SEXUAL ACTIVITY

How can they be taught to resist the normal biological urges of adolescence and the overabundance of sexual stimuli in American culture?

Jeannie I. Rosoff

NO ONE CAN DENY that teenage pregnancy is a serious issue. Births to girls too young to care properly for a baby represent both individual and societal tragedies. Yet, society seems unable to develop realistic responses to the problem. This is due, in part, to the fact that rhetoric often serves to obscure the issue.

Indeed, the claims are confusing, if not downright contradictory. Teenage pregnancies are reported to be "soaring," yet their number has remained relatively stable over the last 10 years or so and is considerably lower than in previous decades. "Babies are having babies," trumpet talk show hosts, yet most births to teenagers are to 18- and 19-year-old women. The public, according to opinion polls, believes that the preponderance of the 1,500,000 abortions that take place each year are to teenage girls and that they account, as well, for the majority of births out of wedlock. However these perceptions have come about, the data show that they are wrong, on both counts. Yet, teenage pregnancy, while a personal and social problem, routinely is cited both as the end result of all that is wrong in American society and as a major source of all social ills.

Teenage pregnancies and births also are held to be the basis of welfare dependency, and politicians currently are trying to outdo each other in their attempts to alleviate the situation. Among the proposed remedies are restoring the value of sexual abstinence, promoting marriage to make out-of-wedlock pregnancies legitimate, and pro-

Ms. Rosoff is president, The Alan Guttmacher Institute, New York.

hibiting public assistance to teenage mothers under the age of 18 who fail to marry. How many young mothers under 18 actually are receiving welfare checks? Not "hundreds of thousands," as claimed recently by one of the country's most respected newspapers, but 32,000 nationwide. This well may be too many, but could "solving" the problem, assuming that the remedies proposed could do the job, truly be expected to put this country "back on the right track"?

Perhaps what is needed, first, is to define the issue. It is not that many more girls are becoming mothers in their teens than in the past. They are not. Is it that, when they do, they often choose not to marry the father? Even if they do, these youthful marriages are likely to be unstable and impermanent. Is it because they failed to use contraception, or contraception failed them? Or is it because they had sex in the first place, or sex out of marriage?

In U.S. society, much sexual activity does occur outside of marriage. Most Americans today engage in sexual relationships prior to marriage, in between marriages, after divorce or widowhood, or when they choose to remain single altogether, although research shows them to be overwhelmingly faithful to their spouses when in a stable union. It also is a fact that accidental pregnancies are extremely common, some among the married, many more among the unmarried. Of the roughly 4,500,000 pregnancies that take place each year, slightly more than half are unplanned and about 1,500,000 are disruptive or unwanted enough to end in abortion. Given the fact that close to 30% of all births—most to adult women, not teenagers—now occur outside of formal wedlock, it also is clear that an increasing number of women choose to become mothers when marriage is not a likely or promising prospect. Because half of all marriages end in divorce, it tends to blur the differences between the life circumstances of children born in or out of wedlock since the result is increasingly the same—a childhood or a good part of childhood in a single-parent family with its attendant financial and social disadvantages. While these trends are disturbing and a legitimate source of concern, they attract relatively little public ire or condemnation. Neither do they prompt the kind of benign or, alternatively, draconian remedies that sexual activity among teenagers seems to elicit.

Children are not adults. They are, at least under the age of 18, still the legal, financial, and moral responsibility of their parents. Not only their parents, but the community as a whole, have, or should have, a vested interest in their getting a good start in life—acquiring an education, obtaining adequate job training, establishing themselves financially, and, eventually, forming families of their own. They are our collective future and we have a collective investment in their well-being. Sexual activity, with its attendant hazards at all ages—including disease and accidental pregnancy—may have particularly destructive consequences for the very young, shaping prematurely the very course of their lives. Thus, public concern is valid and warranted.

Adolescents today, in spite of their occasional experimentations or temporary rebellions, appear to share their parents' values and aspirations for life. Young people increasingly spend part or all of their childhood in single-parent or "blended" families, and research shows that the deleterious consequences on children, including the likelihood of early sexual activity and pregnancy, are higher in each type. Nowadays, both parents usually work and children tend to have less consistent adult assistance and supervision. The role of the media, particularly television, is pervasive, and the depiction of sex and violence is ubiquitous at virtually all hours of the day. Violence is a commonplace experience in many communities, not in the inner city alone. Drugs often are available at high schools or even at junior high schools.

> "Sexual activity, with its attendant hazards at all ages—including disease and accidental pregnancy—may have particularly destructive consequences for the very young, shaping prematurely the very course of their lives."

A large portion—40% of youths aged 15-19—of the country's teenagers live in families that are poor or of low income. Hispanic and black teenagers are substantially more likely than white youths to be at the bottom of the economic ladder, attend substandard schools, fail to graduate from high school, and be unable to pursue further education. Thus, their chances of finding stable and well-paying jobs sometimes are doomed early on. High levels of poverty among children and youths from racial and ethnic minorities, combined with persistent *de facto* segregation in housing and schools, mean that some adolescents, especially African-Americans, grow up in economic and social ghettos where alienation often thrives and education and marriage are not the norm.

It is clear that young people these days are having sex earlier than they did in the past. This has been well-documented in the case of young women on whom information has been collected over the last 20 years. Comparable data for young men and boys is not as plentiful, but, on the whole, they have their first experience with sexual intercourse earlier than girls, a year sooner on average. However, neither are as precocious in their sexual experimentation as the public appears to believe. Still, teenagers are having sex for the first time at younger ages. While initiation of sexual activity during the teenage years has become the norm in the U.S.—as in most developed countries—it should be kept in mind that sex among very young adolescents still is rare and many of the very young girls who have had sex report that they were forced to do so.

Nevertheless, sexual initiation generally has occurred earlier and earlier during the last two decades, with the most significant changes in the behavior of white adolescents. By the end of the 1980s, the differences among youths of different racial, ethnic, and even religious groups had been close to eliminated. This trend toward earlier sexual activity has been accompanied by the gradual postponement of the age of marriage, so that most adolescent sexual activity now occurs outside of marriage. With the median age at marriage approaching 25 for women (and about three years later for men), the interval between the age of puberty and marriage for women has grown from 7.2 years in 1890 to 11.8 years. For men, it is 12.5 years.

The transition from adolescence to full adulthood—usually characterized by entering the labor force full time and setting up one's own household—also has become lengthier. Young people often have to stay in school longer to obtain the same employment opportunities that were available to their parents. There are fewer and poorer job prospects for those who have not completed high school and even for those who have finished high school, but gone no further. Young people who are poor and, within income groups, those who are black or Hispanic, are much less likely than others to graduate from high school on schedule or pursue further education.

So, young people are faced with many contradictory pressures and messages: Get as much education as you can, for as long as you can; establish yourself in a job and achieve financial autonomy; postpone marriage and, at the same time, presumably ignore the biological urges which are normal in adolescence and young adulthood as well as the sexual stimuli that are omnipresent in today's culture. On the whole, young people cope with these conflicting pressures successfully, and without much help from society. On the other hand, clearly, some succeed better than others in delaying sexual activity until relatively mature and avoiding the potentially harmful consequences of unprotected sex.

Within a year, a sexually active teenage girl who does not use contraception has a 90% chance of becoming pregnant. The chances of acquiring a sexually transmitted disease may be even greater since it can result from a single act of intercourse, al-

3. PROBLEMS INFLUENCING PERSONAL GROWTH

though some STDs are transmitted more easily than others. While they may not be totally aware of the risks, two-thirds of adolescents use a contraceptive method (usually the condom) the first time they have intercourse. The older the teenager is at the time of first sexual encounter, the more likely he or she is to use a contraceptive. However, most sexually experienced young women delay for a considerable period of time before they consult a medical professional. Roughly 40% wait 12 months after initiating intercourse before they visit a doctor or clinic and obtain more effective contraceptives than over-the-counter methods. Still, most sexually active teenagers utilize some method of contraception and, in general, pill use increases and condom use decreases with age. There are, however, differences among teenagers from different economic backgrounds. Higher-income adolescents are much more likely than those of lower income to use contraceptives. Black and Hispanic youths are less likely to do so than whites, although the differences between whites and blacks are small.

Contrary to popular belief, although their usage is not always perfect, the large majority of adolescents use contraception successfully. Effective use of most contraceptive methods requires motivation, constant attention, and repeated actions that are difficult even for married adults to maintain. It is obviously even more problematic to achieve for others who are not in a stable, predictable type of relationship. Unmarried teenagers, though, appear to do slightly better in preventing an accidental pregnancy than unmarried women in their early 20s and about as well as women in the next age group, 25-29. At all age groups, however, women who are poor or low-income have more difficulty using contraception successfully and, for adolescents in particular, the consequences of not using a method or of using a method ineffectively can be serious indeed.

Over the last two decades, teenage pregnancy rates have gone both up and down, depending on how they are looked at. Reflecting the dramatic rise in the proportion of young women who have had sexual experience in adolescence, the rate increased about 25% between 1972 (when reliable information first became available on the subject) and 1990. Because these teenage women are using contraception earlier and more effectively, the proportion of those who are sexually experienced who become pregnant accidentally actually has declined. Nearly two-thirds of all teenage pregnancies occur among 18- and 19-year-olds. The proportion of sexually active teenagers who become pregnant increases with age because, as they get older, more adolescents become sexually experienced, tend to have intercourse more frequently than their younger sisters, and are more likely to be married (if Hispanic) and/or to want to become pregnant.

Pregnancy rates also vary with race and ethnicity. Black teenagers have a higher pregnancy rate than their Hispanic or white counterparts, due, partially, to the fact that they are still more likely than whites to have initiated sexual activity a little earlier and to be less likely to use contraception or utilize it effectively.

Most teenagers of any race or background actually do not want to get pregnant; 85% of the pregnancies that do occur are unintended. Teenagers are not alone in experiencing high rates of unplanned pregnancies. More than half of all pregnancies among older women are unexpected or "mistimed." Again, income and race or ethnicity make a difference. Pregnancies among higher-income teenagers are more likely to be unintended than those among the less privileged. Among older women, by contrast, those with higher incomes are less likely to have an unintended pregnancy than those who are poor or of low income. Hispanic teenagers who become pregnant

> **Teenage girls need "practical knowledge and skills to help them cope with the glorification of sex in the media, peer pressure, and advances and blandishments on the part of the opposite sex. . . ."**

are somewhat more likely than either blacks or whites to have wanted to do so, or at least not to have cared whether or not they become pregnant.

Obviously, an unmarried woman or girl has only three ways to deal with a pregnancy if the father refuses to marry her or is not known. She can have the baby and raise it herself, give birth and relinquish the infant for adoption, or have an abortion. The overwhelming majority of teenagers faced with these options choose either abortion or going through with the pregnancy and keeping the child. Fifty-three percent of 15- to 19-year-old teenagers who experience an unintended pregnancy have an abortion, compared with 47% of older women facing the same situation. In general, teenagers who are from families that are better off financially are more likely than those from poorer homes to terminate their pregnancies by abortion. The same is true for teenagers whose parents have more education. Those who have a stronger orientation towards the future, with more hopes and aspirations, are more likely to choose to have an abortion.

The age of the male partner also makes a difference. Among the youngest teenagers, who also have partners under the age of 18, 61% have abortions, almost twice the percentage of those whose partner is over 20. This factor is particularly significant since many of the men involved are considerably older than their teenage girlfriends.

When adolescent women become pregnant unintentionally, the path they follow in resolving their dilemma is determined largely by their income and socioeconomic status. Young women from relatively advantaged families generally have abortions, so they can finish their education, get a job or build a career, and establish themselves before they marry and decide to have children. Poor teenagers frequently have abortions as well, but many are not able to avail themselves of this option for financial and other reasons. They also are more likely to have wanted to become pregnant or, probably, not to have cared very much whether they did or not, and to resign themselves to their fate and have the baby if they become pregnant unintentionally. It bears repeating that more than 80% of teenagers who give birth—as distinct from all those who have sex or even those who become pregnant—either are poor or of marginal incomes.

Society can do much—but on the whole has not—to help teenagers avoid the negative consequences of sexual activity. All teenagers need help in postponing the initiation of intercourse, not simply by exhortation, which has been shown to be of very limited use. They need help in acquiring the practical knowledge and skills to help them cope with the glorification of sex in the media, peer pressure, and advances and blandishments on the part of the opposite sex, particularly from older boys and men. All teenagers, when they become involved sexually—as eight in 10 will before they reach the age of 20—need easy access to low-cost, confidential family planning and STD services. Many also will need easy access to abortion when, as happens so often, contraception fails.

Better coping skills, better and more timely sex education, and improved access to contraceptive, STD, and abortion services will not be sufficient, however, to address the root cause of early childbearing among the disadvantaged teenage women who become parents. For these young women, entrenched poverty, not adolescent pregnancy, is the fundamental issue that must be addressed. Some will have the grit, the inborn talent, and, somehow, garner enough support to escape their circumstances. For most, though, real change in sexual and childbearing behavior will not come unless and until their poverty is alleviated, their schools offer realistic paths to jobs and careers, and their sense of alienation is overcome. In short, it will occur when they develop a sense that their life can, and will if they try, get better. No amount of rhetoric and no laws will change that.

New Passages

Author Gail Sheehy hails the advent of a Second Adulthood after age 45

In the space of one short generation, the whole shape of the life cycle has been fundamentally altered. Since the publication of my book *Passages* in 1976, age norms have shifted and are no longer normative.

Consider: Nine-year-old girls are developing breasts and pubic hair; 9-year-old boys carry guns to school; 16-year-olds can "divorce" a parent; 30-year-old men still live at home with Mom; 40-year-old women are just getting around to pregnancy; 50-year-old men are forced into early retirement; 55-year-old women can have egg donor babies; 60-year-old women start first professional degrees; 70-year-old men reverse aging by 20 years with human growth hormone; 80-year-olds run marathons: 85-year-olds remarry and still enjoy sex; and every day, the "Today" show's Willard Scott says "Happy Birthday!" to more 100-year-old women.

What's going on? There is a revolution in the adult life cycle. People today are leaving childhood sooner, but they are taking longer to grow up and much longer to die. That is shifting all the stages of adulthood ahead—by 10 years. Adolescence is now prolonged for the middle class until the end of the 20s. Today, our First Adulthood only begins at 30. Most baby boomers don't feel fully "grown up" until they are into their 40s. When our parents turned 50, we thought they were old! But today, women and men I've interviewed routinely feel they are five to 10 years younger than the age on their birth certificates. Fifty is what 40 used to be; 60 is what 50 used to be. Middle age has already been pushed far into the 50s—in fact, if you listen to boomers, there is no more middle age. So what's next?

Welcome to Middlescence. It's adolescence the second time around.

The territory of the 50s, 60s and beyond is changing so radically that it now opens up whole new passages leading to stages of life that are nothing like what our parents experienced. An American woman who today reaches age 50 free of cancer and heart disease can expect to see her 92nd birthday. The average man who is 65 today—an age now reached by more than 70 percent of the U.S. population—can expect to live until 81. That amounts to a second adult lifetime.

The average man who is 65 today—an age now reached by more than 70 percent of the U.S. population—can expect to live until 81.

Stop and recalculate. Imagine the day you turn 45 as the old age of your First Adulthood. Fifty then becomes the youth of your Second Adulthood. First Adulthood just happens to you. Second Adulthood, you can custom design. It's a potential rebirth that offers exhilarating new possibilities. But only for those who are aware and who prepare.

For those who are approaching 50, the question increasingly becomes, "How shall we live the rest of our lives?" And the tantalizing dynamic that has emerged in our era is that the second half of adult life is not the stagnant, depressing downward slide we have always assumed it to be.

In the hundreds of interviews I have done with men and women in middle life, especially pacesetters in the educated middle class I have discovered that people are beginning to see there is the exciting potential of a new life to live: one in which they can concentrate on becoming better, stronger, deeper, wiser, funnier, freer, sexier and more attentive to living the privileged moments—even as they are getting older, lumpier, bumpier, slower and closer to the end. Instead of being a dreary tale of decline, our middle life is a progress story, a series of little victories over little deaths.

We now have not one but three adult lives to anticipate: Provisional Adulthood from age 18 to 30, First

3. PROBLEMS INFLUENCING PERSONAL GROWTH

Adulthood from 30 to 45 and Second Adulthood from 45 to 85 and beyond. The most exciting development is that Second Adulthood contains two new territories—an Age of Mastery from 45 to 65 and an Age of Integrity from 65 to 85 and beyond. The startling life changes awaiting all of us are now being charted by path breakers from the World War II generation and the "silent" generation of those who came of age in the 1950s, who are writing new maps for everyone else to follow.

THE FLOURISHING FORTIES

The two generations of baby boomers—the Vietnam generation of the 1960s and the "me" generation of the 1970s—are set to become the longest-living humans in American history. The first of them will officially turn 50 in 1996. A million of them, the Census Bureau predicts, will live past 100. Having indulged themselves in the longest adolescence in history, they betray a collective terror and disgust of aging.

An American woman who today reaches age 50 free of cancer and heart disease can expect to see her 92nd birthday.

Early in life, baby boomers got used to having two things: choice and control. That means that when life's storm clouds threaten, people in their 40s today are likely to feel more out of control than ever. Wally Scott, a participant in one of many "Midlife Passages" group discussions I've attended in recent years, put it this way: "All of a sudden, you have to start listening to the little voices inside: What do I really want to invest my life in? How can I construct a life that fits the me of today as opposed to the me of 15 years ago?"

The Flourishing Forties can be complicated for women by the storms of perimenopause and menopause. Men may face their own version of biological meltdown. Although it is not strictly a male menopause, many men in middle or later life do experience a lapse in virility and vitality and a decline in well-being. About half of American men over 40 have experienced middle-life impotence to varying degrees. This decline can definitely be delayed. It can even be corrected. In the near future, it may even become preventable. But first a man must understand it.

The social arena contains its own challenges as women in their 40s continue to explore new roles, struggle with late child rearing or mourn their lack of children. As couples are forced to renegotiate traditional relationships and medical crises intrude on well-laid plans, men and women in this age group begin to feel their mortality.

Today, smart men and women will use their early 40s as preparation for a custom-designed Second Adulthood. What do you need to learn to maximize your ability to respond quickly to a fluid marketplace? A single, fixed identity is a liability today. Recent research also suggests that developing multiple identities is one of the best buffers against mental and physical illness. When a marriage blows up or the company shuts down or the whole nature of a profession is changed by technology, people with more than one identity can draw upon other sources of self-esteem while they regroup. Such resilience is essential.

SECOND ADULTHOOD

John Guare has been doing exactly what he most loves since he was 9 years old—writing plays. But even the brilliant creator of *Six Degrees of Separation* and *House of Blue Leaves* knows he cannot rest on his laurels. He was 56 when I mentioned to him that I was exploring our Second Adulthood. "I was just saying to my wife, 'I've got to reinvent my life, right now!'" he exploded. "Or we'll be dead. Worse than dead—the walking dead."

That is the challenge of making the passage to Second Adulthood. This new life must be precipitated by a moment of change—the "Aha!" moment. It forces us to look upon our lives differently and to make a transition from survival to mastery. In young adulthood we survive by figuring out how best to please or perform for the powerful ones who will protect and reward us—parents, teachers, lovers, mates, bosses, mentors. It is all about proving ourselves. The transformation of middle life is to move into a more stable psychological state of mastery, where we control much of what happens in our life and can often act on the world rather than react to whatever the world throws at us. Reaching this state of mastery is also one of the best predictors of good mental and psychological functioning in old age.

Second Adulthood takes us beyond the preoccupation with self. We are compelled to search for a greater significance in our engagement in the world. "We are all hungry for connection," said James Sniechowski, a 51-year-old men's group leader in Santa Monica, Calif. *Connection* was a word that came up again and again in my discussions with groups of middle-aged men.

Increasingly, women who have mastered the silent passage through menopause feel a power surge—postmenopausal zest. As family obligations fade away, many become motivated to stretch their independence, learn new skills, return to school, plunge into new careers, rediscover the creativity and adventurousness of their youth and, at last, find their own voices.

THE FLAMING FIFTIES

By the time they reach their Flaming Fifties, most educated women have acquired the skills and self-knowledge to master complex environments and change the conditions around them. Over and over, women who have crossed into their 50s tell me with conviction, "I would not go back to being young again." They remember vividly what it was like to wake up not knowing exactly who they were, to be torn between demands of family and demands of career, to be constantly changing hats (and hairstyles) in the attempt to fit many roles and often losing focus in the blur of it all.

In three major national opinion surveys I have done in the past seven years, I have learned that by Second Adulthood, the dominant influence on a woman's well-being is not income level or social class or marital status. The most decisive factor is age. Older is happier.

"Fifty for me was a time when I really, for the first time, owned my body," said Ginny Ford, a Rochester, N.Y., businesswoman, whose blond hair and dimpled smile evoke Doris Day movies. "I had been very ashamed of my body, and now I love it. Now, there's all this inner stuff going on. I'm probably 10 pounds heavier, my thighs are a little rumply, my arms have flab. Fifteen years ago I would have starved myself. But now I'm enjoying my husband's pasta. I exercise every day, I enjoy myself sexually and I'm proud of this body. It really works!"

For men entering their 50s today, there is no script. It has traditionally been assumed that aging is kinder to men, but a different truth comes out in personal interviews. I found far more uncertainty among men in middle life than among women; indeed, they often appear to be going in opposite directions. Overall, the over-50 men in my surveys don't experience the great transformation from First to Second Adulthood that women do. Most appear to be more resigned to accepting life as it is: Two thirds are not anticipating any major change, and one third feel more concerned about just getting by. Half of these men feel tired and like they're "running out of gas." Their greatest worry is that they can no longer take their health for granted.

Intimate attachments. But among those men I have studied who are well educated, particularly those with an entrepreneurial temperament, a good many are enjoying a sense of mastery. They say the best things about being over 45 are being able to rely on their experience and being clearer about what is truly important in life. Still others find new richness in forging closer, more intimate attachments with their wives or in becoming start-over dads.

How can we make this passage more positively? Find your passion, and pursue it. How do you know where to look? You can start by seeing if it passes the time-flies test. What activity do you do in which time goes by without your even knowing it? What did you most love to do when you were 12 years old? Somewhere in that activity there is a hook to be found that might pull up your dormant self.

Men and women who emerge psychologically healthiest at 50 are those who, as their expectations and goals change with age, "shape a 'new self' that calls upon qualities that were dormant earlier." This was the principal finding of longitudinal studies at the University of California at Berkeley. Men have always been able to start over, and not once but more than once. What is really new is that women now have the option of starting second lives in their mid-40s or 50s, and increasingly they are doing so.

Households headed by someone over 55 control 56 percent of the nation's net worth.

For some that will lead to intellectual pursuits. A remarkable surge is already occurring in higher education among older women. Only 3.2 percent of the women in the World War II generation went back to post-high-school education between the ages of 40 and 54. But fully 11 percent of the "silent" generation of the 1950s went back for some college education in those middle years. In 1991, nearly 1 million women over 40 were enrolled in college nationwide.

This stage brings with it much greater emotional and social license, and a majority of these women have claimed it, becoming more outspoken and less self-conscious. After interviewing 14 women from my national survey who emerged in their 50s with optimum well-being, I learned that they see themselves as survivors. That is not the same as seeing themselves as former victims of terrible physical or emotional abuse, although some do describe overcoming such situations in their lives. What they have "survived" are the economic biases and stereotypical sex roles that threatened to inhibit their development as fully independent adults. They are so strong that they do not expect to feel "old" until they are about 70.

One striking finding among researchers is that men over 50 are becoming somewhat more dependent on their wives, emotionally and financially, and less certain about their future goals. The special stresses of an economy in transition, with its punishing wage declines for non-college-educated workers and corporate downsizing that now robs many college-educated men of identity and meaning, have been added to classic biological stresses, especially the decline of men's physical prowess and, for many, the sagging of their sexual

3. PROBLEMS INFLUENCING PERSONAL GROWTH

performance. Given this new set of conditions, men at middle life probably face the roughest patch of all in mapping the new adult life across time.

"Men over 45 are becoming the new at-risk population for significant problems with anxiety and depression," says Ellen McGrath, a psychologist and author of *When Feeling Bad Is Good*. "And for the first time ever, some of them are acknowledging it and reaching out for help. This is a brand-new trend."

Making a passage to the Age of Mastery often means men are giving up being the master. Alan Alhadeff, a Seattle lawyer of 45, described his "Aha!" moment on a basketball court: "This 20-year-old kid was checking me real hard in the back court. I'm then about 20 pounds heavier than people my height should be. So I pushed him away, somewhat aggressively. I said, 'C'mon. I'm old enough to be your dad.'" The young man looked the older man straight in the eye: "Then get off the court."

"After that day on the basketball court, I mellowed. I realized I don't have to prove myself in physical contests anymore. I don't see that as a negative at all." Indeed, this freed Alhadeff to try other forms of expression he had never entertained before: art, music, gardening, gourmet cooking. "And they're all a lot easier on the knees!"

The real winners among men in middle life do make this shift. Nearly all have developed passions or hobbies that happily occupy and challenge them outside their workaday routines. Such occupations are crucial in offsetting the disenchantment with their profession that polls show is now felt by large numbers of doctors, or the boredom of the accountant defending yet another tax audit of a rich client, or the weariness of the dentist who cannot expect to be wildly stimulated by drilling his billionth bicuspid.

THE SERENE SIXTIES

The 60s have changed just as dramatically as the earlier stages of middle life. What with beta blockers and hip replacements, you're as likely to run into a man of 65 rollerblading in the park as to see him biking with his youngest child, enjoying the adolescent boy in himself as well as the recycled father. Only 10 percent of Americans 65 and over have a chronic health problem that restricts them from carrying on a major physical activity.

Clearly the vast majority of American women and men now in their 60s have reached the stage where maximum freedom coexists with a minimum of physical limitations. And another passage looms: the one from mastery to integrity. Experts in gerontology make a clear distinction between passive aging and successful aging. To engage in successful aging is actually a career choice—a conscious commitment to continuing self-education and the development of a whole set of strategies.

Resilience is probably the most important protection one can have entering the Age of Integrity. An impressive study of the sources of well-being in men at 65 found that the harbinger of emotional health was not a stable childhood or a highflying career. Rather, it was much more important to have developed an ability to handle life's accidents and conflicts without passivity, blaming or bitterness. "It's having the capacity to hold a conflict or impulse in consciousness without acting on it," concludes George Vaillent, a psychiatrist now at Harvard Medical School, who has been scrutinizing—in the Grant Study—the same 173 Harvard men at five-year intervals since they graduated in the early 1940s.

A related finding in the Grant Study: Time does heal. The research shows that even the most traumatic events in childhood had virtually no effect on the well-being of these men by their mid-60s, although severe depression earlier in life did predispose them to continuing problems. Traits that turned out to contribute to happiness in the golden years were not the same ones that had influenced people back in their college days: spontaneity, creative flair and easy sociability. Instead the traits important to smooth functioning as we get older are being dependable, well organized and pragmatic.

Men from the ages of 45 to 64 who live with wives are twice as likely to live 10 years longer than their unmarried counterparts.

The major predictable passage in this period for most people is retirement, though many consider part-time work to help pay for their longer lives and perhaps to handle other family cares like aged parents or the needs of grandchildren. Forty-one percent of retirees surveyed in New York City in 1993 said the adjustment to retirement was difficult. The younger the retiree, the harder the transition. And the higher the status one's work conferred, the steeper the slide to anonymity.

The comfort of mature love is the single most important determinant of older men's outlook on life. Continued excitement about life is the other factor in high well-being for men at this stage. My research with members of the Harvard Business School class of 1949 shows that those who enjoy the highest well-being had reached out for new adventures in half a dozen new directions *before* retiring. They see semi- or full retirement as an enticing opportunity to add richness to their lives.

Grandparenthood can jump-start the transition to the Age of Integrity. For women or men who had to learn, painfully, in First Adulthood how to compartmentalize their nurturing selves and achieving selves, grandparenthood is a particularly welcome second chance to bring all the parts of their lives into harmony.

THE SAGE SEVENTIES

Those who thrive into their 70s and beyond "live very much in the present, but they always have plans for the future," argues Cecelia Hurwich in her doctoral thesis at the Center for Psychological Studies in Albany, Calif. The seventysomethings Hurwich studied had mastered the art of "letting go" of their egos gracefully, so they could focus their attention on a few fine-tuned priorities. These zestful women were not in unusually good physical shape, but believing they still had living to do, they concentrated on what they could do rather than on what they had lost. Every one acknowledged the need for some form of physical intimacy. They found love through sharing a variety of pleasures: music, gardening, hiking, traveling. Several spoke enthusiastically of active and satisfying sex lives.

After that life stage, the most successful octogenarians I have come across seem to share a quality of directness. Robust and unaffected, often hilariously uninhibited in expressing what they really think, they are liable to live with a partner rather than get married or to pick up an old sweetheart and marry despite their kids' disapproval. They have nothing left to lose.

The Age of Integrity is primarily a stage of spiritual growth. Instead of focusing on time running out, we should make it a daily exercise to mark the moment. The present never ages. And instead of trying to maximize our control over our environment, a goal that was perfectly appropriate to the earlier Age of Mastery, now we must cultivate greater appreciation and acceptance of that which we cannot control. Some of the losses of Second Adulthood are inconsolable losses. To accept them without bitterness usually requires making a greater effort to discern the highest spiritual truths that shape the changes and losses of the last passage of life.

Is it normal aging—or Alzheimer's?

Forgetfulness usually doesn't signal senility—and there are ways to bolster a failing memory.

You draw a blank trying to recall an acquaintance's name. You can't recall where you set down the television remote. You misplace your keys—again. Could this be the start of Alzheimer's?

Last November, former President Ronald Reagan's disclosure that he was suffering from Alzheimer's drew national attention to this devastating disease. Then, in May, a large study of elderly people in East Boston, Mass., suggested that Alzheimer's is more common than previously believed, striking nearly one in five people who live to age 80. Of course, that also means that four out of five people who reach the age of 80 do *not* have Alzheimer's disease. At age 70, the researchers figured, only 1 in 20 people will have the disease.

So while memory lapses do tend to become more common with age, they're usually not a sign of Alzheimer's disease. In fact, worrying about whether you're "going senile" is itself a good sign that you're not (see box, Alzheimer's: Tarnishing the Golden Years). In some cases, severe memory loss may be due to an underlying condition that can be remedied. Most of the time, however, occasional forgetfulness is nothing to worry about. And there are a variety of simple strategies that anyone can use to bolster a weak memory.

The aging brain

The overall mental decline that accompanies aging is not as dramatic as many people think. After all, young people forget names and misplace things, too; they just don't suspect Alzheimer's when they do. Forgetfulness in a 30-year-old is considered "spacey," not "senile."

While the average 80-year-old is not as quick-minded as a 30-year-old, the differences are not great. "An elderly person might be able to press a lever in response to a signal just as fast as a younger person can," explains Paul Coleman, Ph.D., director of the Alzheimer's Center at the University of Rochester. "But if the test involves pressing one lever when a *green* light goes on and another lever when a *red* light goes on, an elderly person will respond at a slightly more sluggish pace."

As a practical matter, an older person's experience or perceptiveness can offset that touch of mental sluggishness. In one study, for instance, older typists typed just as fast as younger typists, despite slower reaction times. Puzzled, the researchers investigated and found that the seniors were compensating for their handicap by taking in more words with each glance at the written page.

Age-related memory deficits seem to involve a diminished ability to store *new* information. The ability to retrieve old information tends to remain intact, as anyone knows who has listened to a grandparent recount days of old. In recent studies, for example, scientists from the National Institute on Aging and the National Institute of Mental Health found that older people (aged 64 to 76) had a harder time memorizing new faces than did younger people (aged 23 to 27). Brain scans revealed less activity in the hippocampal region—an area thought to be important in memory storage—among the older volunteers. However, they were just as good as their younger counterparts on perception tests that involved matching identical faces.

Part of the reason that older people tend to do worse than younger people on memory tests may also be that they're tested at the wrong time of day. Duke University researchers have found that older people perform better on tests given in the morning than in the afternoon. So the age-related declines in mental acuity seen in some studies may have been exaggerated.

All told, a debilitating decline in mental powers just doesn't seem to be an inevitable consequence of aging. Ordinarily, the changes that do occur cause

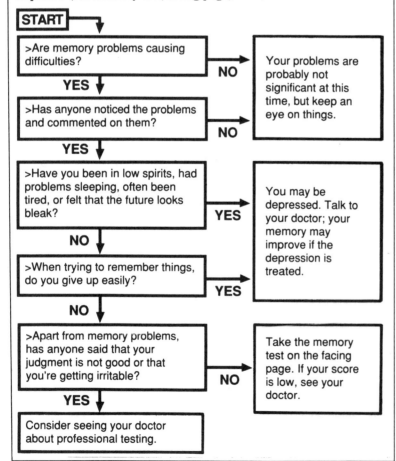

Is poor memory a problem?

Follow the flowchart below to see if a perceived memory problem is really anything to be concerned about. Medical evaluation may be in order if depression appears to be a factor or if memory is seriously impaired (see memory test, facing page).

24. Is It Normal Aging?

only minor problems, if any. When problems with memory or learning skills are severe, they may be the result of an underlying condition other than Alzheimer's. Those include alcohol abuse, depression, severe nutrient deficiencies, sleep disorders, stroke, and thyroid imbalance—all of which can usually be prevented or treated. Mental cloudiness may also be a side effect of medications. Older people, of course, are more likely to be taking medication—often, more than one.

Finally, what appears to be poor memory may reflect poor hearing or failing eyesight, rather than actual memory loss. Those age-related declines can interfere with the ability to receive information—to hear a person's name when introduced, or to see the television remote sitting on the sofa.

Preserve your memories

As we reported in May, regular exercise, a nutritious diet, and other healthy habits may help older people preserve their mental faculties. A study of some 5000 Seattle residents found that those who stayed physically healthy were more likely to remain mentally sharp in their 70s and 80s. One possible explanation is that chronic illnesses such as hypertension, coronary heart disease, and lung disease may reduce the brain's oxygen supply or even cause tiny, unnoticed strokes. Or it may also be that people who feel sick avoid mentally challenging activity. Research suggests that such mental exercise may help preserve the mind, just as physical exercise preserves the body.

It's never too late to become mentally active—learn a language, study a new subject, play chess. Indeed, some studies suggest that becoming mentally active may help older people reverse any decline in memory and other mental abilities. (For more detail, see [Consumer Reports'] May report on healthy habits.)

Clearing the cobwebs

If forgetfulness causes problems in your life, there are ways to give your natural powers an assist, regardless of your age. The most fundamental step is to focus your attention, since memory often fails due to sensory overload—too many things going on at once. Try to limit yourself to one task at a time. Beyond that, studies have found that various mnemonic techniques—tricks for remembering things—do work. Here are some of the most effective techniques for different situations.

To remember names:
- Pause after an introduction and use the person's name. Say "Glad to meet you, Mr. Feltman." Recite the name to yourself. Don't hesitate to ask a new acquaintance to repeat his or her name.
- Try to associate a new name with something distinctive about that person. John Feltman, for example, may have hair like felt. Liz Jones may have eyes like Liz Taylor.
- Before a social gathering, think about who might be there and practice linking names and faces.

A HOME TEST OF FAILING MEMORY

The following test is designed to provide a rough measure of the severity of memory problems. Lower-than-normal scores on this test don't necessarily signal Alzheimer's disease or other forms of dementia. Low scoring can occur for a number of reasons—but medical evaluation may be warranted.

THE PERSON WHO IS GOING TO TAKE THIS TEST SHOULD STOP READING HERE. A close friend or family member can read on to administer the test. Complete all items in turn and add up points at the end. The maximum possible score is 35 points.

20 to 35 points: Normal. No serious memory problem.
15 to 19 points: Borderline. Repeat the test in a few months; if worse, consult a doctor for evaluation.
Below 15 points: Low. Consult a doctor for evaluation.

STOP

1 Examiner: "I'm going to tell you a short story. Remember all you can about it. After the story, I'll ask you to repeat it to me. At the end of this test, I'll ask you to repeat the story again. 'An airplane with 203 people on board left New York for Washington. The experienced pilot became ill but the confident young co-pilot landed the plane safely.'"

Score one point for each of these seven details recalled immediately after story:
- Airplane
- 203 people on board
- From New York
- Washington
- Pilot ill
- Confident co-pilot
- Safe landing

2 Examiner: "I'm going to say three words. I want you to repeat them right after I'm done. I'll ask you the words again in a few minutes. 'CAT, BOOK, PEN.'"

Score one point for each word.

3 Examiner: "I'll now tell you a word and I would like you to spell it backward. The word is 'WORLD.'"

Score one point for each letter in the correct place.

4 Examiner: "Could you now remember the three words that I told you earlier?"

Score one point for each word.

5 Examiner: "Please subtract 7 from 100." (If the answer given is incorrect, go on to question 6. If the answer is correct, ask the subject to continue subtracting 7 from each successive answer until he or she reaches 30 or has given 10 answers. The correct sequence is 93, 86, 79, 72, 65, 58, 51, 44, 37, 30.)

Score one point for each correct answer.

6 Examiner: "Tell me about the story we started with, giving as much detail as you can."

Score one point for each of the seven details listed in question 1. (This is the most important part of the test. Normal recall at this point is four to seven details. But more significant is how many details have been lost since the start of the test; there should be no more than one fewer detail recalled now than had been recalled initially. A person with dementia may recall a total of only one or two details by now.)

Memory test and flowchart courtesy of "Which? Way to Health," a magazine published by Consumers Union's sister organization, Consumers' Association, London, England.

3. PROBLEMS INFLUENCING PERSONAL GROWTH

And don't set out to learn the name of every new face you meet; instead, concentrate on remembering just the ones that might matter most to you.

Summing up

The decline in memory that accompanies aging is usually mild—annoying, not debilitating. Severe memory loss can signal Alzheimer's disease, but it may also be due to medication, depression, or some other underlying condition that can be remedied.

What to do
- If you're concerned about memory loss, follow the flowchart and take the home test to gauge the severity of memory problems and to help determine the need for professional evaluation.
- To shore up a sagging memory, practice the mnemonic techniques for help remembering names, things, actions, and lists and processes.
- Stay physically fit and mentally active to preserve your mind along with your body.

To remember things:
- Set fixed locations for the things you tend to misplace—keys, wallet, television remote. Always return each item to its assigned spot.
- Designate a place near the front door for anything you'll want to take with you. Put each item there as soon as you decide you'll need it.
- Set standard places to put your belongings when you're away from home—such as the front seat of your car, or the left side of your chair in a restaurant.

To remember actions:
- Jot everything down. Record appointments in a pocket calendar. Use adhesive notes, such as *Post-its*. Keep a notebook or even a tape recorder handy.
- Set a watch alarm to help remember appointments. Use a watch or a cooking timer to remind you to follow through on necessary tasks—like turning off the stove when the potatoes are done.
- Do regular chores at the same time every day. Feed the goldfish, for example, right after you've had your breakfast.
- Take medications at the same times every day. Keep pills on your dresser, on the breakfast table, or near anything else you use routinely. To keep track of whether you've taken your pills, fill out a calendar with "P's" for each time you're supposed to take them. Then circle a "P" whenever you do. Or use a multi-compartment pill box, sold in drugstores.
- Focus your attention as you complete tasks that you might wonder about later. Say to yourself, for example, "I'm locking the door now." To help remember you did it *today*, not yesterday, note the weather or what you're wearing as you lock the door.

To remember lists and processes:
- String items together according to their similarities, importance, location, or whatever method fits. For example, if you've got several errands to run, remember them by the route you'll be taking.
- Visualize yourself going through the steps of a new process. Once you've deciphered the instructions on a new VCR, for example, imagine yourself performing all the operations.
- Invent an acronym. For example, FILM (Fred, Irene, Louise, Mark) would help you recall the names of a relative's children. Telephone numbers work especially well as acronyms, using the letters on the push buttons. Even if you can't devise a good word, the attempt itself may fix the items in your mind.

ALZHEIMER'S: TARNISHING THE GOLDEN YEARS

If memory lapses have you worried about Alzheimer's disease, you can probably relax. Fretting and complaining about such lapses and seeking reassurance that they're not a sign of impending senility are normal responses to normal, age-related memory impairment. Experts say that a person with true brain disease is more likely to exhibit signs of denial or to try to hide the deficit.

It takes a battery of physical, neurological, and psychological tests to diagnose Alzheimer's with 80 to 90 percent accuracy. A sure diagnosis can be made only on autopsy. Still, the following signs suggest a serious problem that might indicate Alzheimer's:

- **Severe memory loss.** Anyone can misplace keys. A person with Alzheimer's might not *recognize* keys.
- **Extreme disorientation.** It's easy to get lost when you're away from home; Alzheimer's victims can get lost in their own backyard.
- **Changes in mood or personality.** A person with Alzheimer's may move suddenly from laughter to tears, or may become suspicious for no reason.
- **Speech problems.** An Alzheimer's victim often has trouble finding the right words for things, or mixes up words in a sentence.
- **Loss of reasoning.** This deficit can show up as the inability to generalize from or interpret simple proverbs.
- **Inappropriate behavior.** Anyone might forget to wear gloves in cold weather. Someone with Alzheimer's can forget a coat or even pants.

There's clearly a genetic component to Alzheimer's disease; this summer, researchers reported several breakthroughs in the discovery of genes that appear to play a key role in the development of the disease in some people. Aluminum, long suspected of promoting Alzheimer's, apparently doesn't, judging by reviews of dozens of studies covering every kind of exposure to aluminum. Now zinc has come under suspicion. But there are as yet no solid data to justify avoiding that important nutrient.

Recent studies have hinted that the risk of developing Alzheimer's disease may be lower in women on estrogen replacement therapy and in people who regularly use non-steroidal anti-inflammatory drugs, typically prescribed for arthritis. Those findings have provided researchers with interesting leads to pursue, but the evidence is far too preliminary to suggest preventive regimens.

The only drug specifically approved for Alzheimer's disease is tacrine (*Cognex*), which can improve brain function somewhat in anywhere from 5 to 40 percent of patients, though it won't halt the disease. Several other drugs are being tested. For details on clinical trials, or for more information on Alzheimer's, including a referral to services in your area, call the Alzheimer's Association at 800-272-3900. Or contact your county or state department of health.

The Mystery of Suicide

The road to self-destruction starts with depression and ends in the grave. But who chooses to die and why? Is it stress? Brain chemistry? A despair rotting the soul? The answers are as varied as the weapons.

David Gelman

They inhabit a strange pantheon of the suicidal, prowled by brilliant, troubled ghosts. Some came to grief in the nightfall of acclaimed careers, some in the withering, high-noon glare of public adulation. There are Hemingway and Plath, Monroe and Garland, dead by premeditation or by cumulative acts of self-destruction. There are Presley, Morrison, Hendrix and Joplin, all of them fatally overdosed on drugs and fame. Some are noted almost as much for the manner of their deaths as for the impact of their lives. Last summer a depression-prone White House counsel named Vincent Foster burst into unwelcome national prominence with his final act, a self-inflicted gunshot wound to the head. And last week police in Seattle found the bloodied body of Kurt Cobain, leader of the hugely popular group Nirvana, sprawled in his home. He had apparently killed himself at least a day earlier, the police said, with the shotgun they found resting against him.

Once again, the rock world was shaken by the death of one of its gifted young artists, a tragedy that seems endemic to the pop-music scene. To many it was all too predictable. "The whole thing reeks of cliché: 'Pop icon commits suicide'," said Chris Dorr, a 23-year-old Seattle college student. "It makes you wonder if our icons are genetically programmed to self-destruct in their late 20s."

But Cobain's death hit hardest in Seattle. Thousands of grieving callers bombarded local radio stations, prompting the stations to broadcast crisis-hot-line numbers and organize a candlelight vigil for Sunday. Meanwhile, dozens of mourners gathered outside his house, leaving flowers and carting off mementos.

Suicides always take their own portion of mystery with them, as President Bill Clinton suggested after Foster, his close friend and aide, killed himself. For all the recent advances in the study of behavior, there's still much that doctors don't understand about the persistent phenomenon of people taking their own lives. "We can't talk with the person who committed suicide, so we can only piece together the data," says psychiatrist George Murphy, of Washington University in St. Louis. But researchers are making a determined effort to chart the process, and what they're finding, especially on the cutting edge of brain science, may help bring down the annual toll of suicide deaths.

That toll, of course, takes its full measure on those left behind. Suicides don't simply give up on life: they leave a smear of nullity behind them. Their private act of negation attacks our own often tenuous sense of a meaning in existence. It's a kind of desertion, making everyone feel a little less defended against nothingness. "The suicide does not play the game, does not observe the rules," wrote the novelist Joyce Carol Oates in a 1978 meditation on the subject. "He leaves the party too soon, and leaves the other guests painfully uncomfortable."

In life, Cobain was often in pain. Until his death, he was scarcely known outside the youth culture. But his band, most of whose bitter-edged lyrics he wrote and sang, had become the authentic voice of the 20-plus generation. In the few years since its formation, Nirvana helped establish grunge rock as the sound and style of '90s disillusionment. Its 1991 album, "Nevermind," sold nearly 10 million copies, and one of its songs, "Smells Like Teen Spirit," has become a virtual anthem for the rebellious young.

Besieged: Cobain's life began unraveling not long after his band hit the charts, bringing him attention he couldn't seem to handle. He felt besieged by fans and critics. Between bouts of heroin abuse, he was subject to episodes of depression. Yet friends described him as gentle and caring, not really prone to the violence that surrounds much of the rock culture. Small and almost frail-looking, he wrote music that was oddly melodic despite the abrasiveness of its lyrics. But in the end, by some process still unknown, the sadness of life led him to put a shotgun to his head.

In most instances, suicide seems an enormously selfish act. One of the strongest arguments against it is the harm it can do to others, especially the shattering legacy of guilt and grief it bequeaths to the family of the deceased. Many people reacting to Cobain's death expressed concern about what it might do to his 19-month-old daughter, Frances Bean, the only issue of his troubled marriage to singer Courtney Love.

On the other hand, libertarians and others posit a "right" to suicide, especially for the elderly and the ill. Some argue that such suicides, while tragic, may be "rational"—a proposition that Michigan's Dr. Jack Kevorkian is testing in the courts. "There's an honest debate going on, especially on the front of physician-assisted suicides," says clinical psychologist David Jobes, of Catholic University in Washington, D.C. "Should we continue to uphold the principle that suicide is never acceptable? That's the hottest evolving area in the field."

Whatever the ethics of suicide, researchers are digging closer to its roots. The 19th-century French founder of sociology, Emile Durkheim, thought the source lay in the ups and downs of

3. PROBLEMS INFLUENCING PERSONAL GROWTH

society itself. Modern researchers put more emphasis on genes and neurotransmitters. Nor do all agree with assertions that the primary cause is "life stress." Says Dr. David Clark, director of the Center for Suicide Research and Prevention at Chicago's Rush-Presbyterian-St. Luke's Medical Center: "That's the lay public assumption and that's what drives a lot of suicide-prevention work. And it simply doesn't hold water."

Researchers know, says Clark, that there's as much suicide among the rich as there is among the poor and the middle class. They cite a wide range of potential suicide triggers, from loss of employment or loved ones to aging and physical impairment. But, in almost all cases, they agree there is an underlying psychiatric illness—primarily depression, followed by alcoholism and substance abuse. Clinically depressed people are at a 50 percent greater risk of killing themselves. But the doctors can't agree on whether suicidal depression itself is a state of mind or a result of chemical deficiency.

The good news, if there can be any about suicide, is that it's a relatively rare event: 99.9 percent of Americans don't kill themselves; for better or worse, they stick to the rules—the unspoken "covenant" we all have with each other to affirm life even, perhaps, when there's little left to affirm. The figures tend to climb and fall in waves, but they've remained stable in this country since the end of World War II: at the latest count, around 30,000 people took their own lives in 1991. Gender differences have remained fairly steady as well. Females, by around 3 to 1, attempt suicide more often than males, but males, partly because they employ more violent means, are four times more likely to die. It's estimated there are 20 persons who try suicide for every person who tries successfully.

Violence and despair: The rate for teenagers, after climbing steeply for two decades, began leveling off in the mid-1970s—although it's still not dropping as experts had hoped. The only groups going against the grain are black males and the elderly, especially white men over 65—many of them perhaps victims of the loss of status and income incurred with retirement. The increase among blacks, some demographers guess, might be because suicide is part of the continuum of violence and despair that surrounds many of them. The old are getting older and healthier; their suicide rate dropped through much of the century after 1933. Yet since about 1980, the rate has begun climbing to higher levels. Yeates Conwell, a geriatric psychiatrist at the University of Rochester, conjectures that as they live longer, people are also growing frailer, more isolated, and harder to find and rescue. The suicide rate for the elderly is higher all over the world than it is for teenagers and young adults, says Conwell. "But it is in the U.S. that we find more elderly men committing suicide."

No profile of likely suicides has emerged. However, there are some typical signs to watch for. According to Clark, for instance, in about two thirds of cases there is usually some form of suicidal communication before the actual attempt. Edwin Shneidman, emeritus professor of thanatology at UCLA, who founded the American Association of Suicidology, was also the leading developer of the "psychological autopsy," aimed, among other things, at finding such patterns. Reviewing several years' worth of postmortems, Shneidman and his colleagues at UCLA found that around 90 percent of the suicides left clear behavioral and verbal clues, such as giving away possessions.

Shneidman, although one of the pioneers in the field, has also become one of its mavericks. He objects, for instance, to the emphasis that mainstream suicide researchers place on psychiatric illness, preferring, he says, the Oxford English Dictionary to psychiatry's diagnostic manual. No one dies of depression, he says. "It's not a tenable entry on the death certificate."

As with much of psychiatry these days, the real cutting edge of suicide research is in biochemistry. In the past few years there have been some exciting advances in studies of serotonin, the ubiquitous neurotransmitter that modulates the action of other brain chemicals. A variety of violent, impulsive behaviors have been associated with low levels of serotonin. And Dr. Frederick Goodwin, head of the National Institute of Mental Health, reports that 22 of 22 autopsy studies of brains and body fluid have also connected low levels of the chemical with suicide. Since the newer antidepressant medications, like Prozac and Zoloft, are aimed specifically at boosting serotonin, Goodwin says, doctors may eventually have a selective way to treat depressions associated with suicidal behavior.

Greater risk: Lately, researchers studying particular types of serotonin-related suicide have discovered they tend to be the more serious attempts—those characterized by careful planning and greater medical damage. According to psychiatrist J. John Mann, head of the NIMH research center at the University of Pittsburgh School of Medicine, studies in Sweden of hospitalized depressives with low serotonin levels found that about 20 percent committed suicide within the year. In another group with normal levels, between 1 and 2 percent killed themselves. "That's a tenfold greater risk," says Mann. It remains unclear why some people have low serotonin levels. Mann believes the reasons could be genetic, developmental or environmental. Not surprisingly, he notes, men tend to have lower levels than women. That may be one of the reasons why two or three men complete suicides

Suicide Weapon

% OF TOTAL NUMBER OF SUICIDES IN U.S. IN 1990

Firearms	61.0
Hanging & Strangulation	14.5
Gas Poisoning	7.5
Other Poisoning	10.0
Other	7.0

SOURCE: BUREAU OF THE CENSUS

Suicide by Race

RATES PER 100,000 IN 1970

White Male	18.0
Black Male	8.0
White Female	7.1
Black Female	2.6

DEATH RATES IN 1980

White Male	19.9
Black Male	10.3
White Female	5.9
Black Female	2.2

DEATH RATES IN 1990

White Male	22.0
Black Male	12.0
White Female	5.3
Black Female	2.3

SOURCE: BUREAU OF THE CENSUS

compared with women. We don't know if it has any relationship to [unsuccessful] attempts."

What researchers do know, says Mann, is that a person's serotonin level reveals "some sort of vulnerability" to suicide. "This is the biggest leap we've made in terms of identifying people at high risk, as well as offering meaningful intervention." The serotonin connection points the way not only to a potential screening technique, but to treatment. By raising serotonin levels, as the newer antidepressants do, researchers believe they can raise the threshold for acting on suicidal impulses. "It's similar to the way we're treating epilepsy today, by raising the threshold at which seizures occur," says Mann. "In the short term, our hypothesis is that antidepressants may reduce your chances of acting on suicidal thoughts. We believe the antisuicidal effects occur before the antidepressant effects kick in."

But some treatment may actually increase the risk of suicide. "When a person is profoundly depressed," says Goodwin, "what protects them is, they can't figure out how to kill themselves. Suicide requires energy, and they don't have it." With treatment, the first thing that comes back is energy and functional capacity. "When they become activated and are still depressed, that is a very dangerous period," he says, "so drugs have to be carefully monitored."

While science tries to piece together the suicide puzzle, other forces seem determined to muddle it. Goodwin is irked by such opportunistic books as the best-selling "Final Exit," a kind of how-to manual for would-be suicides, although the way the book was snatched up suggests many people saw no reason to shun such advice. He thinks, also, that the attention given to Kevorkian's suicide machine "trivializes" suicide and ignores the fact that in Western culture it is not looked on as a normal practice. Rather, he says, "people go to enormous lengths to stay alive, even under the worst possible conditions."

On the whole, we *are* life-affirming, but it's an affirmation that often needs boostering. "Every one . . . is bound to preserve himself," wrote the 17th-century English philosopher John Locke, "and not to quit his station willfully." Locke was talking about an obligation to the Creator, but it's also a duty we owe to ourselves, our families and the society we live in.

With MARY HAGER *and* PAT WINGERT *in Washington,* VICKI QUADE *in Chicago,* TESSA NAMUTH *in New York and* JEANNE GORDON *in Los Angeles*

Relating to Others

People in groups can be seen everywhere: couples in love, parents with their children, teachers and students, gatherings of friends, church groups, theatergoers. People have much influence on one another when they congregate in groups.

Groups spend a great deal of time communicating with members and nonmembers. The communication can be intentional and forceful, such as when protesters demonstrate against a totalitarian regime in a far-off land. Or communication can be more subtle, for example, when fraternity brothers reject a prospective brother who refuses to wear the symbols of pledging.

In some groups the reason a leader emerges is clear—perhaps the most skilled individual in the group is elected leader by the group members. In other groups, for example, during a spontaneous nightclub fire, the qualities of the rapidly emerging, perhaps self-appointed, leader are less apparent. Nonetheless, the followers flee unquestioningly in the leader's direction. Even in dating couples, one person may seem to lead or be dominant over the other.

Some groups, such as corporations, issue formal rules in writing; discipline for rule breaking is also formalized. Other groups, families or trios of friends, for example, possess fewer, less formal rules and disciplinary codes, but their rules are still quickly learned by and are important to all unit members.

Some groups are large but seek more members, such as nationalized labor unions. Other groups seek to keep their groups small and somewhat exclusive, such as teenage cliques. Groups exist that are almost completely adversarial with other groups. Conflict between youth gangs is receiving much media attention today. Other groups pride themselves on their ability to remain cooperative, such as neighbors who band together in a community crime watch.

Psychologists are so convinced that interpersonal relationships are important to the human experience that they have intensively studied them. There is ample evidence that contact with other people is a necessary part of human existence. Research has shown that most individuals do not like being isolated from other people. In fact, in laboratory experiments where subjects experience total isolation for extended periods, subjects begin to hallucinate the presence of others. In prisons, solitary confinement is often used as a form of punishment because it is so aversive. Other research has shown that people who must wait under stressful circumstances prefer to wait with others, even if the others are total strangers, rather than wait alone. This unit examines intimate groups, groups of friends, dating partners, and married couples. The next unit examines the effects of larger groups, in fact, of society at large.

First, a new and hot issue is examined: emotional intelligence or EQ. Daniel Goleman's pioneering book on this topic suggests that emotional intelligence is more important to our success in life than any other aspect of our being. He claims that EQ determines how many friends we have, how successful we are in school and on the job, and other important parts of our interpersonal relationships. Here, some of the myths that have grown up around his concept of EQ are dispelled.

The second article in this unit pertains to friendships. In "The Enduring Power of Friendship," Susan Davis probes adult friendships, which are far less studied than childhood friendships. She also queries why adult friendships end. Interestingly, they do not end catastrophically, as do some adult intimate relationships. Most adult friendships fizzle out when life circumstances change.

Next is a companion piece. Some individuals have difficulty establishing friendships because they are shy. There is now an abundance of research on this topic. The results of this research are shared with the reader in "Are You Shy?" There are a variety of different causes, as you will see.

Another reason friendships end or people do not become friends in the first place is that some individuals are hotheads. That is, they are often hostile to others around them. In fact, Edward Dolnick suggests that chronic hostility toward others is actually detrimental to our health in that it causes heart attacks.

Should we find ourselves in a position where we have blemished our friendship, the next selection explores how and when to apologize. A well-placed apology can go a long way toward mending broken friendships. This is the topic of "Go Ahead, Say You're Sorry."

Then we examine very close, romantic relationships. In "The Heart and the Helix," Jeffrey Kluger suggests in a humorous way that there are different love styles. Finding a mate with the same style seems to be what happy relationships are all about. On the other hand, other authors contend that in our society we are too obsessed with love

UNIT 4

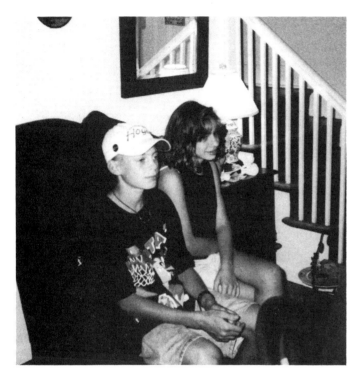

and intimacy. This is the main point of "Back Off!" by Geraldine Piorkowski. When we are so obsessed with close relationships, we simply expect too much of them; hence, many close, romantic relationships do not last in our society.

A close, romantic relationship often turns into a marriage proposal, but today nearly half of all marriages end in divorce. "Preventing Failure in Intimate Relationships" examines reasons for divorce. Methods for keeping close, romantic relationships solid are also highlighted.

Sometimes love and marriage become destructive, as in domestic violence where spouses batter one another. "Patterns of Abuse" discloses who is abused, who the abuser is, why abuse occurs, and other important matters.

We move finally to a special close relationship, the one between brothers and sisters. In "The Secret World of Siblings," Erica Goode explores how siblings interact with each other and how in modern society sibling relations are becoming more important.

Looking Ahead: Challenge Questions

What is emotional intelligence? How does it develop; how can we tell if we possess it? What are some of the myths about emotional intelligence?

What are friends for? Why do friendships last? Are special types of friendships, say between homosexuals, better or different from typical friendships? What methods are there for saving a failing friendship? How can a wounded friendship be mended? When would a friendship not be worth salvaging?

How can you tell if you are shy? What are the causes of shyness? How do others perceive shy individuals? What can a shy person do to overcome shyness?

Why is hostility toward others so destructive? Is it destructive only to the opponent? Describe the hostile personality. How can hostility kill us? How can we overcome hostility and cynicism against others?

What is an apology? What are the elements of a sincere apology, one that would have the effect of reestablishing trust and friendship?

Love has emotional components, but what physical components does love have? Why do people fall in love? Discuss whether or not there are sex differences in loving relationships, and whether or not it is important to find someone with the same love style.

Discuss whether or not love is found only in our society. How do individuals in other societies express love to each other? Discuss why you agree or disagree that our society is obsessed with intimacy and love.

What is it that happy couples do right? Do you agree or disagree that true love makes couples happy? Why? Do you agree or disagree that it is possible to find happiness by oneself (without an intimate partner)? Why? What are the benefits of an intimate relationship? What are the disadvantages? What do couples need to do to develop positive, friendly relationships? If a couple you know were contemplating marriage, what advice would you give them? What are some of the myths surrounding divorce? Why do people divorce?

What causes domestic violence? Is any type of person or social class immune to it? Explain. Who are the abusers? Who are the victims? What can be done to intervene in abusive relationships?

Do you think adult siblings or childhood siblings bicker more? Explain. What causes friction between siblings? How can sibling rivalries be better managed? What positive consequences are there to sibling relationships? How has the role of siblings changed?

The unit examines close relationships including siblings, friends, and lovers. For each, which factors make the relationship better, and which make it worse? Explain whether or not the same social processes are operative in all close relationships. What interpersonal relationships and processes besides the ones discussed in this anthology would be important to study?

The EQ Factor

New brain research suggests that emotions, not IQ, may be the true measure of human intelligence

NANCY GIBBS

IT TURNS OUT THAT A SCIENTIST can see the future by watching four-year-olds interact with a marshmallow. The researcher invites the children, one by one, into a plain room and begins the gentle torment. You can have this marshmallow right now, he says. But if you wait while I run an errand, you can have two marshmallows when I get back. And then he leaves.

Some children grab for the treat the minute he's out the door. Some last a few minutes before they give in. But others are determined to wait. They cover their eyes; they put their heads down; they sing to themselves; they try to play games or even fall asleep. When the researcher returns, he gives these children their hard-earned marshmallows. And then, science waits for them to grow up.

By the time the children reach high school, something remarkable has happened. A survey of the children's parents and teachers found that those who as four-year-olds had the fortitude to hold out for the second marshmallow generally grew up to be better adjusted, more popular, adventurous, confident and dependable teenagers. The children who gave in to temptation early on were more likely to be lonely, easily frustrated and stubborn. They buckled under stress and shied away from challenges. And when some of the students in the two groups took the Scholastic Aptitude Test, the kids who had held out longer scored an average of 210 points higher.

When we think of brilliance we see Einstein, deep-eyed, woolly haired, a thinking machine with skin and mismatched socks. High achievers, we imagine, were wired for greatness from birth. But then you have to wonder why, over time, natural talent seems to ignite in some people and dim in others. This is where the marshmallows come in. It seems that the ability to delay gratification is a master skill, a triumph of the reasoning brain over the impulsive one. It is a sign, in short, of emotional intelligence. And it doesn't show up on an IQ test.

For most of this century, scientists have worshipped the hardware of the brain and the software of the mind; the messy powers of the heart were left to the poets. But cognitive theory could simply not explain the questions we wonder about most: why some people just seem to have a gift for living well; why the smartest kid in the class will probably not end up the richest; why we like some people virtually on sight and distrust others; why some people remain buoyant in the face of troubles that would sink a less resilient soul. What qualities of the mind or spirit, in short, determine who succeeds?

The phrase "emotional intelligence" was coined by Yale psychologist Peter Salovey and the University of New Hampshire's John Mayer five years ago to describe qualities like understanding one's own feelings, empathy for the feelings of others and "the regulation of emotion in a way that enhances living." Their notion is about to bound into the national conversation, handily shortened to EQ, thanks to a new book, *Emotional Intelligence* (Bantam; $23.95) by Daniel Goleman. Goleman, a Harvard psychology Ph.D. and a New York *Times* science writer with a gift for making even the chewiest scientific theories digestible to lay readers, has brought together a decade's worth of behavioral research into how the mind processes feelings. His goal, he announces on the cover, is to redefine what it means to be smart. His thesis: when it comes to predicting people's success, brainpower as measured by IQ and standardized achievement tests may actually matter less than the qualities of mind once thought of as "character" before the word began to sound quaint.

At first glance, there would seem to be little that's new here to any close reader of fortune cookies. There may be no less original idea than the notion that our hearts hold dominion over our heads. "I was so angry," we say, "I couldn't think straight." Neither is it surprising that "people skills" are useful, which amounts to saying, it's good to be nice. "It's so true it's trivial," says Dr. Paul McHugh, director of psychiatry at Johns Hopkins University School of Medicine. But if it were that simple, the book would not be quite so interesting or its implications so controversial.

This is no abstract investigation. Goleman is looking for antidotes to restore "civility to our streets and caring to our communal life." He sees practical applications everywhere for how companies should decide whom to hire, how couples can increase the odds that their marriages will last, how parents should raise their children and how schools should teach them. When street gangs substitute for families and schoolyard insults end in stabbings, when more than half of marriages end in divorce, when the majority of the children murdered in this country are killed by parents and stepparents, many of whom say they were trying to discipline the child for behavior like blocking the TV or crying too much, it suggests a demand for remedial emotional education. While children are still young, Goleman argues, there is a "neurological window of opportunity" since the brain's prefrontal circuitry, which regulates how we act on what we feel, probably does not mature until mid-adolescence.

And it is here the arguments will break out. Goleman's highly popularized conclusions, says McHugh, "will chill any veteran scholar of psychotherapy and any neuroscientist who worries about how his research may come to be applied." While many researchers in this relatively new field are glad to see emotional issues finally taken seriously, they fear that a notion as handy as EQ invites misuse. Goleman admits the danger of suggesting that you can assign a numerical yardstick to a person's character as well as his intellect; Goleman never even uses the phrase EQ in his book. But he (begrudgingly) approved an "unscientific" EQ test in *USA Today* with choices like "I am aware of even subtle feelings as I have them," and "I can sense the pulse of a group or relationship and state unspoken feelings."

"You don't want to take an average of your emotional skill," argues Harvard psychology professor Jerome Kagan, a pioneer in child-development research. "That's what's wrong with the concept of intelligence for mental skills too. Some people handle anger well but can't handle fear. Some people can't take joy. So each emotion has to be viewed differently."

EQ is not the opposite of IQ. Some people are blessed with a lot of both, some with little of either. What researchers have been trying to understand is how they complement each other; how one's ability to handle stress, for instance, affects the ability to concentrate and put intelligence to use. Among the ingredients for success, researchers now generally agree that IQ counts for about 20%; the rest depends on everything from class to luck to the neural pathways that have developed in the brain over millions of years of human evolution.

It is actually the neuroscientists and evolutionists who do the best job of explaining the reasons behind the most unreasonable behavior. In the past decade or so, scientists have learned enough about the brain to make judgments about where emotion comes from and why we need it. Primitive emotional responses held the keys to survival: fear drives the blood into the large muscles, making it easier to run; surprise triggers the eyebrows to rise, allowing the eyes to widen their view and gather more information about an unexpected event. Disgust wrinkles up the face and closes the nostrils to keep out foul smells.

Emotional life grows out of an area of the brain called the limbic system, specifically the amygdala, whence come delight and disgust and fear and anger. Millions of years ago, the neocortex was added on, enabling humans to plan, learn and remember. Lust grows from the limbic system; love, from the neocortex. Animals like reptiles that have no neocortex cannot experience anything like maternal love; this is why baby snakes have to hide to avoid being eaten by their parents. Humans, with their capacity for love, will protect their offspring, allowing the brains of the young time to develop. The more connections between limbic system and the neocortex, the more emotional responses are possible.

It was scientists like Joseph LeDoux of New York University who uncovered these cerebral pathways. LeDoux's parents owned a meat market. As a boy in Louisiana, he first learned about his future specialty by cutting up cows' brains for sweetbreads. "I found them the most interesting part of the cow's anatomy," he recalls. "They were visually pleasing—lots of folds, convolutions and patterns. The cerebellum was more interesting to look at than steak." The butchers' son became a neuroscientist, and it was he who discovered the short circuit in the brain that lets emotions drive action before the intellect gets a chance to intervene.

A hiker on a mountain path, for example, sees a long, curved shape in the grass out of the corner of his eye. He leaps out of the way before he realizes it is only a stick that looks like a snake. Then he calms down; his cortex gets the message a few milliseconds after his amygdala and "regulates" its primitive response.

Without these emotional reflexes, rarely conscious but often terribly powerful, we would scarcely be able to function. "Most decisions we make have a vast number of possible outcomes, and any attempt to analyze all of them would never end," says University of Iowa neurologist Antonio Damasio, author of *Descartes' Error: Emotion, Reason and the Human Brain*. "I'd ask you to lunch tomorrow, and when the appointed time arrived, you'd still be thinking about whether you should come." What tips the balance, Damasio contends, is our unconscious assigning of emotional values to some of those choices. Whether we experience a somatic response—a gut feeling of dread or a giddy sense of elation—emotions are helping to limit the field in any choice we have to make. If the prospect of lunch with a neurologist is unnerving or distasteful, Damasio suggests, the invitee will conveniently remember a previous engagement.

When Damasio worked with patients in whom the connection between emotional brain and neocortex had been severed because of damage to the brain, he discovered how central that hidden pathway is to how we live our lives. People who had lost that linkage were just as smart and quick to reason, but their lives often fell apart nonetheless. They could not make decisions because they didn't know how they felt about their choices. They couldn't react to warnings or anger in other people. If they made a mistake, like a bad investment, they felt no regret or shame and so were bound to repeat it.

If there is a cornerstone to emotional intelligence on which most other emotional skills depend, it is a sense of self-awareness, of being smart about what we feel. A person whose day starts badly at home may be grouchy all day at work without quite knowing why. Once an emotional response comes into awareness—or, physiologically, is processed through the neocortex—the chances of handling it appropriately improve. Scientists refer to "metamood," the ability to pull back and recognize that "what I'm feeling is anger," or sorrow, or shame.

Metamood is a difficult skill because emotions so often appear in disguise. A person in mourning may know he is sad, but he may not recognize that he is also angry at the person for dying—because this seems somehow inappropriate. A parent who yells at the child who ran into the street is expressing anger at disobedience, but the degree of anger may owe more to the fear the parent feels at what could have happened.

In Goleman's analysis, self-awareness is perhaps the most crucial ability because it allows us to exercise some self-control. The idea is not to repress feeling (the reaction that has made psychoanalysts rich) but rather to do what Aristotle considered the hard work of the will. "Anyone can become angry—that is easy," he wrote in the *Nicomachean Ethics*. "But to be angry with the right person, to the right degree, at the right time, for the right purpose, and in the right way—that is not easy."

Some impulses seem to be easier to control than others. Anger, not surprisingly, is one of the hardest, perhaps because of its evolutionary value in priming people to action. Researchers believe anger usually arises out of a sense of being trespassed against—the belief that one is being robbed

4. RELATING TO OTHERS

of what is rightfully his. The body's first response is a surge of energy, the release of a cascade of neurotransmitters called catecholamines. If a person is already aroused or under stress, the threshold for release is lower, which helps explain why people's tempers shorten during a hard day.

Scientists are not only discovering where anger comes from; they are also exposing myths about how best to handle it. Popular wisdom argues for "letting it all hang out" and having a good cathartic rant. But Goleman cites studies showing that dwelling on anger actually increases its power; the body needs a chance to process the adrenaline through exercise, relaxation techniques, a well-timed intervention or even the old admonition to count to 10.

Anxiety serves a similar useful purpose, so long as it doesn't spin out of control. Worrying is a rehearsal for danger; the act of fretting focuses the mind on a problem so it can search efficiently for solutions. The danger comes when worrying blocks thinking, becoming an end in itself or a path to resignation instead of perseverance. Overworrying about failing increases the likelihood of failure; a salesman so concerned about his falling sales that he can't bring himself to pick up the phone guarantees that his sales will fall even further.

But why are some people better able to "snap out of it" and get on with the task at hand? Again, given sufficient self-awareness, people develop coping mechanisms. Sadness and discouragement, for instance, are "low arousal" states, and the dispirited salesman who goes out for a run is triggering a high arousal state that is incompatible with staying blue. Relaxation works better for high-energy moods like anger or anxiety. Either way, the idea is to shift to a state of arousal that breaks the destructive cycle of the dominant mood.

The idea of being able to predict which salesmen are most likely to prosper was not an abstraction for Metropolitan Life, which in the mid-'80s was hiring 5,000 salespeople a year and training them at a cost of more than $30,000 each. Half quit the first year, and four out of five within four years. The reason: selling life insurance involves having the door slammed in your face over and over again. Was it possible to identify which people would be better at handling frustration and take each refusal as a challenge rather than a setback?

The head of the company approached psychologist Martin Seligman at the University of Pennsylvania and invited him to test some of his theories about the importance of optimism in people's success. When optimists fail, he has found, they attribute the failure to something they can change, not some innate weakness that they are helpless to overcome. And that confidence in their power to effect change is self-reinforcing. Seligman tracked 15,000 new workers who had taken two tests. One was the company's regular screening exam, the other Seligman's test measuring their levels of optimism.

One Way to Test Your EQ

UNLIKE IQ, WHICH IS GAUGED BY THE FAMOUS STANFORD-Binet tests, EQ does not lend itself to any single numerical measure. Nor should it, say experts. Emotional intelligence is by definition a complex, multifaceted quality representing such intangibles as self-awareness, empathy, persistence and social deftness.

Some aspects of emotional intelligence, however, can be quantified. Optimism, for example, is a handy measure of a person's self-worth. According to Martin Seligman, a University of Pennsylvania psychologist, how people respond to setbacks—optimistically or pessimistically—is a fairly accurate indicator of how well they will succeed in school, in sports and in certain kinds of work. To test his theory, Seligman devised a questionnaire to screen insurance salesmen at MetLife.

In Seligman's test, job applicants were asked to imagine a hypothetical event and then choose the response (A or B) that most closely resembled their own. Some samples from his questionnaire:

You forget your spouse's (boyfriend's/girlfriend's) birthday.
A. I'm not good at remembering birthdays.
B. I was preoccupied with other things.

You owe the library $10 for an overdue book.
A. When I am really involved in what I am reading, I often forget when it's due.
B. I was so involved in writing the report, I forgot to return the book.

You lose your temper with a friend.
A. He or she is always nagging me.
B. He or she was in a hostile mood.

You are penalized for returning your income-tax forms late.
A. I always put off doing my taxes.
B. I was lazy about getting my taxes done this year.

You've been feeling run-down.
A. I never get a chance to relax.
B. I was exceptionally busy this week.

A friend says something that hurts your feelings.
A. She always blurts things out without thinking of others.
B. My friend was in a bad mood and took it out on me.

You fall down a great deal while skiing.
A. Skiing is difficult.
B. The trails were icy.

You gain weight over the holidays, and you can't lose it.
A. Diets don't work in the long run.
B. The diet I tried didn't work.

Seligman found that those insurance salesmen who answered with more B's than A's were better able to overcome bad sales days, recovered more easily from rejection and were less likely to quit. People with an optimistic view of life tend to treat obstacles and setbacks as temporary (and therefore surmountable). Pessimists take them personally; what others see as fleeting, localized impediments, they view as pervasive and permanent.

The most dramatic proof of his theory, says Seligman, came at the 1988 Olympic Games in Seoul, South Korea, after U.S. swimmer Matt Biondi turned in two disappointing performances in his first two races. Before the Games, Biondi had been favored to win seven golds—as Mark Spitz had done 16 years earlier. After those first two races, most commentators thought Biondi would be unable to recover from his setback. Not Seligman. He had given some members of the U.S swim team a version of his optimism test before the races; it showed that Biondi possessed an extraordinarily upbeat attitude. Rather than losing heart after turning in a bad time, as others might, Biondi tended to respond by swimming even faster. Sure enough, Biondi bounced right back, winning five gold medals in the next five races.

—*By Alice Park*

Among the new hires was a group who flunked the screening test but scored as "superoptimists" on Seligman's exam. And sure enough, they did the best of all; they outsold the pessimists in the regular group by 21% in the first year and 57% in the second. For years after that, passing Seligman's test was one way to get hired as a MetLife salesperson.

Perhaps the most visible emotional skills, the ones we recognize most readily, are the "people skills" like empathy, graciousness, the ability to read a social situation. Researchers believe that about 90% of emotional communication is nonverbal. Harvard psychologist Robert Rosenthal developed the PONS test (Profile of Nonverbal Sensitivity) to measure people's ability to read emotional cues. He shows subjects a film of a young woman expressing feelings—anger, love, jealousy, gratitude, seduction—edited so that one or another nonverbal cue is blanked out. In some instances the face is visible but not the body, or the woman's eyes are hidden, so that viewers have to judge the feeling by subtle cues. Once again, people with higher PONS scores tend to be more successful in their work and relationships; children who score well are more popular and successful in school, even then their IQs are quite average.

Like other emotional skills, empathy is an innate quality that can be shaped by experience. Infants as young as three months old exhibit empathy when they get upset at the sound of another baby crying. Even very young children learn by imitation; by watching how others act when they see someone in distress, these children acquire a repertoire of sensitive responses. If, on the other hand, the feelings they begin to express are not recognized and reinforced by the adults around them, they not only cease to express those feelings but they also become less able to recognize them in themselves or others.

Empathy too can be seen as a survival skill. Bert Cohler, a University of Chicago psychologist, and Fran Stott, dean of the Erikson Institute for Advanced Study in Child Development in Chicago, have found that children from psychically damaged families frequently become hypervigilant, developing an intense attunement to their parents' moods. One child they studied, Nicholas, had a horrible habit of approaching other kids in his nursery-school class as if he were going to kiss them, then would bite them instead. The scientists went back to study videos of Nicholas at 20 months interacting with his psychotic mother and found that she had responded to his every expression of anger or independence with compulsive kisses. The researchers dubbed them "kisses of death," and their true significance was obvious to Nicholas, who arched his back in horror at her approaching lips—and passed his own rage on to his classmates years later.

Empathy also acts as a buffer to cruelty, and it is a quality conspicuously lacking in child molesters and psychopaths. Goleman cites some chilling research into brutality by Robert Hare, a psychologist at the University of British Columbia. Hare found that psychopaths, when hooked up to electrodes and told they are going to receive a shock, show none of the visceral responses that fear of pain typically triggers: rapid heartbeat, sweating and so on. How could the threat of punishment deter such people from committing crimes?

It is easy to draw the obvious lesson from these test results. How much happier would we be, how much more success-

---

Square Pegs in the Oval Office?

IF A HIGH DEGREE OF EMOTIONAL INTELLIGENCE IS A PREREQUISITE FOR OUTstanding achievement, there ought to be no better place to find it than in the White House. It turns out, however, that not every man who reached the pinnacle of American leadership was a gleaming example of self-awareness, empathy, impulse control and all the other qualities that mark an elevated EQ.

Oliver Wendell Holmes, who knew intelligence when he saw it, judged Franklin Roosevelt "a second-class intellect, but a first-class temperament." Born and educated as an aristocrat, F.D.R. had polio and needed a wheelchair for most of his adult life. Yet, far from becoming a self-pitying wretch, he developed an unbridled optimism that served him and the country well during the Depression and World War II—this despite, or because of, what Princeton professor Fred Greenstein calls Roosevelt's "tendency toward deviousness and duplicity."

Even a first-class temperament, however, is not a sure predictor of a successful presidency. According to Duke University political scientist James David Barber, the most perfect blend of intellect and warmth of personality in a Chief Executive was the brilliant Thomas Jefferson, who "knew the importance of communication and empathy. He never lost the common touch." Richard Ellis, a professor of politics at Oregon's Willamette University who is skeptical of the whole EQ theory, cites two 19th century Presidents who did not fit the mold. "Martin Van Buren was well adjusted, balanced, empathetic and persuasive, but he was not very successful," says Ellis. "Andrew Jackson was less well adjusted, less balanced, less empathetic and was terrible at controlling his own impulses, but he transformed the presidency."

Lyndon Johnson as Senate majority leader was a brilliant practitioner of the art of political persuasion, yet failed utterly to transfer that gift to the White House. In fact, says Princeton's Greenstein, L. B. J. and Richard Nixon would be labeled "worst cases" on any EQ scale of Presidents. Each was touched with political genius, yet each met with disaster. "To some extent," says Greenstein, "this is a function of the extreme aspects of their psyches; they are the political versions of Van Gogh, who does unbelievable paintings and then cuts off his ear."

History professor William Leuchtenburg of the University of North Carolina at Chapel Hill suggests that the 20th century Presidents with perhaps the highest IQs—Wilson, Hoover and Carter—also had the most trouble connecting with their constituents. Woodrow Wilson, he says, "was very high strung [and] arrogant; he was not willing to strike any middle ground. Herbert Hoover was so locked into certain ideas that you could never convince him otherwise. Jimmy Carter is probably the most puzzling of the three. He didn't have a deficiency of temperament; in fact, he was too temperate. There was an excessive rationalization about Carter's approach."

That was never a problem for John Kennedy and Ronald Reagan. Nobody ever accused them of intellectual genius, yet both radiated qualities of leadership with an infectious confidence and openheartedness that endeared them to the nation. Whether President Clinton will be so endeared remains a puzzle. That he is a Rhodes scholar makes him certifiably brainy, but his emotional intelligence is shaky. He obviously has the knack for establishing rapport with people, but he often appears so eager to please that he looks weak. "As for controlling his impulses," says Willamette's Ellis, "Clinton is terrible." —By Jesse Birnbaum.
Reported by James Carney/Washington and Lisa H. Towle/Raleigh

4. RELATING TO OTHERS

ful as individuals and civil as a society, if we were more alert to the importance of emotional intelligence and more adept at teaching it? From kindergartens to business schools to corporations across the country, people are taking seriously the idea that a little more time spent on the "touchy-feely" skills so often derided may in fact pay rich dividends.

In the corporate world, according to personnel executives, IQ gets you hired, but EQ gets you promoted. Goleman likes to tell of a manager at AT&T's Bell Labs, a think tank for brilliant engineers in New Jersey, who was asked to rank his top performers. They weren't the ones with the highest IQs; they were the ones whose E-mail got answered. Those workers who were good collaborators and networkers and popular with colleagues were more likely to get the cooperation they needed to reach their goals than the socially awkward, lone-wolf geniuses.

When David Campbell and others at the Center for Creative Leadership studied "derailed executives," the rising stars who flamed out, the researchers found that these executives failed most often because of "an interpersonal flaw" rather than a technical inability. Interviews with top executives in the U.S. and Europe turned up nine so-called fatal flaws, many of them classic emotional failings, such as "poor working relations," being "authoritarian" or "too ambitious" and having "conflict with upper management."

At the center's executive-leadership seminars across the country, managers come to get emotionally retooled. "This isn't sensitivity training or Sunday-supplement stuff," says Campbell. "One thing they know when they get through is what other people think of them." And the executives have an incentive to listen. Says Karen Boylston, director of the center's team-leadership group: "Customers are telling businesses, 'I don't care if every member of your staff graduated with honors from Harvard, Stanford and Wharton. I will take my business and go where I am understood and treated with respect.'"

Nowhere is the discussion of emotional intelligence more pressing than in schools, where both the stakes and the opportunities seem greatest. Instead of constant crisis intervention, or declarations of war on drug abuse or teen pregnancy or violence, it is time, Goleman argues, for preventive medicine. "Five years ago, teachers didn't want to think about this," says principal Roberta Kirshbaum of P.S. 75 in New York City. "But when kids are getting killed in high school, we have to deal with it." Five years ago, Kirshbaum's school adopted an emotional literacy program, designed to help children learn to manage anger, frustration, loneliness. Since then, fights at lunchtime have decreased from two or three a day to almost none.

Educators can point to all sorts of data to support this new direction. Students who are depressed or angry literally cannot learn. Children who have trouble being accepted by their classmates are 2 to 8 times as likely to drop out. An inability to distinguish distressing feelings or handle frustration has been linked to eating disorders in girls.

Many school administrators are completely rethinking the weight they have been giving to traditional lessons and standardized tests. Peter Relic, president of the National Association of Independent Schools, would like to junk the SAT completely. "Yes, it may cost a heck of a lot more money to assess someone's EQ rather than using a machine-scored test to measure IQ," he says. "But if we don't, then we're saying that a test score is more important to us than who a child is as a human being. That means an immense loss in terms of human potential because we've defined success too narrowly."

This warm embrace by educators has left some scientists in a bind. On one hand, says Yale psychologist Salovey, "I love the idea that we want to teach people a richer understanding of their emotional life, to help them achieve their goals." But, he adds, "what I would oppose is training conformity to social expectations." The danger is that any campaign to hone emotional skills in children will end up teaching that there is a "right" emotional response for any given situation—laugh at parades, cry at funerals, sit still at church. "You can teach self-control," says Dr. Alvin Poussaint, professor of psychiatry at Harvard Medical School. "You can teach that it's better to talk out your anger and not use violence. But is it good emotional intelligence not to challenge authority?"

SOME PSYCHOLOGISTS GO further and challenge the very idea that emotional skills can or should be taught in any kind of formal, classroom way. Goleman's premise that children can be trained to analyze their feelings strikes Johns Hopkins' McHugh as an effort to reinvent the encounter group: "I consider that an abominable idea, an idea we have seen with adults. That failed, and now he wants to try it with children? Good grief!" He cites the description in Goleman's book of an experimental program at the Nueva Learning Center in San Francisco. In one scene, two fifth-grade boys start to argue over the rules of an exercise, and the teacher breaks in to ask them to talk about what they're feeling. "I appreciate the way you're being assertive in talking with Tucker," she says to one student. "You're not attacking." This strikes McHugh as pure folly. "The author is presuming that someone has the key to the right emotions to be taught to children. We don't even know the right emotions to be taught to adults. Do you really think a child of eight or nine really understands the difference between aggressiveness and assertiveness?"

The problem may be that there is an ingredient missing. Emotional skills, like intellectual ones, are morally neutral. Just as a genius could use his intellect either to cure cancer or engineer a deadly virus, someone with great empathic insight could use it to inspire colleagues or exploit them. Without a moral compass to guide people in how to employ their gifts, emotional intelligence can be used for good or evil. Columbia University psychologist Walter Mischel, who invented the marshmallow test and others like it, observes that the knack for delaying gratification that makes a child one marshmallow richer can help him become a better citizen or—just as easily—an even more brilliant criminal.

Given the passionate arguments that are raging over the state of moral instruction in this country, it is no wonder Goleman chose to focus more on neutral emotional skills than on the values that should govern their use. That's another book—and another debate. —*Reported by Sharon E. Epperson and Lawrence Mondi/New York, James L. Graff/Chicago and Lisa H. Towle/Raleigh*

The Enduring Power of Friendship

Susan Davis

Susan Davis is a writer in San Francisco.

A few years ago one of my best friends suddenly stopped returning my calls. There had been some tension between us for about a year. We'd all but stopped seeing each other. Given our long history, I figured we would pick up again soon. But for her, it was time to end the friendship.

It was a hard pill for me to swallow. In the 12 years we'd known each other, Kelly and I had gone through a lot together. We shared a house in Boston, traveled cross-country and talked endlessly of our rural roots, our families and our dreams of the future. We wept when I moved to California for graduate school, but we stayed close through letters, phone calls and visits. "We're best friends forever," Kelly used to say. "We'll grow old together on a porch somewhere."

I always agreed. But when Kelly came to California to start a new life several years after I had, something was out of kilter. I had begun a career and met the man I wanted to marry; she wanted neither a "real" job nor a husband. I wanted to talk about my new feelings. She acted as if I'd betrayed her by even having them.

When Kelly finally stopped speaking to me, I was devastated. We had shared everything. Now my confidante was gone. Worse, she no longer even liked me. I felt unsure and exposed, as if we were schoolgirls on a playground and she were telling stories about me.

Does everyone go through what I went through? As it turns out, many of us do. For years sociologists and psychologists have focused primarily on friendships in childhood and adolescence, because it's during these rich periods that we learn to approach and interact with others. Now they're realizing that the long decades of adulthood are equally vital. With job demands and "downsizing" increasing our mobility and divorce rates still sky high, family ties are strained to their limits. That means adult friendships are perhaps more important than ever. We learn to make friends in our early years, researchers say, but as adults we learn to depend on these essential links.

It isn't always easy. We like to think friendships are warm, casual, fairly simple affairs. In reality they're more complicated. "Friendships involve a good deal of ambiguity and ambivalence," says Dr. William Rawlins, an interpersonal communications expert at Purdue University in West Lafayette, Ind., and author of *Friendship Matters*. Every friendship entails subtle, usually silent negotiations over such fundamental questions as whether we're "just" friends, "good" friends or "best" friends and how generous we'll be with our time. Friction occurs when one friend wants more, gives more or even reveals more than the other.

Unfortunately, guidance on nurturing friendships is sparse. Dr. Diane Prusank, a specialist in interpersonal communications at the University of Hartford (Conn.), looked at scores of articles in eight magazines for women and teenage girls published between 1974 and 1990. She found 125 stories on romantic relationships and families and only nine on friendship. "Our culture is obsessed with romance," says Prusank. "Friendship is secondary; no one thinks it has to be talked about."

4. RELATING TO OTHERS

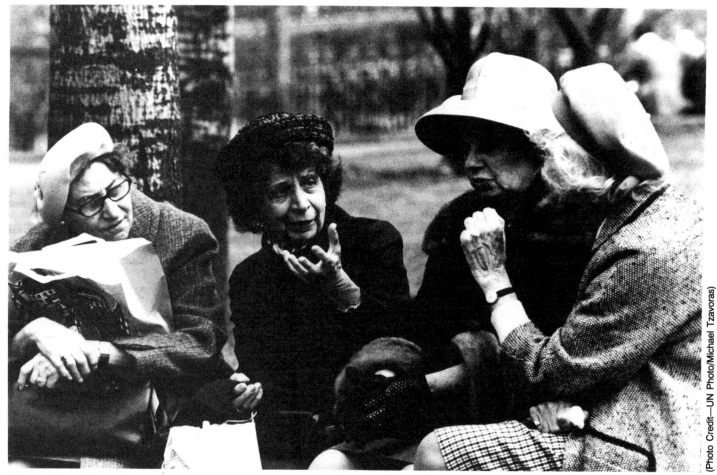

Most adults tend to make new friends. Many people are comfortable casually meeting others, while some feel the need to join some structured club or other social group.

It should be. Friendships provide varying degrees of indispensable support, from the agreeable neighbor who lends you his hedge clipper to the former college roommate you can call at any hour of the night for advice or commiseration. But since friendships are voluntary, unbound by obligations of law or kinship, they're especially susceptible to life's ups and downs, particularly when one friend's life changes in a way that the other's does not. Whether it's marriage, divorce or a career switch, these "developmental transitions" make us see ourselves—and our friends—in a new light.

"Sometimes it's something major, like having children," says study author Dr. Donald Pannen, a psychologist at the University of Puget Sound in Tacoma, Wash. "Other times it's just a little thing like a disagreement about a political candidate. But these changes can create barriers and awkward feelings. They can make it more difficult to maintain the friendship." In fact, according to one study of 17- to 64-year-olds who had recently ended friendships, 77% said life changes precipitated the rift.

People have always gone through developmental transitions, but these days two people rarely hit the same transition at the same time. It's quite conceivable, for instance, for a 35-year-old woman to be a stay-at-home mom with two children while her close friend of the same age works 60-hour weeks and goes out on dates.

Certain developmental transitions are more disruptive than others. Career success—and the envy it provokes—can turn even the closest friendship sour. Some friendships may falter simply because two people no longer share the same values, say, about money or politics. Marriage poses one of the biggest threats to friendship, especially for women. Spousal intimacy may weaken a woman's need for a best friend, says Prusank. This seeming abandonment can be hard on the single friends who are left behind.

The hectic pace of modern life also makes keeping up with friends difficult. The new friendships we make on the job are often tenuous, because of the unstable nature of corporate life today. Not only do we leave jobs more often, but we also compete more with our coworkers to hang on to the jobs we have. Add children, hobbies and volunteer or religious activities to the mix, and our social contacts get spread pretty thin. "It used to be that everyone lived and worked and socialized in the same town," says Pannen. "But it takes much more effort to keep friends in today's fragmented society."

It's rare too for an adult to have a single best friend. Most of us have several "very good" friends in different circles. "The bond between adult best friends just isn't the same as in childhood," says Prusank. "The tight connection is diluted by many activities and obligations."

Trouble is, few of us actually acknowledge these pressures, much less discuss them with our friends. "Most people are afraid to burden a friendship with too much talk," says Dr. Julia T. Wood, an expert in communication at the University of North Carolina at Chapel Hill. "If you speak up about what's bothering you, there's a risk that the other person will shy away."

That reticence often continues to the bitter end. Unlike romantic relationships, which tend to break apart with a bang, friendships typically dissolve with barely a whimper. In the Puget Sound study, only 13% of subjects said their friendships ended abruptly, and just 15% managed to have an open discussion of the relationship's problems. "We have no language for describing friendship difficulties," says Prusank. "We don't have 'breakup' conversations, and we don't give back the objects we exchanged. Without these symbolic displays of finality—for example, returning gifts or photographs—it can be difficult to move on."

Both men and women take the loss of a pal hard: Six months after their friendships ended, 70% of the Puget Sound subjects said they felt ambivalent about their conflicts, 50% admitted to still feeling sad and 14% felt angry; only 17% said they were happy to have the friend out of their life.

And once we lose a few friends, whether it's due to work changes, moving, having children or death, it gets harder to approach new people. "Go through a lot of these transitions and you become wary," says Wood. "Older people often **withdraw because they have endured so many losses.**"

Still, most adults tend to make new friends, though often they have to take active measures to do so. "Many people join groups, like local political clubs, or even move to a new neighborhood or city specifically to meet people," says Dr. Rosemary Blieszner, a gerontologist at Virginia Polytechnic Institute and State University in Blacksburg, Va., and coauthor of *Adult Friendships*. If you're shy, try giving yourself "homework assignments," such as approaching two new people a week or reapproaching someone you've met recently and asking them to join you for a cup of coffee.

Of course, low self-esteem or lack of trust in others can make even these minor social interactions difficult. Simply deciding to embark on a friend-making campaign won't make these impediments go away, though a professional counselor can often help.

Much has happened since Kelly and I parted. I've switched jobs, married the man I fell in love with and become closer to my family. I'm sorry that Kelly hasn't been able to share these developments with me. But to endure, adult friendships need to be flexible. And that, say researchers, may be a rare quality.

"Part of what makes a friendship resilient is a mutual ability to weather changes and tolerate shifting demands on your friend's life," says Wood. If your best friend suddenly meets the man of her dreams, for instance, the wisest course of action might be to let her go for a while. To maintain a friendship, you need to be willing to come back and rejuvenate it after a period of less contact. "If you always think the silence stems from a lack of affection or care," says Wood, "the bond becomes less stable."

Then again, part of being a good friend is knowing when to let go. One instance, Purdue's Rawlins says, is when an unforgivable betrayal occurs, for example if a friend sleeps with your spouse or damages your reputation. Another is when a friend makes you feel bad about yourself. "There's a value to being able to let go as we take on new roles," says Wood. "This ability to adapt and change is healthy."

I'm not ready to say the breakup of my own friendship was healthy. I still miss Kelly too much. But perhaps my mother, listening to me moan yet again about the loss of my friend, put it best: "You met when you were girls," she said. "You laughed and cried together as girls. Now you're not girls anymore."

ARE YOU SHY?

You have lots of company. Nearly one of two Americans claims to be shy. What's more, the incidence is rising, and technology may be turning ours into a culture of shyness.

Bernardo J. Carducci, Ph.D., with Philip G. Zimbardo, Ph.D.

In sharp contrast to the flamboyant lifestyle getting under way at dance clubs across the country, another, quieter, picture of Americans was emerging from psychological research. Its focus: those on the sidelines of the dance floor. In 1975 *Psychology Today* published a groundbreaking article by Stanford University psychologist Philip Zimbardo, Ph.D., entitled "The Social Disease Called Shyness." The article revealed what Zimbardo had found in a survey conducted at several American colleges: An astonishing 40 percent of the 800 questioned currently considered themselves to be shy.

In addition to documenting the pervasiveness of shyness, the article presented a surprising portrait of those with the condition. Their mild-mannered exterior conceals roiling turmoil inside. The shy disclosed that they are excessively self-conscious, constantly sizing themselves up negatively, and overwhelmingly preoccupied with what others think of them. While everyone else is meeting and greeting, they are developing plans to manage their public impression (*If I stand at the far end of the room and pretend to be examining the painting on the wall, I'll look like I'm interested in art but won't have to talk to anybody*). They are consumed by the misery of the social setting (*I'm having a horrible time at this party because I don't know what to say and everyone seems to be staring at me*). All the while their hearts are pounding, their pulses are speeding, and butterflies are swarming in their stomach—physiological symptoms of genuine distress.

The article catalogued the painful consequences of shyness. There are social problems, such as difficulty meeting people and making new friends, which may leave the shy woefully isolated and subject to loneliness and depression. There are cognitive problems; unable to think clearly in the presence of others, the shy tend to freeze up in conversation, confusing others who are trying to respond to them. They can appear snobbish or disinterested in others, when they are in fact just plain nervous. Excessively egocentric, they are relentlessly preoccupied with every aspect of their own appearance and behavior. They live trapped between two fears: being invisible and insignificant to others, and being visible but worthless.

The response to the article was overwhelming. A record number of letters to the editor screamed HELP ME!, surprising considering that then, as now, PT readers were generally well-educated, self-aware, and open-minded—not a recipe for shyness.

The article launched a whole new field of study. In the past 20 years, a variety of researchers and clinicians, including myself, have been scrutinizing shyness. To celebrate the 20th anniversary of PT's epochal report, we decided to spotlight recent advances in understanding this social disease:

• Research in my laboratory and elsewhere suggests that, courtesy of changing cultural conditions, the incidence of shyness in the U.S. may now be as high as 48 percent—and rising.

• Most shyness is hidden. Only a small percentage of the shy appear to be obviously ill at ease. But all suffer internally.

• Some people are born with a temperamental tilt to shyness. But even that inheritance doesn't doom one to a life of averting others' eyes. A lot depends on parenting.

• Most shyness is acquired through life experiences.

• There is a neurobiology of shyness. At least three brain centers that mediate fear and anxiety orchestrate the whole-body response we recognize as shyness. Think of it as an over-generalized fear response.

• The incidence of shyness varies among countries. Israelis seem to be the least shy inhabitants of the world. A major contributing factor: cultural styles of assigning praise and blame to kids.

• Shyness has huge costs to individuals at all ages, especially in Western cultures.

• Shyness does have survival value.

• Despite the biological hold of shyness, there are now specific and well-documented ways to overcome its crippling effects.

Shy on the Sly

How is it possible that 40 to 50 percent of Americans—some of your friends, no doubt—are shy? Because while some people are obviously, publicly shy, a much larger percentage are privately shy. Their shyness, and its pain, is invisible to everyone but themselves.

Only 15 to 20 percent of shy people actually fit the stereotype of the ill-at-ease person. They use every excuse in the book to avoid social events. If they are unlucky enough to find themselves in casual conversation, they can't quite manage to make eye contact, to reply to questions without stumbling over their words, or to keep up their end of the conversation; they seldom smile. They are easy to pick out of a crowd because their shyness is expressed behaviorally.

The other 80 to 85 percent are privately shy, according to University of Pittsburgh psychologist Paul Pilkonis, Ph.D. Though their shyness leaves no behavioral traces—it's felt subjectively—it wreaks personal havoc. They feel their shyness in a pounding heart and pouring sweat. While they may seem at ease and confident in conversation, they are actually engaging in a self-deprecating inner dialogue, chiding themselves for being inept and questioning whether the person they are talking to really likes them. "Even though these people do fairly well socially, they have a lot of negative self-thought going on in their heads," explains Pilkonis. Their shyness has emotional components as well. When the conversation is over, they feel upset or defeated.

"There are a lot of people who have private aspects of shyness who are willing to say they are shy but don't quite gibe with the people we can see trembling or blushing," notes Pilkonis.

Shyness can lurk in unlikely hosts—even those of the talk show variety. Take David Letterman, king of late-night TV. Although his performance in front of a live studio audience and countless viewers seems relaxed and spontaneous, Letterman is known to be relentless in the planning and orchestration of each nightly performance down to the last detail. Like Johnny Carson, he spends little time socializing outside a very small circle of friends and rarely attends social functions.

Letterman is the perfect example of what Zimbardo calls the shy extrovert: the cool, calm, and collected type whose insides are in fact churning. A subset of the privately shy, shy extroverts may be politicians, entertainers, and teachers. They have learned to act outgoing—as long as they are in a controlled environment. A politician who can speak from a prepared script at a mass political rally really may get tongue-tied during a question-and-answer period. A professor may be comfortable as long as she is talking about her area of expertise; put in a social gathering where she may have to make small talk, she clams up.

Zimbardo's short list of notable shy extroverts: funny lady Carol Burnett, singer Johnny Mathis, television reporter Barbara Walters, and international opera star Joan Sutherland. These stars are not introverts, a term often confused with shyness. Introverts have the conversational skills and self esteem necessary for interacting successfully with others but prefer to be alone. Shy people want very much to be with others but lack the social skills and self-esteem.

What unites the shy of any type is acute self-consciousness. The shy are even self-conscious about their self-consciousness. Theirs is a twisted egocentricity. They spend so much time focusing on themselves and their weaknesses, they have little time or inclination to look outward.

Wired for Shyness?

According to developmental psychologist Jerome Kagan, Ph.D., and colleagues at Harvard University, up to a third of shy adults were born with a temperament that inclined them to it. The team has been able to identify shyness in young infants before environmental conditions make an impact.

In his longitudinal studies, 400 four-month-old infants were brought into the lab and subjected to such stimuli as moving mobiles, a whiff of a Q-Tip dipped in alcohol, and a tape recording of the human voice. Then they were brought back at a later age for further study. From countless hours of observation, rerun on videotapes, Kagan, along with Harvard psychologists Nancy Snidman, Ph.D, and Doreen Arcus, Ph.D., have nailed down the behavioral manifestations of shyness in infants.

About 20 percent of infants display a pattern of extreme nervous-system reactivity to such common stimuli. These infants grow distressed when faced with unfamiliar people, objects, and events. They momentarily extend their arms and legs spastically, they vigorously wave their arms and kick their legs, and, on occasion, arch their backs. They also show signs of distress in the form of excessive fretting and crying, usually at a high pitch and sustained tension that communicates urgency. Later on, they cling to their parents in a new play situation.

In contrast, 40 percent of all infants exposed to the same stimuli occasionally move an arm or leg but do not show the motor outbursts or fretting and crying typical of their highly reactive brethren. When the low-reactive infants do muster up a crying spell, it is nothing out of the ordinary.

Lab studies indicate that highly reactive infants have an easily excitable sympathetic nervous system. This neural network regulates not only many vital organs, including the heart, but the brain response of fear. With their high-strung, hair-trigger temperament, even the suggestion of danger—a stranger, a new environment—launches the psychological and physiologic arousal of fear and anxiety.

One of the first components of this reaction is an increased heart rate. Remarkably, studies show that high-reactive infants have a higher-than-normal heart rate—and it can be detected even before birth, while the infant is still *in utero*. At 14 months, such infants have over-large heart rate acceleration in response to a neutral stimulus such as a sour taste.

Four years later, the same kids show another sign of sympathetic arousal—a cooler temperature reading in their right ring finger than in their left ring finger while watching emotionally evocative film clips. Too, as children they show more brain wave activity in the right frontal lobe; by contrast, normally reactive children display more brain wave activity in the left frontal area. From other studies it is known that the right side of the brain is more involved in the expression of anxiety and distress.

The infant patterns point to an inborn variation in the response threshold of the

---

The Natural History of Shyness

Shyness has not always been a source of pain. Being shy or inhibited serves a very protective function: It breeds caution. No doubt shyness has pulled *H. sapiens* out of some pretty tight spots over the eons.

Originally, shyness served as protective armor around the physical self. After all, only after an animal has fully acquainted itself with a new environment is it safe to behave in a more natural, relaxed manner and explore around. The process of habituation is one of the most fundamental characteristics of all organisms.

As conscious awareness has increased, the primary threat is now to the psychological self—embarrassment. Most people show some degree of social inhibition; they think about what they are going to say or do beforehand, as well as the consequences of saying or doing it. It keeps us from making fools of ourselves or hurting the feelings of others.

According to Wellesley psychologist Jonathan Cheek, Ph.D., situational shyness "can help to facilitate cooperative living; it inhibits behaviors that are socially unacceptable." So, a little bit of shyness may be good for you and society. But too much benefits no one.

amygdala, an almond-shaped brain structure linked to the expression of fear and anxiety (see "The Shy Brain"). This neural hypersensitivity eventually inclines such children to avoid situations that give rise to anxiety and fear—meeting new people or being thrown into new environments. In such circumstances they are behaviorally inhibited.

Though it might sound strange, there may even be a season for shyness—specifically early fall. Kagan and Harvard sociologist Stephen Gortmaker, Ph.D., have found that women who conceive in August or September are particularly likely to bear shy children. During these months, light is waning and the body is producing increasing amounts of melatonin, a hormone known to be neurally active; for example, it helps set our biological clocks. As it passes through the placenta to the developing fetal brain, Kagan surmises, the melatonin may act on cells to create the hyperaroused, easily agitated temperament of the shy.

Further evidence of a biological contribution to shyness is a pattern of inheritance suggesting direct genetic transmission from one generation to the next. Parents and grandparents of inhibited infants are more likely to report being shy as children than the relatives of uninhibited children, Snidman found in one study. Kagan and company are looking for stronger proof—such as, say, an elevated incidence of panic disorder (acute episodes of severe anxiety) and depression in the parents of inhibited children. So far he has found that among preschool children whose parents were diagnosed with panic attack or depression, one-third showed inhibited behavior. By contrast, among children whose parents experience neither panic disorder nor depression, only about five percent displayed the inhibited reactive profile.

Are inhibited infants preordained to become shy adults? Not necessarily, Doreen Arcus finds. A lot has to do with how such children are handled by their parents. Those who are overprotected, she found from in-home interviews she conducted, never get a chance to find some comfortable level of accommodation to the world; they grow up anxious and shy. Those whose parents do not shield them from stressful situations overcome their inhibition.

Snidman, along with Harvard psychiatrist Carl Schwartz, M.D., examined the staying power of shyness into adolescence. They observed 13- and 14-year-olds who were identified as inhibited at two or three years of age. During the laboratory interview, the adolescents with a history of inhibition tended to smile less, made fewer spontaneous comments, and reported being more shy than those who were identified as uninhibited infants.

Taken over a lifetime, gender doesn't figure much into shyness. Girls are more apt to be shy from infancy through adolescence, perhaps because parents are more protective of them than boys, who are encouraged to be more explorative. Yet in adolescence, boys report that shyness is more painful than do girls. This discomfort is likely related to sex-role expectations that boys must be bold and outgoing, especially with girls, to gear up for their role as head of family and breadwinner. But once into adulthood, gender differences in shyness disappear.

Bringing Biology Home

If only 15 to 20 percent of infants are born shy and nearly 50 percent of us are shy in adulthood, where do all the shy adults come from? The only logical answer is that shyness is acquired along the way.

One powerful source is the nature of the emotional bond parents forge with their children in the earliest years of life. According to Paul Pilkonis, children whose parenting was such that it gave rise to an insecure attachment are more likely to end up shy. Children form attachments to their caregivers from the routine experiences of care, feeding, and caressing. When caretaking is inconsistent and unreliable, parents fail to satisfy the child's need for security, affection, and comfort, resulting in insecure bonds. As the first relationship, attachment becomes the blueprint for all later relationships. Although there are no longitudinal studies spotlighting the development of shyness from toddlerhood to adulthood, there is research showing that insecure early attachment can predict shyness later on.

"The most damnable part of it is that this insecure attachment seems to become self-fulfilling," observes Pilkonis. Because of a difficult relationship to their parents, children internalize a sense of themselves as having problems with all relationships. They generalize the experience—and come to expect that teachers, coaches, and peers won't like them very much.

These are the narcissistically vulnerable—the wound to the self is early and deep, and easily evoked. They are quick to become disappointed in relationships, quick to feel rejection, shame, ridicule. They are relentlessly self-defeating, interpreting even success as failure. "They have negative perceptions of themselves and of themselves in relation to others that they hold onto at all costs," says Pilkonis. The narcissistically vulnerable are among the privately shy—they are seemingly at ease socially but torture themselves beneath the surface. Theirs is a shyness that is difficult to ameliorate, even with psychotherapy.

Shyness can also be acquired later on, instigated at times of developmental transition when children face new challenges in their relationships with their peers. For instance, entering the academic and social whirl of elementary school may leave them feeling awkward or inept with their peers. Teachers label them as shy and it sticks; they begin to see themselves that way—and act it.

Adolescence is another hurdle that can kick off shyness. Not only are adolescents' bodies changing but their social and emotional playing fields are redefining them. Their challenge is to integrate sexuality and intimacy into a world of relationships that used to be defined only by friendship and relatives. A complicated task!

Nor are adults immune. Shyness may re-

Helping Others Beat Shyness

You may not be shy, but one out of two people are. Be sensitive to the fact that others may not be as outgoing and confident. It's your job to make others comfortable around you. Be a host to humanity.

• Make sure no one person at a social gathering—including yourself—is the focus of attention. That makes it possible for everyone to have some of the attention some of the time.

• Like the host of any party, make it your job to bring out the best in others, in any situation. At school, teachers should make it a point to call on kids who are reluctant to speak up. At work, bosses should seek out employees who don't comment in meetings; encouragement to express ideas and creativity will improve any company. At parties, break the ice by approaching someone who is standing alone.

• Help others put their best foot forward. Socially competent people feel comfortable because they tend to steer conversation to their own interests. Find out what the shy person next to you is interested in; introduce the topic.

• Help others keep the conversation going. Shy people often don't speak up in ongoing conversations. Ask a shy person his or her opinion next time you are in a lively discussion.

sult from tail-spinning life upheavals. Divorce at mid-life might be one. "A whole new set of problems kick in with a failure of a relationship, especially if you are interested in establishing new relationships," says Pilkonis. For highly successful, career-defined people, being fired from a long-held job can be similarly debilitating, especially in the interviewing process.

Count in the Culture

Biology and relationship history are not the sole creators of shyness. Culture counts, too. Shyness exists universally, although it is not experienced or defined the same way from culture to culture. Even Zimbardo's earliest surveys hinted at cultural differences in shyness: Japanese and Taiwanese students consistently expressed the highest level of shyness, Jewish students the lowest. With these clues, Zimbardo took himself to Japan, Israel, and Taiwan to study college students. The cross-cultural studies turned up even greater cultural differences than the American survey. In Israel, only 30 percent of college-age students report being shy—versus 60 percent in Japan and Taiwan.

From conversations with foreign colleagues and parents, Zimbardo acquired unprecedented insights into how culture shapes behavior in general, and more specifically the cultural roots of shyness. The key is in the way parents attribute blame or praise in the performance of their children. When a child tries and fails at a task, who gets the blame? And when a child tries and succeeds, who gets the credit?

In Japan, if a child tries and succeeds, the parents get the credit. So do the grandparents, teachers, coaches, even Buddha. If there's any left over, only then is it given to the child. But if the child tries and fails, the child is fully culpable and cannot blame anyone else. An "I can't win" belief takes hold, so that children of the culture never take a chance or do anything that will make them stand out. As the Japanese proverb states, "the nail that stands out is pounded down." The upshot is a low-key interpersonal style. Kids are likely to be modest and quiet; they do little to call attention to themselves. In fact, in studies of American college students' individuation tendencies—the endorsement of behaviors that will make a person stand out, unique, or noticed—Asian students tend to score the lowest. They are much less likely to speak or act up in a social gathering for fear of calling attention to themselves.

In Israel, the attributional style is just the opposite. A child who tries gets rewarded, regardless of the outcome. Consider the

We Shall Overcome

1. Overcoming the Anxiety: To tame your racing heart and churning stomach, learn how to relax. Use simple breathing exercises that involve inhaling and exhaling deeply and slowly.

You can ride out the acute discomfort by staying around for a while. If you give into your distress and flee a party after only five minutes, you guarantee yourself a bad time. Stick around.

2. Getting Your Feet Wet: Nothing breeds success like success. Set up a nonthreatening social interaction that has a high probability of success and build from there. Call a radio show with a prepared comment or question. Call some sort of information line.

3. Face to Face: Then tackle the art of very, very small talk face-to-face. Start a casual, quick exchange with the person next to you, or the cashier, in the supermarket checkout line. Most people in such situations would be very responsive to passing the time in light conversation. Since half the battle is having something to say, prepare. Scan the newspaper for conversation topics, and practice what you are going to say a few times.

5. Smile and Make Eye Contact: When you smile you project a benign social force around you; people will be more likely to notice you and smile back. If you frown or look at your feet, you don't exist for people, or worse, you project a negative presence. Once you have smiled and made eye contact, you have opened up a window for the casual "This elevator is so slow"–type comment. Always maintain eye contact in conversation; it signals that you are listening and interested.

6. Compliment: The shortest route to social success is via a compliment. It's a way to make other people feel good about themselves and about talking to you. Compliment someone every day.

7. Know How to Receive Compliments: Thank the person right away. Then return the compliment: "That's great coming from you, I've always admired the way you dress." Use this as a jumping-off point for a real conversation. Elaborate, ask him where he gets his ties or shops for suits.

8. Stop Assuming the Worst: In expecting the worst of every situation, shy people undermine themselves—they get nervous, start to stutter, and forget what they wanted to say. Chances are that once you actually throw yourself into that dreaded interaction it will be much easier than you thought. Only then will you realize how ridiculous your doomsday predictions are. Ask your workmate if he likes his job. Just do it.

9. Stop Whipping Yourself: Thoughts about how stupid you sound or how nobody really likes you run through your head in every conversation. No one would judge your performance as harshly as you do. Search for evidence to refute your beliefs about yourself. Don't get upset that you didn't ask someone to dance; focus on the fact that you talked to a woman you wanted to meet.

Don't overgeneralize your social mishaps. Say you start to stutter in conversation with someone at a party. Don't punish yourself by assuming that every other interaction that night or in your life will go the same way.

10. Lose the Perfectionism: Your jokes have to be hilarious, your remarks insightful and ironic. Truth is, you set standards so impossible they spawn performance anxiety and doom you to failure. Set more realistic standards.

11. Learn to Take Rejection: Rejection is one of the risks *everyone* takes in social interaction. Try not to take it personally; it may have nothing to do with you.

12. Find Your Comfort Zone: Not all social situations are for everybody. Go where your interests are. You might be happier at an art gallery, book club, or on a volleyball team than at a bar.

13. Comfort Is Not Enough: The goal in overcoming shyness is to break through your self-centeredness. In an interaction, focus on the other person. Make other people's comfort and happiness your main priority. If people think to themselves, "I really enjoyed being with her," when they leave you, then you have transformed your shyness into social competence. Congratulations.

4. RELATING TO OTHERS

Yiddish expression *kvell*, which means to engage in an outsize display of pride. If a child tries to make a kite, people *kvell* by pointing out what a great kite it is. And if it doesn't fly, parents blame it on the wind. If a child tries and fails in a competitive setting, parents and others might reproach the coach for not giving the child enough training. In such a supportive environment, a child senses that failure does not have a high price—and so is willing to take a risk. With such a belief system, a person is highly likely to develop *chutzpah*, a type of audacity whereby one always take a chance or risk—with or without the talent. Children of such a value system are more apt to speak up or ask someone to dance at a party without overwhelming self-consciousness.

Shyness, then, is a relative, culture-bound label. It's a safe bet that a shy Israeli would not be considered shy in Japan. Nancy Snidman brings the point home. In studying four-month-olds in Ireland and the U.S., she found no differences in degree of nervous system reactivity. But at age five, the Irish kids did not talk as much nor were they as loud as the American kids. The difference lies in the cultural expectations expressed in child-rearing. Using American norms of social behavior as the standard of comparison, the normal Irish child would be labeled shy. But, in their own culture, with their own norms of behavior, they are not. By the same token, American kids may be perceived as boorish by the Irish.

The Scarlet S

Shyness is un-American. We are, after all, the land of the free and the home of the brave. From the first settlers and explorers who came to the New World 500 years ago to our leadership in space exploration, America has always been associated with courageous and adventurous people ready to boldly go where others fear to tread. Our culture still values rugged individualism and the conquering of new environments, whether in outer space or in overseas markets. Personal attributes held high in our social esteem are leadership, assertiveness, dominance, independence, and risk-taking. Hence a stigma surrounding shyness.

The people given the most attention in our society are expressive, active, and sociable. We single out as heroes actors, athletes, politicians, television personalities, and rock stars—people expert at calling attention to themselves: Madonna, Rosanne, Howard Stern. People who are most likely to be successful are those who are able to obtain attention and feel comfortable with it.

What shy people don't want, above all

The Shy Brain

We all take time to get used to (or habituate to) a new stimulus (a job interview, a party) before we begin to explore the unfamiliar. After all, a novel stimulus may serve as a signal for something dangerous or important. But shy individuals sense danger where it does not exist. Their nervous system does not accommodate easily to the new. Animal studies by Michael Davis, Ph.D., of Yale University, indicate that the nerve pathways of shyness involve parts of the brain involved in the learning and expression of fear and anxiety.

Both fear and anxiety trigger similar physiologic reactions: muscle tension, increased heart rate, and blood pressure, all very handy in the event an animal has to fight or flee sudden danger. But there are important differences. Fear is an emotional reaction to a specific stimulus; it's quick to appear, and just as quick to dissipate when the stimulus passes. Anxiety is a more generalized response that takes much longer to dissipate.

Studies of cue conditioning implicate the **amygdala** as a central switchboard in both the association of a specific stimulus with the emotion of fear and the expression of that fear. Sitting atop the brain stem, the amygdala is crucial for relaying nerve signals related to emotions and stress. When faced with certain stimuli—notably strangers, authority figures, members of the opposite sex—the shy associate them with fearful reactions.

In contrast to such "explicit" conditioning is a process of "contextual" conditioning. It appears more slowly, lasts much longer. It is often set off by the context in which fear takes place. Exposure to that environment then produces anxiety-like feelings of general apprehension. Through contextual conditioning, shy people come to associate general environments—parties, group discussions where they will be expected to interact socially—with unpleasant feelings, even before the specific feared stimulus is present.

Contextual conditioning is a joint venture between the amygdala and the **hippocampus**, the sea horse–shaped cell cluster near the amygdala, which is essential to memory and spatial learning. Contextual conditioning can be seen as a kind of learning about unpleasant places.

But a crucial third party participates in contextual conditioning. It's the **bed nucleus of the stria terminalis (BNST)**. The long arms of its cells reach to many other areas of the brain, notably the **hypothalamus** and the brain stem, both of which spread the word of fear and anxiety to other parts of the body. The BNST is principally involved in the generalized emotional-behavioral arousal characteristic of anxiety. The BNST may be set off by the neurotransmitter corticotropin releasing factor (CRF).

Once alerted, the hypothalamus triggers the sympathetic nervous system, culminating in the symptoms of inner turmoil experienced by the shy—from rapid heartbeat to sweaty paleness. Another pathway of information, from the amygdala to the brain stem, freezes movement of the mouth.

The shy brain is not different in structure from yours and mine; it's just that certain parts are more sensitive. Everyone has a "shyness thermostat," set by genes and other factors. The pinpointing of brain structures and neurochemicals involved in shyness holds out the promise that specific treatment may eventually be developed to curb its most debilitating forms.

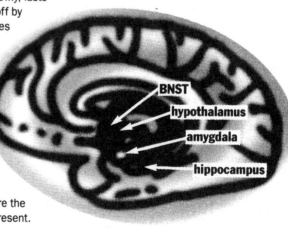

else, is to be the focus of attention. Thus, in elementary school, the shy child may not even ask the teacher for help. In college, the shy student is reluctant to ask a question in class. In adulthood, the shy employee is too embarrassed to make a formal presentation to those who grant promotions. In every cases, shyness undermines the ability to access the attention of others who would increase the likelihood of success. In a culture where everybody loves a winner, shyness is like entering a foot race with lead insoles.

Consider the findings of Stanford Business School professor Thomas Harrell. To figure out the best predictors of success in business, he gathered the records of Stanford B-School graduates, including their transcripts and letters of recommendation. Ten years out of school, the graduates were ranked from most to least successful based on the quality of their jobs. The only consistent and significant variable that could predict success (among students who were admittedly bright to start with) was verbal fluency—exactly what the typically tongue-tied shy person can't muster. The verbally fluent are able to sell themselves, their services, and their companies—all critical skills for running a corporation; think of Lee Iacocca. Shy people are probably those behind the scenes designing the cars, programs, and computers—impressive feats, but they don't pay as much as CEO.

The costs of shyness cut deeper than material success, and they take on different forms over a lifetime.

• A shy childhood may be a series of lost opportunities. Think of the child who wants so much to wear a soccer uniform and play just like all the other kids but can't muster the wherewithal to become part of a group. And if the parents do not find a way to help a child overcome feelings of nervousness and apprehension around others, the child may slip into more solitary activities, even though he really wants to be social. The self-selection into solitary activities further reduces the likelihood of the child developing social skills and self-confidence.

• Shy kids also have to endure teasing and peer rejection. Because of their general disposition for high reactivity, shy children make prime targets for bullies. Who better to tease and taunt than someone who gets scared easily and cries?

• Whether inherited or acquired, shyness predisposes to loneliness. It is the natural consequence of decades spent shunning others due to the angst of socializing. Reams of research show that loneliness and isolation can lead to mental and physical decline, even a hastened death.

• Without a circle of close friends or relatives, people are more vulnerable to risk. Lacking the opportunity to share feelings and fears with others, isolated people allow them to fester or escalate. What's more, they are prone to paranoia; there's no one around to correct their faulty thinking, no checks and balances on their beliefs. We all need someone to tell us when our thinking is ridiculous, that there is no Mafia in suburban Ohio, that no one is out to get you, that you've just hit a spate of bad luck.

• Shyness brings with it a potential for abusing alcohol and drugs as social lubricants. In Zimbardo's studies, shy adolescents report feeling greater peer pressure to drink or use drugs than do less shy adolescents. They also confide that they use drugs and alcohol to feel less self-conscious and to achieve a greater sense of acceptance.

• Call it the Hugh Grant Effect. Shyness is linked to sexual, uh, difficulties. Shy people have a hard time expressing themselves to begin with; communicating sexual needs and desires is especially difficult. Shy men may turn to prostitutes just to avoid the awkwardness of intimate negotiations. When Zimbardo asked them to describe their typical client, 20 San Francisco prostitutes said that the men who frequented them were shy and couldn't communicate their sexual desires to wives or girlfriends. And the shy guys made distinctive customers. They circled a block over and over again in their car before getting the nerve to stop and talk to the prostitute. To shy men, the allure of a prostitute is simple—she asks what you want, slaps on a price, and performs. No humiliation, no awkwardness.

Performance anxiety may also make the prospect of sex overwhelming. And because shy people avoid seeking help, any problems created by embarrassment or self-doubt will likely go untreated.

• Another cost—time. Shy people waste time deliberating and hesitating in social situations that others can pull off in an instant. Part of their problem is that they don't live in the present, observes Zimbardo, who is currently focusing on the psychology of time perspective. "Shy people live too much in their heads," obsessed with the past, the future, or both. A shy person in conversation is not apt to think about what is being said at the moment, but about how past conversations have initially gone well and then deteriorated—just as the current one threatens to. Says Zimbardo: "These are people who cannot enjoy that moment because everything is packaged in worries from the past—a Smithsonian archive of all the bad—that restructure the present."

28. Are You Shy?

Or shy people may focus all their thoughts and feelings on future consequences: If I say this, will he laugh at me? If I ask him something simple like where he is from, he'll be bored and think I'm a lousy conversationalist, so why bother anyway? The internal decision trees are vast and twisted. "Concern for consequences always makes you feel somewhat anxious. And that anxiety will impair the shy person's performance," says Zimbardo.

Factoring in past and future is wise, but obsession with either is undermining. Shy people need to focus on the now—the person you are talking to or dancing with—to appreciate any experience. "Dancing is a good example of being completely of the moment," comments Zimbardo. "It is not something you plan, or that you remember, you are just doing it." And enjoying it.

If the costs of shyness are paid by shy people, the benefits of shyness are reaped by others—parents, teachers, friends, and society as a whole.

Yet shy people are often gifted listeners. If they can get over their self-induced pressures for witty repartee, shy people can be great at conversation because they may actually be paying attention. (The hard part comes when a response is expected.) According to Harvard's Doreen Arcus, shy kids are apt to be especially empathic. Parents of the children she studies tell her that "even in infancy, the shy child seemed to be sensitive, empathic, and a good listener. They seem to make really good friends and their friends are very loyal to them and value them quite a bit." Even among children, friendships need someone who will talk and someone who will listen.

For any society to function well, a variety of roles need to be played. There is a place for the quiet, more reflective shy individual who does not jump in where angels fear to tread or attempt to steal the limelight from others. Yet as a culture we have devalued these in favor of boldness and expressiveness as a means of measuring worth.

The Future of Shyness

To put it bluntly, the future of shyness is bleak. My studies have documented that since 1975 its prevalence has risen from 40 percent to 48 percent. There are many reasons to expect the numbers to climb in the decades ahead.

Most significantly, technology is continually redefining how we communicate. We are engaging in a diminishing number of face-to-face interactions on a daily basis. When was the last time you talked to a bank teller? Or a gas station attendant? How often do you call friends or colleagues when you know they aren't in just so you can leave a message on their machine? Voice mail, faxes, and E-mail give us the illusion of being "in touch," but what's to touch but the keyboard? This is not a Luddite view of technology, but a sane look at its deepest costs.

The electronic age was supposed to give us more time, but ironically it has stolen it from us. Technology has made us time-efficient—and redefined our sense of time and its value. It is not to be wasted, but to be used quickly and with a purpose.

Office encounters have become barren of social interaction. They are information-driven, problem-oriented, solution-based. No pleasantries. No backs slapped. We cut to the chase: I need this from you. Says Zimbardo, "You have to have an agenda." Some people don't even bother to show at the office at all; they telecommute.

The dwindling opportunities for face-to-face interaction put shy people at an increasing disadvantage. They no longer get to practice social skills within the comfort of daily routine. Dropping by a colleague's office to chat becomes increasingly awkward as you do it less and less. Social life has shrunk so much it can now be entirely encapsulated in a single, near-pejorative phrase: "face time," denoting the time employees may engage in eyeball-to-eyeball conversation. It's commonly relegated to morning meetings and after 4:00 P.M.

Electronic hand-held video games played solo now crowd out the time-honored social games of childhood. Even electronically simulated social interactions can't substitute—they do not permit people to learn the necessary give and take that is at the heart of all interpersonal relationships.

Technology is not the only culprit. The rise of organized sports for kids and the fall of informal sidewalk games robs kids of the chance to learn to work out their own relationship problems. Instead, the coach and the referee do it.

If technology is ushering in a culture of shyness, it is also the perfect medium for the shy. The Internet and World Wide Web are conduits for the shy to interact with others; electronic communication removes many of the barriers that inhibit the shy. You prepare what you want to say. Nobody knows what you look like. The danger, however, is that technology will become a hiding place for those who dread social interaction.

The first generation to go from cradle to grave with in-home computers, faxes, and the Internet is a long way from adulthood.

Helping Shy Kids

Infants with a touchy temperament are not necessarily doomed to become shy adults. Much depends on the parenting they receive.

Do not overprotect or overindulge: Although it may sound counterintuitive, you can help you child cope more effectively with shyness by allowing him or her to experience moderate amounts of anxiety in response to challenges. Rather than rush to your child's aid to soothe away every sign of distress, provide indirect support. Gradually expose your child to new objects, people, and places so that the child will learn to cope with his own unique level of sensitivity to novelty. Nudge, don't push, your child to continue to explore new things.

Show respect and understanding: Your children have private emotional lives separate from yours. It is important to show your shy child that you can understand and sympathize with her shyness, by talking with the child about her feelings of nervousness and being afraid. Then talk with her about what might be gained by trying new experiences *in spite of* being afraid. Revealing related experiences from your own childhood is a natural way to start the ball rolling. Overcoming fears and anxieties is not an easy process; the feelings may remain even after specific shy behaviors have been overcome. Key ingredients are sympathy, patience, and persistence.

Ease the tease: Shy children are especially sensitive to embarrassment. Compared to other children, they need extra attention, comfort, and reassurance after being teased and more encouragement to develop positive self-regard.

Help build friendships: Invite one or two playmates over to let the child gain experience in playing with different kids in the security of familiar surroundings. But allow them as much freedom as possible in structuring play routines. Shy kids sometimes do better when playing with slightly younger children.

Talk to teachers: Teachers often overlook a shy child or mistake quietness and passivity for disinterest or a lack of intelligence. Discuss what measure might be taken in the classroom or playground.

Prepare the child for new experiences: You can help to reduce fears and anxieties by helping your child get familiar with upcoming novel experiences. Take the child to a new school before classes actually start. Help rehearse activities likely to be performed in new situations, such as practicing for show-and-tell. Also role play with the child any anticipated anxiety-provoking situations, such as how to ask someone to dance at a party (if they'll let you) or speak up in a group at summer camp.

Find appropriate activities: Encourage your child to get involved in after-school activities as a means of developing a network of friends and social skills.

Provide indirect support: Ask the child the degree to which he wants you to be involved in his activities. For some kids, a parent cheering in the bleachers is humiliating. Better is indirect support—discussing the child's interests with him and letting him know of your pleasure and pride in him for participating.

Fit not fight: It's not as important to overcome shyness as to find a comfort zone consistent with your child's shyness. Rather than try to make your daughter outgoing, help her find a level of interaction that is comfortable and consistent with her temperament.

Own your temperament: Think how your own personality or interaction style operates in conjunction with your child's. If you aren't shy, understand that your child may need more time to feel comfortable before entering a novel situation or joining a social group. If you are shy, you may need to address your own shyness as a bridge to helping your child with hers.

Bottom Line: Talk, listen, support, and love shy children for who they are, not how outgoing you would like them to be.

We will have to wait at least another 20 years to accurately assess shyness in the wake of the new electronic age. But to do so, we must find a group of infants—shy and non-shy—and follow them through their life, rather than observe different people, from different generations, in different periods of their lives. Only then will we see the course of shyness over a lifetime. Stay tuned for **PT**'s next shyness article, in 2015.

hotheads
and heart attacks

Blowing your stack—or even seething silently—can put your heart at risk. So what are you supposed to do about it? Take a deep breath and read on

Edward Dolnick

Jaw clenched, voice rising, short, sturdy finger jabbing furiously as if to impale her victim, Mary Brown pauses momentarily to catch her breath. "She's my grandmother, for God's sake!" she yells at the nursing home supervisor. "We're paying all this money, and nobody even checks on her? Don't you tell me you can't do it. You went into this business to take care of people. If you can't do it, get out of the business!"

The anger is real, but little else in the scene is genuine. Brown, though she seems to have forgotten it, is a volunteer in a study designed to gauge the impact of anger on the heart. Hooked up to a blood pressure cuff and heart monitors in a physiology lab at Baltimore's v.a. hospital, she is simply acting a role, though it helps that her own grandmother was once neglected by the staff at a nearby nursing home.

Brown has focused all her attention on the young man playing the role of the nursing supervisor. She has ignored the true source of her torment, a small figure standing quietly at the edge of the room. He is Aron Siegman, a soft-spoken 66-year-old psychologist with a slight paunch and a fringe of white hair.

His mild appearance to the contrary, Siegman spends his days stirring up trouble—coaxing a college student to recall a spouse's adulterous affair, for example, or repeatedly interrupting a volunteer's answer to a question he has posed about her aging father. A connoisseur of anger, he is as caught up in the nuances of his favorite subject as any wine collector. The reason is simple: A host of studies seem to show that we have become a nation of Rumplestiltskins, so much more likely to lose our cool than we were even a few decades ago that we have pushed our bodies to the breaking point.

It's not a pretty picture. Too many of us overreact to the countless provocations of everyday life—traffic jams and surly clerks and brutish bosses—by boiling over. Heart pounding, blood pressure skyrocketing, adrenaline surging, we are doing ourselves in prematurely, the experts say, by pushing our bodies beyond what they can take. One of the leading proponents of this new theory summarizes it with a succinctness more common on bumper stickers than in science. Current wisdom, declares Duke University stress researcher Redford Williams, is that "anger kills."

Fortunately, a simple remedy may be at hand. Siegman is now testing a theory that anger in itself isn't bad for your heart; the unhealthy consequences only kick in, he says, if you act out that anger. If he is right, the cry from the sixties to "let it all hang out" had it exactly backwards. It's perfectly okay, says the University of Maryland psychologist, to think that the nitwit who just turned left from the right lane shouldn't be let outdoors without a keeper; what's not okay is to scream at him and pound the steering wheel.

The Mary Brown experiment, for example, has two halves. First, Siegman wants to show that expressing anger sets the heart racing and blood pressure soaring. The lab's recording devices make that clear. Her blood pressure alone, normally 176/75, has skyrocketed to 213/98 since her tirade began. The experiment's second half involves coaxing Brown to replay the same infuriating scene, but this time without any outward displays of anger. What physiological changes do the various monitors reveal when a person feels angry but chooses not

4. RELATING TO OTHERS

A study that looked at 118 lawyers found that of those who scored in the top quarter for hostility, one in five was dead by age 50.

to express it? "Virtually nothing," says Siegman. "We don't get anything."

Here no news truly is good news. Heart disease is the nation's leading killer, and anger is emerging as a risk factor as important as smoking or high cholesterol or any of the other well-known villains. If Siegman is right that anger can be tamed, and tamed fairly simply, he's on to something big.

THE KIND OF HOSTILE personality that may put people at especially high risk for heart disease does not yet have a name. For the moment, let's call it Type H, for hostility, and to acknowledge its link to the famous Type A personality.

Type A behavior is a mix of impatience, aggressiveness, anger, and competitiveness. Mix Donald Trump with Margaret Thatcher, stir in Murphy Brown, and you have a Type A. For decades, everyone living this high-strung, fast-paced life was seen as a heart attack waiting (impatiently) to happen.

By 1981, the Type A theory had earned an official stamp of approval. An all-star panel appointed by the National Heart, Lung, and Blood Institute to evaluate the evidence had come back with a hearty endorsement.

This was major news. Medicine had long paid lip service to the idea that the mind affects the body—no one who has ever blushed could deny it—but this was more. After years in the shadows, psychology had suddenly leapt onstage. In predicting heart disease, a psychological trait seemed as important as any biological measure.

But no sooner had the experts committed their enthusiasm for Type A to print than a slew of new and authoritative studies appeared. Their message: Type A's faced no higher risk of heart disease than anyone else. Two studies that looked at patients who already had heart disease came to an even more unwelcome conclusion. Type A's, it seemed, fared *better* than their laid-back counterparts.

Oops!

The Type H theory salvages something important from that wreckage. Indeed, it seems Type A theorists weren't entirely off the mark, after all. Type A was a package, and though most of its ingredients were irrelevant to heart disease, one component—hostility—may truly be toxic. Impatience and competitiveness, on the other hand, seem to have been innocents who got a bad reputation by hanging out with the wrong crowd.

Type H theory rests on some compelling findings. In one study, for example, 255 doctors who had taken a standard personality test while attending the University of North Carolina's medical school were tracked down 25 years later. Those whose hostility scores had been in the top half were four to five times as likely to have developed heart disease in the intervening decades as were those whose hostility scores had been in the lower half.

A similar study that looked at 118 lawyers found equally striking results. Of those lawyers who had scored in the top quarter for hostility, nearly one in five was dead by age 50. Of those in the lowest quarter, only one in 25 had died.

What's more, say the Type H proponents, such findings have a straightforward biological explanation. Evolution, they note, has designed the human body to respond to acutely stressful situations with a cascade of changes. In crises, your heart pumps faster and harder, arteries that carry blood to your muscles dilate so that blood flow increases still more, your platelets become stickier so that you are less likely to bleed to death if an attacker takes a bite out of you.

It's a fine system if you're running from a lion. If you start the whole process up every time the elevator is late, though, everyday life will soon lay you low. As blood surges through your arteries and stress hormones pour from your adrenal glands, once-smooth artery walls begin to scar and pit. Then fatty cells clump on that pocked surface, like mineral deposits in an old water pipe. Arteries narrow, blood flow decreases, and your body is starved of oxygen. The downward spiral eventually ends in chest pain or strokes or heart attacks.

The mechanism behind Type A, in contrast, was a good deal harder to picture. Exactly how would competitiveness, say, put the body at risk? Even in its heyday, Type A had other problems, as well. For one, it seemed to call for a personality transplant. To teach his frazzled patients mellowness, for example, one Type-A pioneer had them wait in the longest line at the bank and drive all day in the right-hand lane. It sounds brutal, the brainstorm of a malicious researcher who had grown bored with harassing rats and was looking for bigger game.

"With the original Type A," says David Krantz, a psychologist at Uniformed Services University of the Health Sciences, in Bethesda, Maryland, "people would say, 'You're telling me I can't be competitive? I shouldn't meet deadlines? How am I going to explain that to my boss?' Now the message is more manageable: 'Ambition is not the problem. Aggressiveness is not the problem. *Hostility* is the problem.'

"What your boss wants is for you to get a hell of a lot of work done," Krantz adds. "He doesn't necessarily want you to act like a son of a bitch."

The Type H theory differs from its forebear in one other important way—it specifically includes women. In theory, Type A did, too, but in practice it focused heavily on males. In part, the reason was a matter of convenience for the researchers: Most men have their heart attacks ten years earlier than women; in larger part, the reason was that when scientists thought Type A, the stereotype that came to mind was a male executive.

They might have thought of Mary Brown instead. She is a delightful woman, lively and down-to-earth and a good storyteller. It's just that, as the Pompeians said about Vesuvius, there is this one, tiny quirk. Brown is in her sixties now and works hard to keep her temper in bounds, but for as long as she can remember she has erupted at the slightest provocation. "I'm real proud if I can go two days without getting upset," she says. "I blow up. I know it's terrible, but I just do."

If someone cuts ahead of her in the supermarket line, Brown tells them off. "I'd like to see someone try to butt in front of me," she boasts. If they venture into the express line with a dozen items rather than the legal ten, Brown dresses them down and makes sure the cashier knows of their sin, too. On the freeway, preparing to exit, she sticks close to the car in front of her so that no one else can cut in. "I'm not going to let you in," she snarls at anyone trying it. "You should have moved in way back there."

Mary Brown is no tyrant. She's funny, and, once the storm has passed, she can laugh at her tirades. She has been married to the same man for 50 years. "It's incredible, some of what he's had to put up with," she says with a rueful smile. And she is close to her son and daughter.

Outsiders are more at risk. Brown cannot abide injustice, and she sees it in every driver who runs a yellow light, in every shopper with an extra can of soup. "To me," she says, "silence is acceptance. If I don't say anything, I'm agreeing with something that's wrong, and"—she hammers out the last words, like a general exhorting the troops to defend their homeland—"that cannot happen."

THE MEDICAL ESTABLISHMENT tends to wrinkle its nose in distaste at this whole subject. Many cardiologists concede that a diseased heart can be undone by such sudden stresses as winning the lottery or getting robbed at gunpoint; in ways that are not well understood, stress somehow sets the heart's ventricles to chaotic quivering. But they question whether chronic stress

Men, Women, and Anger

Is a fiery display of temper as common in a woman as it is in a man? Lately psychologists have begun to fill in the hostility picture.

WE ALL GET ANGRY

According to a number of studies, women and men tend to get angry equally often (about six or seven times a week), equally intensely, and for more or less the same reasons. Tests designed to reveal aggressive feelings, hidden anger, or hostility turned inward haven't discovered any sex differences at all.

MEN EXPLODE, WOMEN MOSTLY SEETHE

Some angry women do shout and pound their fists, of course—just as some men do. But in general, studies show, women and men have very different styles when it comes to getting angry. Women are more likely to express anger by crying, for example, or to keep their anger under wraps. "Women have cornered the market on the seething, unspoken fury that is always threatening to explode," says Anne Campbell, a psychologist at England's Durham University. Women are also more likely to express their anger in private. They might get angry at a boss or coworker, but chances are they'll wait until they're alone or with a spouse or close friend to show their anger.

IN WOMEN, AN ANGRY OUTBURST, THEN REGRET

Surveys show that anger itself means different things to men than it does to women. Men's anger tends to be uncomplicated by restraint and guilt, says Campbell. It is straightforwardly about winning and losing. Women are more likely to feel embarrassed when they show anger, equating it with a loss of control, she says. Women are also more likely than men to believe their anger is out of proportion to the events that caused it. "After an outburst," she says, "women tell themselves, 'Whoa! Get a grip.' Men say, 'That ought to show him.'" According to one study, the more furious a woman gets, the longer it takes her to get over the episode. That's not true for men—at least not to the same degree.

The way women and men view crying is different, too. According to Campbell and other researchers, men often see women's crying as a sign of remorse or contrition—or as a tactic used to win a fight. Women are more likely to view crying as a sign of frustration or rage—a way to release tension. According to one study, 78 percent of women who cried during fights did so out of frustration.

So what does all this mean for women's risk of heart disease? Researchers say that whether anger is expressed through clenched teeth or raised voices, in public or in private, it appears to wreak the same havoc on the heart. —*E.D.*

4. RELATING TO OTHERS

in general, or hostility in particular, can undo a healthy heart.

Look again, for example, at the study that showed a high number of deaths among hostile lawyers. It's tempting, critics say, to conclude that hostility gradually undermined their healthy hearts. But maybe not. Maybe heart disease strikes randomly at the hostile and the pleasant alike, and hostility serves only to speed up the dying process in those who are already vulnerable. In large measure, this is simply "show me" skepticism. Where, doubters ask, is clear-cut proof?

Part of the problem is that a theory based on hostility is harder to pin down than one based on something as easy to measure as blood pressure. Even Siegman concedes that the case for Type H is far from airtight. "Look," he says, "it's a complicated story. It was the same with cholesterol. That started out, Cholesterol is bad. Then somebody found out cholesterol levels alone didn't predict so well, and then there was HDL and LDL, and then the ratio between them. It's an ongoing story."

But even if Siegman and his colleagues are right that hostility is bad for the heart, is there anything we can do about it?

To begin with, everyone agrees that we cannot banish anger. Even if we wanted to, we could no more stop getting angry than we could stop getting hungry. But who would want to? Anger has its place. There is injustice in the world, after all, and righteous indignation is an honorable emotion.

In a rare lyric moment, psychologists have dubbed the real problem free-floating hostility. An occasional flash of temper is fine, they say; a permanent snarl is not. Hostile people are perpetually suspicious, wary, and snappish, forever tense and on edge. They see every sales clerk as determined to linger on the phone for hours, every compliment as a dig in disguise, every colleague as a rival in waiting.

That's bad for two reasons, says Timothy Smith, a psychologist at the University of Utah in Salt Lake City. First, hostility is harmful for all the Type H reasons. Second, hostility feeds on itself, typically leaving its "victims" precariously alone. That's worrisome because a variety of studies have shown that people with friends and families, or even pets, fare better than those without such support.

So what is a hostile person to do? The advice from the experts is surprisingly straightforward: Relax, take a deep breath, decide whether this latest injustice really merits a battle. Give in to your anger, they say, and you become all the more angry. Resist it, by keeping your voice down or your teeth ungritted, and the anger seeps away.

"Anger is not just emotion, it's physiology, too," Siegman says. "Your blood pressure goes up, your voice gets loud, you clench your jaws"—he has worked himself into a mini-tirade, bellowing at the top of his voice, windmilling his arms, thrusting his chin out belligerently—"but then, if you lower your voice, speak more slowly, relax your muscles"—he has followed his own instructions and collapsed weakly into his seat, like a balloon with a slow leak—"if you do that, if you eliminate any part of the cycle, then you weaken the whole performance, and you can't sustain the feelings of anger."

Siegman's experiments seem to support this theory. In its own way, Hollywood has tested the same idea. Audiences watching an actor in a supposed rage see and hear all the familiar signs of anger—we recognize *bad* acting precisely because there is a dissonance between spoken words and body language—and actors, by their own report, feel the emotions they simulate. Similarly, studies on laughter and smiling have shown that simulated merriment offers the same benefits—increased blood flow, reduced levels of hormones that create stress, reduced pain perception—as the genuine article.

But even among those who believe that Type H's are putting themselves at risk, Siegman's strategy for taming anger is controversial. "What if your anger is unresolved?" asks Lynda Powell, a psychologist at Chicago's Rush-Presbyterian-Saint Luke's Medical Center. "What if it's inside and you haven't dealt with it? Sometimes when you express it, you get it out and get beyond it. If you've just stuffed it inside, then the question is, Could that do just as much damage to your heart?"

Siegman is impatient with such objections, which he sees as smacking of an outdated Freudianism. "The psychoanalysts thought that anger was like physical energy," he complains. "They thought it couldn't be dissipated—the only choice was to

Give in to your anger,
Siegman says, and you become all the more angry. Resist it, and the anger seeps away.

express it or to repress it. But anger is not like physical energy," he says. "An angry person who chooses to divert his attention will no longer be angry. We have a lot of evidence to show that."

Siegman tries to head off the doubters by making a distinction between suppressing the outward expressions of anger, which he favors, and repress-

29. Hotheads and Heart Attacks

ing anger itself, which he warns against. The difference, he says, is that people who repress their anger don't merely stifle it; they hide it so well that they themselves are unaware of it. The person who follows Siegman's advice walks a middle road; she neither denies her rage nor gives in to it. Instead she simply decides that the matter isn't worth the theatrical fireworks—whether expressed in pounded fists and shouting or in the seething language of gritted teeth—and calmly talks it out or lets it go. The result is that the anger neither festers nor explodes, but gradually loses its hold.

DESPITE SKEPTICS' OBJECTIONS, the hostility–heart disease connection is undeniably tantalizing. For one thing, it seems suspicious that so many studies of heart disease in the past few years have fingered hostility as a culprit. Where there's smoke, there's ire.

So if we are a long way from proof beyond a reasonable doubt, we may still have enough evidence to justify a small bet.

What seems called for, in fact, is a mundane version of Pascal's wager. The French philosopher opted to believe in God, on the grounds that he had everything to gain if he was right and nothing to lose by being wrong.

When it comes to hostility, there doesn't seem to be much downside in taking the experts' advice to ease up a bit. This is unusual. With most medical advice—quit eating chocolate cake, say—the risks are considerable. Giving up cake cuts out part of life's pleasure, first of all, and the loss could be even worse. In five years, researchers might come back and say, "It turns out we had it wrong. It's really, The more cake the better. Sorry about that."

Here, the experts' advice amounts to every grandmother's list of maxims: Take a deep breath and count to ten, look on the bright side, don't say anything if you can't say anything nice, and so on. What's the risk? At best, you'll live longer and better. At worst, you'll be better company.

Are You Too Angry for Your Own Good?

THE TEST

Gauging your hostility quotient isn't as simple as measuring blood pressure or cholesterol. But the following 12 questions—supplied by Redford Williams, director of behavioral research at Duke University and the author of *Anger Kills*—could indicate whether a hostile temperament is getting the best of you.

1. Have you ever been so angry at someone that you've thrown things or slammed a door?
2. Do you tend to remember irritating incidents and get mad all over again?
3. Do little annoyances have a way of adding up during the day, leaving you frustrated and impatient?
4. Stuck in a long line at the express checkout in the grocery store, do you often count to see if anyone ahead of you has more than ten items?
5. If the person who cuts your hair trims off more than you wanted, do you fume about it for days afterward?
6. When someone cuts you off in traffic, do you flash your lights or honk your horn?
7. Over the past few years, have you dropped any close friends because they just didn't live up to your expectations?
8. Do you find yourself getting annoyed at little things your spouse does that get under your skin?
9. Do you feel your pulse climb when you get into an argument?
10. Are you often irritated by other people's incompetence?
11. If a cashier gives you the wrong change, do you assume he's probably trying to cheat you?
12. If someone doesn't show up on time, do you find yourself planning the angry words you're going to say?

To gauge your level of hostility, add up your yes responses. If you scored three or less, consider yourself one cool cucumber. A score of four to eight is a warning sign that anger may be raising your risk of heart disease. A score of nine or more puts you squarely in the hot zone for hostility, significantly increasing your risk of dying prematurely.

THE CURE

A few simple strategies can cool down even the hottest temper. First, when you feel yourself getting angry, stop long enough to ask yourself three questions: Is this really serious enough to get worked up over? Am I justified in getting angry? And is getting angry going to make any difference? If the answer to all three is yes, experts say, go ahead and get mad—it just might make you feel better. If not—if the answer to any of the questions is no—cool out. Often, just asking reasonable questions is enough to take the edge off anger. But if you're still simmering, distract yourself by picking up a magazine, turning on music, taking a walk. Or simply close your eyes and concentrate on your breathing. —*Peter Jaret*

Go Ahead, Say You're Sorry

We tend to view apologies as a sign of weak character. But in fact, they require great strength. And we better learn how to get them right, because it's increasingly hard to live in the global village without them.

Aaron Lazare, M. D.

Aaron Lazare, M. D., is chancellor/dean of the University of Massachusetts Medical Center in Worcester. He has authored 66 articles and written or edited six books.

A genuine apology offered and accepted is one of the most profound interactions of civilized people. It has the power to restore damaged relationships, be they on a small scale, between two people, such as intimates, or on a grand scale, between groups of people, even nations. If done correctly, an apology can heal humiliation and generate forgiveness.

Yet, even though it's such a powerful social skill, we give precious little thought to teaching our children how to apologize. Most of us never learned very well ourselves.

Despite its importance, apologizing is antithetical to the ever-pervasive values of winning, success, and perfection. The successful apology requires empathy and the security and strength to admit fault, failure, and weakness. But we are so busy winning that we can't concede our own mistakes.

The botched apology—the apology intended but not delivered, or delivered but not accepted—has serious social consequences. Failed apologies can strain relationships beyond repair or, worse, create life-long grudges and bitter vengeance.

As a psychiatrist who has studied shame and humiliation for eight years, I became interested in apology for its healing nature. I am perpetually amazed by how many of my friends and patients—regardless of ethnicity or social class—have long-standing grudges that have cut a destructive swath through their own lives and the lives of family and friends. So many of their grudges could have been avoided altogether or been reconciled with a genuine apology.

In my search to learn more about apologies, I have found surprisingly little in the professional literature. The scant research I've unearthed is mostly in linguistics and sociology, but little or nothing touches on the expectations or need for apologies, their meaning to the offender and offended, and the implications of their failure.

Religious writings, however, in both Christian and Jewish traditions, are a rich source of wisdom on the subject, under such headings as absolution, atonement, forgiveness, penance, and repentance. The *Talmud*, in fact, declares that God created repentance before he created the universe. He wisely knew humans would make a lot of mistakes and have a lot of apologizing to do along the way.

What makes apologies work is an exchange of shame and power between offender and offended.

No doubt the most compelling and common reason to apologize is over a personal offense. Whether we've ignored, belittled, betrayed, or publicly humiliated someone, the common denominator of any personal offense is that we've diminished or injured a person's self-concept. The self-concept is our story about ourselves. It's our thoughts and feelings about who we are, how we would like to be, and how we would like to be perceived by others.

If you think of yourself first and foremost as a competent, highly valued professional and are asked tomorrow by your boss to move into a cramped windowless office, you would likely be personally offended. You might be insulted and feel hurt or humiliated. No matter whether the interpersonal wound is delivered in a professional, family, or social setting, its depth is determined by the meaning the event carries to the offended party, the relationship between offender and offended, and the vulnerability of the offended to take things personally.

No-shows at family funerals, disputes over wills, betrayals of trust—whether in love or friendship—are situations ripe for wounds to the self-concept. Events of that magnitude put our self-worth on the line, more so for the thin-skinned. Other events people experience as personal offenses include being ignored, treated unfairly, embarrassed by someone else's behavior, publicly humiliated, and having one's cherished beliefs denigrated.

So the personal offense has been made, the blow to the self-concept landed, and an apology is demanded or expected. Why bother? I count four basic motives for apologizing:

- **The first is to salvage or restore the relationship.** Whether you've hurt someone you love, enjoy, or just plain need as your ally in an office situation, an apology may well rekindle the troubled relationship.
- **You may have purely empathic reasons for apologizing.** You regret that you have caused someone to suffer and you apologize to diminish or end their pain.

The last two motives are not so lofty:

- **Some people apologize simply to escape punishment,** such as the criminal who apologizes to his victim in exchange for a lesser plea.
- **Others apologize simply to relieve themselves of a guilty conscience.** They feel so ashamed of what they did that, even though it may not have bothered you that much, they apologize profusely. A long letter explaining why the offender was a half hour late to dinner would be such an occasion. And in so doing, they are trying to maintain some self-respect, because they are nurturing an image of themselves in which the offense, lack of promptness, violates some basic self-concept.

Whatever the motive, what makes an apology work is the exchange of shame and power between the offender and the offended. By apologizing, you take the shame of your offense and redirect it to yourself. You admit to hurting or diminishing someone and, in effect, say that you are really the one who is diminished—I'm the one who was wrong, mistaken, insensitive, or stupid. In acknowledging your shame you give the offended the power to forgive. The exchange is at the heart of the healing process.

ANATOMY OF AN APOLOGY

But in practice, it's not as easy as it sounds. There's a right way and a wrong way to apologize. There are several integral elements of any apology and unless they are accounted for, an apology is likely to fail.

First, you have to acknowledge that a moral norm or an understanding of a relationship was violated, and you have to accept responsibility for it. You must name the offense—no glossing over in generalities like, "I'm sorry for what I have done." To be a success, the apology has to be specific—"I betrayed you by talking behind your back" or "I missed your daughter's wedding."

You also have to show you understand the nature of your wrongdoing and the impact it had on the person—"I know I hurt you and I am so very sorry."

This is one of the most unifying elements of the apology. By acknowledging that a moral norm was violated, both parties affirm a similar set of values. The apology reestablishes a common moral ground.

The second ingredient to a successful apology is an explanation for why you committed the offense in the first place. An effective explanation makes the point that what you did isn't representative of who you are. You may offer that you were tired, sick, drunk, distracted, or in love—and that it will not happen again. Such an explanation protects your self-concept.

A recent incident widely reported in the news provides an excellent, if painful, illustration of the role of an apology in protecting the offender's self-concept. An American sailor apologized at his court-martial for brutally beating to death a homosexual shipmate: "I can't apologize enough for my actions. I am not trying to make any excuses for what happened that night. It was horrible, but I am not a horrible person."

Another vital part of the explanation is to communicate that your behavior wasn't intended as a personal affront. This lets the offended person know that he should feel safe with you now and in the future.

A good apology also has to make you suffer. You have to express genuine, soul-searching regret for your apology to be taken as sincere. Unless you communicate guilt, anxiety, and shame, people are going to question the depth of your remorse. The anxiety and sadness demonstrate that the potential loss of the relationship matters to you. Guilt tells the offended person that you're distressed over hurting him. And shame communicates your disappointment with yourself over the incident.

YOU OWE ME AN APOLOGY

When there's the matter of settling debt. The apology is a reparation of emotional, physical, or financial debt. The admission of guilt, explanation, and regret are meant, in part, to repair the damage you did to the person's self-concept. A well-executed apology may even the score, but sometimes words are just not enough. An open offer of, "Please let me know if there is anything I can do?" might be necessary. Some sort of financial compensation, such as replacing an object you broke, or reimbursing a friend for a show you couldn't make it to, could be vital to restoring the relationship. Or, in long-term close relationships, an unsolicited gift or favor may completely supplant the verbal apology—every other dimension of the apology may be implicit.

Reparations are largely symbolic. They are a way of saying, "I know who you are, what you value, and am thoughtful about your needs. I owe you." But they don't always have to be genuine to be meaningful. Say your boss wrongfully accused you in front of the whole office. A fair reparation would require an apology-in front of the whole office. His questionable sincerity might be of secondary importance.

Ultimately, the success of an apology rests on the dynamics between the two parties, not on a pat recipe. The apology is an interactive negotiation process in which a deal has to be struck that is emotionally satisfactory to both involved parties.

Nor is the need for an apology confined to intimates. Used strategically, it has great social value within the public domain. The apology is, after all, a social contract of sorts. It secures a common moral ground, whether between two people or within a nation. Present in all societies, the apology is a statement that the harmony of the group is more important than the victory of the individual. Take a look at what will certainly go down in history as one of the world's greatest apologies, F.W. de Klerk's apology to all South Africans for his party's imposition of apartheid.

A successful apology also has to make you suffer. You must express soul-searching regret.

On April 29, 1993, during a press conference, de Klerk *acknowledged* that apartheid led to forced removals of people from their homes, restrictions on their freedom and jobs, and attacks on their dignity.

He *explained* that the former leaders of the party were *not vicious people* and, at the time, it seemed that the policy of separate nations was better than the colonial policies. "It was not our intention to deprive people of their rights and to cause misery, but eventually apartheid led to just that. Insofar as that occurred, we deeply regret it."

"*Deep regret,*" de Klerk continued, "goes further than just saying you are sorry. Deep regret says that if I could turn the clock back, and if I could do anything about it, I would have liked to have avoided it."

4. RELATING TO OTHERS

In going on to describe a new National Party logo, he said: "It is a statement that we have broken with that which was wrong in the past and are not afraid to say we are deeply sorry that our past policies were wrong." He promised that the National Party had scrapped apartheid and opened its doors to all South Africans.

De Klerk expressed all the same ingredients and sentiments essential in interpersonal apologies. He enumerated his offenses and explained why they were made. He assured himself and others that the party members are not vicious people. Then he expressed deep regret and offered symbolic reparations in the form of his public apology itself and the new party logo.

In fact, as the world becomes a global village, apologies are growing increasingly important on both national and international levels. Communications, the media, and travel have drawn the world ever closer together. Ultimately we all share the same air, oceans, and world economy. We are all upwind, downstream, over the mountains, or through the woods from one another. We can't help but be concerned with Russia's failing economy, Eastern Bloc toxic waste, Middle Eastern conflicts, and the rain forest, whether it be for reasons of peace, fuel, or just plain oxygen.

In this international community, apologies will be vital to peaceful resolution of conflicts. Within the last several years alone Nelson Mandela apologized for atrocities committed by the African National Congress in fighting against apartheid; Exxon for the *Valdez* spill; Pope John Paul II "for abuses committed by Christian colonizers against Indian peoples"; former Japanese Prime Minister Morihiro Hosokawa for Japanese aggression during World War II; and Russian President Boris Yeltsin apologized for the massacre of 15,000 Polish army officers by Soviet forces during World War II. And that's only the start of it.

But apologies are useful only if done right. There are in the public arena ample examples of what not to do—stunning portraits of failed apologies. They typically take the form of what I call "the pseudoapology"—the offender fails to admit or take responsibility for what he has done. Recent history furnishes two classics of the genre.

Reel back to August 8, 1974—President Richard Nixon's resignation speech. "I regret deeply any injuries that may have been done in the course of events that have led to this decision. I would say only that if some of my judgments were wrong, and some were wrong, they were made in what I believed at the time to be in the best interest of the nation." Unlike de Klerk, Nixon never acknowledges or specifies his actual offense, nor does he describe its impact. By glossing over his wrongdoing he never takes responsibility for it.

Consider, too, the words of Senator Bob Packwood, who was accused of sexually harassing at least a dozen women during his tenure in Congress. His 1994 apology outfails even Nixon's: "I'm apologizing for the conduct that it was alleged that I did." No acceptance of responsibility or accounting for his alleged offense to be found. An *alleged* apology, not even named.

'The apology is a show of strength. It's an act of generosity, because it restores the self-concept of those we offended.'

The most common cause of failure in an apology—or an apology altogether avoided—is the offender's pride. It's a fear of shame. To apologize, you have to acknowledge that you made a mistake. You have to admit that you failed to live up to values like sensitivity, thoughtfulness, faithfulness, fairness, and honesty. This is an admission that our own self-concept, our story about ourself, is flawed. To honestly admit what you did and show regret may stir a profound experience of shame, a public exposure of weakness. Such an admission is especially difficult to bear when there was some degree of intention behind the wrongdoing.

Egocentricity also factors into failed or avoided apologies. The egocentric is unable to appreciate the suffering of another person; his regret is that he is no longer liked by the person he offended, not that he inflicted harm. That sort of apology takes the form of "I am sorry that you are upset with me" rather than "I am sorry I hurt you." This offender simply says he is bereft—not guilty, ashamed, or empathic.

Another reason for failure is that the apology may trivialize the damage incurred by the wrongdoing—in which case the apology itself seems offensive. A Japanese-American who was interned during World War II was offended by the U.S. government's reparation of $20,000. He said that the government stole four years of his childhood and now has set the price at $5,000 per year.

Timing can also doom an apology. For a minor offense such as interrupting someone during a presentation or accidentally spilling a drink all over a friend's suit, if you don't apologize right away, the offense becomes personal and grows in magnitude. For a serious offense, such as a betrayal of trust or public humiliation, an immediate apology misses the mark. It demeans the event. Hours, days, weeks, or even months may go by before both parties can integrate the meaning of the event and its impact on the relationship. The care and thought that goes into such apologies dignifies the exchange.

For offenses whose impact is calamitous to individuals, groups, or nations, the apology may be delayed by decades and offered by another generation. Case in point: The apologies now being offered and accepted for apartheid and for events that happened in WWII, such as the Japanese Imperial Army's apology for kidnapping Asian women and forcing them into a network of brothels.

Far and away the biggest stumbling block to apologizing is our belief that apologizing is a sign of weakness and an admission of guilt. We have the misguided notion we are better off ignoring or denying our offenses and hope that no one notices.

In fact the apology is a show of strength. It is an act of honesty because we admit we did wrong; an act of generosity, because it restores the self-concept of those we offended. It offers hope for a renewed relationship and, who knows, possibly even a strengthened one. The apology is an act of commitment because it consigns us to working at the relationship and at our self-development. Finally, the apology is an act of courage because it subjects us to the emotional distress of shame and the risk of humiliation, rejection, and retaliation at the hands of the person we offended.

All dimensions of the apology require strength of character, including the conviction that, while we expose vulnerable parts of ourselves, we are still good people.

The Heart and the Helix

When you're looking for love, are your chromosomes the compass?

JEFFREY KLUGER

FOR MOST PEOPLE, LEARNING THE ways of romance can be a tricky business. For me, it was even harder. On the whole, I blame Camp Comet.

Camp Comet, as the name suggests, was a "space age" summer camp established in the early 1960s, during the just-post-Sputnik era. The announced purpose of the place was to provide American boys with a better grounding in both sports and twentieth-century technologies so that they could better catch up with their presumably vigorous, presumably satellite-savvy Soviet counterparts. The thinking evidently was that if the United States was lagging behind in aerospace engineering, we could still thump the Russians but good in the cutting-edge fields of tetherball technology and moccasin switching.

What Camp Comet had to offer those of us who spent our summers there, however, was not science or sports or even the opportunity to pick on Edgar Weiner from the beginning of July to the end of August. What Camp Comet had to offer us was Camp Wohelo. Located on the opposite side of a moatlike lake, Camp Wohelo was a tantalizingly close all-girls' camp that, as a federal statute at the time apparently required, bore a vaguely Native American name.

For those of us on the boys' side of the watery divide, the presence of Camp Wohelo was, at best, a distraction. Put 200 boys with a median age of 15 anywhere near an equal number of girls, and you create a level of sexual tension that can be picked up on NORAD missile-tracking systems. To prevent a hormonal meltdown that would threaten at least three outlying counties, the elders of the two camps would periodically schedule what they called "socials"—highly elegant affairs in which the entire boys' camp, dressed in white T-shirts, blue shorts, and regulation penny loafers, would travel to the girls' camp for an evening of socializing.

For midteens, of course, socializing can be a clumsy business, and in general the hours the two camps spent together involved little more than a group of boys and a group of girls standing on opposite sides of a recreation hall while somebody played "Na Na Hey Hey (Kiss Him Goodbye)" on a Close' n' Play for two or three hours. Occasionally, one or two of my more courageous friends would ask one or two horrified girls to dance, but a 15-year-old male trying to lambada while dressed like the Campbell's Soup boy is not a pretty picture, and for most of the night the gulf between the two groups remained unbridgeable.

What effect, I've often wondered in the years since my last summer at camp, did such an awkward introduction to the art of romance have on me? Can a bad social in your early years make you *less* social in your later years? Do teenage romantic lessons determine adult romantic patterns? Is it our experiences that determine our courtship capabilities, our passion potential, or, as with other aspects of our personalities, is it our genes? Niels Waller and Phillip Shaver think they might know.

Waller and Shaver are psychologists at the University of California at Davis, and in 1990 they decided to study just what it is that makes some people lucky in love, while others are unable to locate Cupid with a Filofax and an E-mail address. The roots of human personality are elusive at best, however, and no one has ever determined whether it is nature or nurture that makes us the complicated beings we are. Nevertheless, over the years there *have* been some indications that our character dice are genetically cast before we even get into the game. Research has at least suggested that children born to depressive parents but raised by adoptive parents tend to grow up gloomy themselves. Similarly, shy parents often seem to produce equally diffident issue, hyperkinetic parents yield frantic issue, and even such obscure traits as vocational interests, social attitudes, and religiousness appear to be encoded in advance on the hard disk of our chromosomes. According to Waller and Shaver, however, love is the exception to this preordination rule.

4. RELATING TO OTHERS

"You would think that something this fundamental would have genetic roots," Waller says. "Every psychological variable I've studied has always had a strong heritable part. The fact that genes played almost no role is surprising."

WALLER AND SHAVER BEGAN THEIR exploration of the roots of romance five years ago by studying one of nature's most enduring curiosities: twins. If most of us give any thought at all to twins, it doesn't go much beyond Castor and Pollux, Patty and Cathy, and Harmon Killebrew. For geneticists and behavioral scientists, however, twins amount to nothing short of a walking control experiment.

Identical twins occur when a fertilized egg splits in two within the first 14 days after conception, creating a pair of viable zygotes and transforming an already cozy womb for one into a hopelessly cramped nine-month share. Since the two babies-to-be originate from the same egg and sperm, their genetic makeup is identical down to the last strand of DNA, and so too will be their eventual appearances and temperaments. Nature creates human twins sparingly, making these chromosomal carbon copies in only three out of every thousand births. While it's tempting to wish such fetal fission happened more often—imagine a scat-singing quartet made up of two Sarah Vaughans and a pair of Mel Tormés, or an FDR-FDR presidential ticket—it's probably just as well that it doesn't. Would you want to live in a world with a Stan and Ollie North able to commit perjury before both houses of Congress simultaneously? A Tad and Ted Koppel able to have two bad hair days on two networks at once? A Ringo and Bingo Starr *both* trying to sing?

More common than identical twins are fraternal twins, occurring in about eight out of every thousand births. Fraternal twins are created when two ova are released into the womb and are fertilized by two different sperm. Genetically, the siblings created by this most primal of double dates are no more alike than any other pair of brothers or sisters, sharing about 50 percent of the DNA that makes them who they are. Temperamentally, however, they're often quite similar. Spending your first nine months with a sibling who's in your face before you even *have* a face creates a closeness that defies measurement. After birth, the onetime wombmates often move through childhood in lockstep, going to the same schools, making the same friends, and generally forging a lifelong bond that makes the Smith Brothers look estranged.

Waller, like most behavioral psychologists, has long been fascinated by both types of twin—so much so that he has devoted a large part of his career to studying them. "My training was at the University of Minnesota, and I worked on twin studies there," he says. "When I moved to the University of California, I decided to create a twin registry out here. So far we have approximately 3,000 pairs of fraternal and identical twins on file, ranging in age from one day old to 92 years."

In their effort to crack the code of romance, Waller and Shaver figured this preexisting sibling list would be just the thing. If the courtship figure we cut depends more on our genes than our jeans, they figured, the identical twins in their directory should have fairly similar relationship patterns—far more alike certainly than those of fraternal twins. If the answer lies instead in what we learn, the siblings built from the same genetic schematic should be no more alike than the siblings built from two different ones.

In order to take their subjects' amorous measures, Waller and Shaver relied on a model created by psychologist J. A. Lee in 1988. Lee defined a number of romantic personality types, all of which are found in every one of us to different degrees and in different combinations. In a world in which women and men increasingly need the assistance of Madeleine Albright and a UN peacekeeping force before they can so much as meet for coffee, you would think we had enough interpersonal differences. Lee, however, insisted that things are even trickier than we dreamed, describing no fewer than six romantic temperaments, all of which take their names from the Greek, and each of which can make for a formidable dinner date. Composing Lee's role call of romantic temperaments are:

Eros: Enjoy intimacy, fall in love quickly, consider themselves hopeless romantics; least likely to believe in extended imprisonment for the person who wrote the lyric "Someone left the cake out in the rain."

Ludus: Prefer fun and excitement in relationships, often with multiple serial partners; consider no evening complete without an arraignment.

Storge: Value friendship, companionship, and reliable affection at the expense of passion. Sex symbols: Leon Panetta, Camilla Parker-Bowles.

Pragma: Highly pragmatic; enter relationships only if practical needs such as financial stability are met. Most likely to shop for lingerie in the Land's End catalog.

Agape: Consider other people's needs above their own; more oriented toward what they can give than what they can receive. Make excellent parents, grandparents, major-organ donors.

Manic: Desperate and conflicted about romance; yearn intensely for love but see it as a source of pain, jealousy, anxiety, and obsession. This category includes every species on the face of the planet with the exception of a few recently discovered arachnids.

Armed with these personality profiles, Waller and Shaver assembled a sample group of 345 pairs of identical twins and 100 pairs of fraternal twins. Additionally, they randomly selected the spouses of 172 of the individuals from both groups. All 1,062 subjects were then asked to complete two personality surveys. The first, designed specifically to measure romantic styles, required respondents to indicate whether they agreed or disagreed with such statements as "I fall in love at first sight," "I try to keep my partner uncertain about our commitment," and "I frequently fantasize about former directors of the Office of Management and Budget." The second questionnaire, intended to measure overall personality, elicited subjects' responses to a series of more general questions on everything from family relationships to job satisfaction to World Geography for $100.

All of this Q&A was expected to yield a lot, and in fact it did. To study gene-linked traits in any two family members, psychologists try to figure statistically how likely it is that a temperamental or physical characteristic that manifests itself in someone will also manifest itself in a close relative. The higher the number, the likelier it is that the trait is genetically based. Identical twins are 50 percent concordant for schizophrenia, for example—a probable sign that genes are involved—and 90 percent concordant for autism, an all-but-certain one. Absolute overlap of any characteristic is extremely rare, but on occasion it does occur. Large singing families from Salt Lake City, for example, appear to be 100 percent concordant for dirigible-size hairstyles; British royal families that can trace their lineage back before the Magna Carta seem genetically required to manifest the personality of couscous. In the case of love styles, things were not so clear.

Tallying their data, Waller and Shaver found that on a number of scales, identical twins were not only not very similar to each other but were actually less similar than fraternal twins. For psychologists, this kind of finding is the reddest of red flags, indicating that genes play a small role, if any, in a behavior being studied. In the Storge category, for example, the responses to the questionnaires suggested that only 11 percent of the similarities or differences between any two twins—whether identical or fraternal—was attributable to their genes; the rest was attributable to experiences that had occurred after birth. In the Pragma group, the heritability was even lower, factoring out to just 8 percent; in Eros, it was only 5.

Low as these numbers were, Waller and Shaver were even more surprised when they computed the results from the Ludus and Agape categories, in which the genetic component was just about zero. The only time the researchers saw any significant overlap at all was when they looked at the figures from the Manic group. As the apparent heritability of depression, obsessive-compulsiveness, and other psychological conditions suggests, emotional disorders may be bequeathed to us, at least in part, by our chromosomes. The Manic group, characterized by anxiety, unpredictability, and conflict, seemed to confirm this, with a comparatively high figure of 17 percent.

If the majority of non-Manic twins seemed to have almost nothing romantically in common, however, spouses turned out to be quite another story. Members of even the most incompatible couples can be surprisingly similar, with many husbands and wives finding that they can predict each other's thoughts, finish each other's sentences, and occasionally pose for each other's driver's license photos. To be sure, this is not always a good thing. If you're Mrs. Sam Nunn, you may not *want* to think that you're destined to develop the charisma of a saltine. If you're Mrs. Sam Donaldson, you may not *want* Leonard Nimoy's eyebrows. While these traits may or may not be shared by partners, love styles clearly are.

"Our study," Waller says, "shows that people do pick their mates based on love styles." Using a statistical correlation formula in which higher numbers indicate greater temperamental similarity and lower numbers indicate less, Waller and Shaver compared spouses' romantic personalities as well as other shared traits. Measuring, for example, husbands' and wives' sense of general well-being, the researchers came up with a low correlation figure—only .04. Measuring social effectiveness, they came up with a similarly modest .05. In love styles, however, things were much closer, with the Eros trait, for example, showing a .36 correlation, Pragma a .29, and Storge a .22. This phenomenon, Waller explains professorially, is known as assortative mating and shows, he adds more folksily, "that birds of a feather choose each other."

Persuasive as Waller and Shaver's findings are, of course, they are by no means conclusive. Just because environment trounces heredity in this round of the love wars doesn't mean that the mystery of human romance is solved, and other researchers armed with other methods will no doubt continue to seek other answers. What is it, for example, that makes a man on a first date think that a woman wants to spend at least 20 minutes listening to his imitation of Sonny Corleone? What is it that makes a woman think that the sixtieth minute of the seventh game of the Knicks-Bulls playoff is the right time to begin discussing caulking the guest bathroom? What is it that makes a couple as a whole think that a living room full of party guests really *hoped* to see their upholstery swatches? Until these questions are answered, romance science will remain incomplete. *Le coeur* may have *ses raisons*, but a good research grant wouldn't hurt either.

> **What makes some people lucky in love, while others can't locate Cupid with a Filofax?**

BACK OFF!

We're putting way too many expectations on our closest relationships. It's time to retreat a bit. Consider developing same-sex friendships. Or cultivating a garden. Whatever you do, take a break from the relentless pursuit of intimacy.

Geraldine K. Piorkowski, Ph.D.

You can't miss it. It's the favorite topic of Oprah and all the other talk shows. It's the suds of every soap opera. And I probably don't have to remind you that it's the subject of an extraordinary number of self-help books. Intimate relationships. No matter where we tune or turn, we are bombarded with messages that there is a way to do it right, certainly some way of doing it better—if only we could find it. There are countless books simply on the subject of how to communicate better. Or, if it's not working out, to exit swiftly.

We are overfocused on intimate relationships, and I question whether our current preoccupation with intimacy isn't unnatural, not entirely in keeping with the essential physical and psychological nature of people. The evidence suggests that there is a limit to the amount of closeness people can tolerate and that we need time alone for productivity and creativity. Time alone is necessary to replenish psychological resources and to solidify the boundaries of the self.

All our cultural focus on relationships ultimately has, I believe, a negative impact on us. It causes us to look upon intimate relationships as a solution to all our ills. And that only sets us up for disappointment, contributing to the remarkable 50 percent divorce rate.

Our overfocus on relationships leads us to demand too much of intimacy. We put all our emotional eggs in the one basket of intimate romantic relationships. A romantic partner must be all things to us—lover, friend, companion, playmate, and parent.

We approach intimate relationships with the expectation that this new love will make up for past letdowns in life and love. The expectation that this time around will be better is bound to disappoint, because present-day lovers feel burdened by demands with roots in old relationships.

We expect unconditional love, unfailing nurturance, and protection. There is also the expectation that the new partner will make up for the characteristics we lack in our own personality—for example, that he or she will be an outgoing soul to compensate for our shyness or a goal-oriented person to provide direction in our messy life.

If the personal ads were rewritten to emphasize the emotional expectations we bring to intimacy, they would sound like this. "WANTED: Lively humorous man who could bring joy to my gloomy days and save me from a lifetime of depression." Or, "WANTED: Woman with self-esteem lower than mine. With her, I could feel superior and gain temporary boosts of self-confidence from the comparison."

From my many years as a clinical psychologist, I have come to recognize that intimacy is not an unmitigated good. It is not only difficult to achieve, it is treacherous in some fundamental ways. And it can actually harm people.

The potential for emotional pain and upset is so great in intimate relationships because we are not cloaked in the protective garb of maturity. We are unprotected, exposed, vulnerable to hurt; our defenses are down. We are wide open to pain.

Intuitively recognizing the dangers involved, people normally erect elaborate barriers to shield themselves from closeness. We may act superior, comical, mysterious, or super independent because we fear that intimacy will bring criticism, humiliation, or betrayal—whatever an earlier relationship sensitized us to. We develop expectations based on what has happened in our lives with parents, with friends, with a first love. And we often act in anticipation of these expectations, bringing about the result we most want to avoid.

The closer we get to another person, the greater the risks of intimacy. It's not just that we are more vulnerable and defenseless. We are also more emotionally unstable, childish, and less intelligent than in any other situation. You may be able to run a large company with skill and judgment, but be immature, ultrasensitive, and needy at home. Civilized rules of conduct often get suspended. Intimacy is both unnerving and baffling.

HEALTHY RETREATS

Once our fears are aroused in the context of intimacy, we tend to go about calming them in unproductive ways. We make excessive demands of our partner, for affection, for unconditional regard. The trouble is, when people feel demands are being made of them, they tend to retreat and hide in ways that hurt their partner. They certainly do not listen.

Fears of intimacy typically limit our vulnerability by calling defensive strategies into play. Without a doubt, the defense of choice against the dangers of intimacy is withdrawal. Partners tune out. One may retreat into work. One walks out of the house, slamming the door. Another doesn't call for days. Whatever the way, we spend a great deal of time avoiding intimacy.

After many years of working with all kinds of couples, I have come to believe that human nature dictates that intimate relationships have to be cyclical.

When one partner unilaterally backs off, it tends to be done in a hurtful manner. The other partner feels rejected, uncared about, and unloved. Typically, absolutely nothing gets worked out.

However, avoidance is not necessarily unhealthy. Partners can pursue a time out, where one or both work through their conflict in a solitary way that is ultimately renewing. What usually happens, however, is that when partners avoid each other, they are avoiding open warfare but doing nothing to resolve the underlying conflicts.

Fears of intimacy can actually be pretty healthy, when they're realistic and protective of the self. And they appear even in good relationships. Take the fears of commitment that are apt to surface in couples just before the wedding. If they can get together and talk through their fears, then they will not scare one another or themselves into backing off permanently.

After many years of working with all kinds of couples, I have come to believe that human nature dictates that intimate relationships have to be cyclical. There are limitations to intimacy and I think it is wise to respect the dangers. Periods of closeness have to be balanced with periods of distance. For every two steps forward, we often need to take one step back.

An occasional retreat from intimacy gives individuals time to recharge. It offers time to strengthen your sense of who you are. Think of it as constructive avoidance. We need to take some emphasis off what partners can do for us and put it on what we can do for ourselves and what we can do with other relationships. Developing and strengthening same-sex friendships, even opposite-sex friendships, has its own rewards and aids the couple by reducing the demands and emotional expectations we place on partners.

In our culture, our obsession with romantic love relationships has led us to confuse all emotional bonds with sexual bonds, just as we confuse infatuation with emotional intimacy. As a result, we seem to avoid strong but deeply rewarding emotional attachments with others of our own sex. But having recently lost a dear friend of several decades, I am personally sensitive to the need for emotionally deep, same-sex relationships. They can be shared as a way of strengthening gender identity and enjoying rewarding companionship. We need to put more energy into nonromantic relationships as well as other activities.

One of the best ways of recharging oneself is to take pleasure in learning and spiritual development. And there's a great deal to be said for spending time solving political, educational, or social ills of the world.

Distance and closeness boundaries need to be calibrated and constantly readjusted in every intimate relationship. Such boundaries not only vary with each couple, they change as the relationship progresses. One couple may maintain their emotional connection by spending one evening together a week, while another couple needs daily coming together of some sort. Problems arise in relationships when partners cannot agree on the boundaries. These boundaries must be jointly negotiated or the ongoing conflict will rob the relationship of its vitality.

S.O.S. SIGNALS

When you're feeling agitated or upset that your partner is not spending enough time with you, consider it a signal to step back and sort out internally what is going on. Whether you feel anxiety or anger, the emotional arousal should serve as a cue to back off and think through where the upset is coming from, and to consider whether it is realistic.

That requires at least a modest retreat from a partner. It could be a half hour, or two hours. Or two days—whenever internal clarity comes. In the grip of emotion, it is often difficult to discriminate exactly which emotion it is and what its source is. "What is it I am concerned about? Is this fear realistic considering Patrick's behavior in the present? He's never done this to me before, and he's been demonstrating his trustworthiness all over the place, so what am I afraid of? Is it coming from my early years of neglect with two distant parents who never had time for me? Or from my experiences with Steve, who dumped me two years ago?"

Introspective and self-aware people already spend their time thinking about how they work, their motives, what their feelings mean. Impulsive people will have a harder time with the sorting-out process. The best way to sort things out is to pay attention to the nature of the upset. Exactly what you are upset about suggests what your unmet need is, whether it's for love, understanding, nurturance, protection, or special status. And once you identify the need, you can figure out its antecedents.

The kinds of things we get upset about in intimacy tend to follow certain themes. Basically, we become hurt or resentful because we're getting "too much" or "too little" of something. Too many demands, too much criticism, too much domination. Or the converse, too little affectional, conversational, or sexual attention (which translates into "you don't feel I'm important" or "you don't love me"). Insufficient empathy is usually voiced as "you don't understand me," and too little responsibility translates into failure to take on one's share of household and/or financial tasks. All these complaints require some attention, action, or retreat.

4. RELATING TO OTHERS

SHIFTING GEARS

It's not enough to identify the source of personal concern. You have to present your concerns in a way your partner can hear. If I say directly to my partner, "I'm afraid you're going to leave me," he has the opportunity to respond, "Darling, that's not true. What gave you that idea?" I get the reassurance I need. But if I toss it out in an argument, in the form of "you don't care about me," then my partner's emotional arousal keeps him from hearing me. And he is likely to back away—just when I need reassurance most.

If people were aware that intimate relationships are by nature characterized by ambivalence, they would understand the need to negotiate occasional retreats. They wouldn't feel so threatened by the times when one partner says, "I have to be by myself because I need to think about my life and where I'm going." Or "I need to be with my friends and spend time playing." If people did more backing off into constructive activities, including time to meditate or to play, intimate relationships would be in much better shape today.

If couples could be direct about what they need, then the need for retreat would not be subject to the misrepresentation that now is rampant. The trouble is, we don't talk to each other that openly and honestly. What happens is, one partner backs off and doesn't call and the partner left behind doesn't know what the withdrawal means. But he or she draws on a personal history that provides room for all sorts of negative interpretations, the most common being "he doesn't care about me."

No matter how hard a partner tries to be all things to us, gratifying all of another's needs is a herculean task—beyond the human calling. Criticism, disappointment, and momentary rejection are intrinsic parts of intimate life; developing a thicker skin can be healthy. And maintaining a life apart from the relationship is necessary. Energy invested in other people and activities provides a welcome balance.

GOOD-ENOUGH INTIMACY

Since our intimate partner will never be perfect, what is reasonable to expect? The late British psychiatrist D. W. Winnicott put forth the idea of "good-enough mothering." He was convinced that mothering could never be perfect because of the mother's own emotional needs. "Good-enough mothering" refers to imperfect, though adequate provision of emotional care that is not damaging to the children.

In a similar vein, I believe there is a level of imperfect intimacy that is good enough to live and grow on. In good-enough intimacy, painful encounters occasionally occur, but they are balanced by the strength and pleasures of the relationship. There are enough positives to balance the negatives. People who do very well in intimate relationships don't have a perfect relationship, but it is good enough.

The standard of good-enough intimacy is essentially subjective, but there are some objective criteria. A relationship must have enough companionship, affection, autonomy, connectedness, and separateness, along with some activities that partners engage in together and that they both enjoy. The relationship meets the needs of both partners reasonably well enough, both feel reasonably good about the relationship. If one person is unhappy in the relationship, then by definition it is not good enough for them.

People looking for good-enough intimacy are bound to be happier than those seeking perfect intimacy. Their expectations are lower and more realistic. Time and time again, those who examine the intricacies of happiness have found the same thing—realistic expectations are among the prime contributors to happiness.

Preventing Failure in Intimate Relationships

Disrespect, mistrust, and alienation can create a brick wall between a couple. Forgiveness can tear it down.

J. Earl Thompson Jr.

Dr. Thompson is professor of pastoral psychology and family studies, Andover Newton Theological School, Newton Centre, Mass.

WE LIVE in a time when domestic violence is rampant and divorce is common. Every 15 seconds, according to the FBI, a woman is battered by her husband or lover. Domestic abuse is the leading cause of injury to women and accounts for more physical harm to them than automobile accidents, rape, and muggings combined. A conservative estimate is that at least 20% of the women in the U.S. are likely to be the victims of severe violence at the hands of men at least once in their lifetimes, a figure that has remained constant for the last decade.

One-half of first and 60% of second marriages end in divorce. Why does love turn sour? What causes marriages to fail? What factors lead to couple disaffection and the breakdown of committed relationships? Why is there so much violence in intimate relationships? Is there any hope for people to create and sustain non-violent relationships that animate and fulfill them?

Fascination with the dynamics of intimate relationships is rife. There is a veritable flood of popular and scholarly books, articles, and TV talk shows about family and couple relationships. Self-proclaimed relationship gurus claim to have the answer to what makes for a good marriage. The degree of concern with this subject seems to be a direct response to the spread of domestic violence and the breakdown of marriages in American society, one which seldom has been grounded in and informed by solid empirical research.

A lot more is known about why intimate relationships fail than in the past. Then, knowledge about marital disaffection was based mainly upon ideological convictions, clinical intuition, structured interviews, or surveys. Thanks to researchers such as cognitive-behavioral psychologist John Gottman and sociologists of emotions Suzanne Retzinger and Thomas Scheff, there now is a trustworthy foundation of empirical evidence that solves many of the puzzles and clarifies much of the confusion about the causes of alienation and even violence in couple relationships.

Gottman studied 2,000 couples over 20 years and followed 484 of them for as long as a decade. While doing laboratory interviewing of the couples about neutral, positive, and negative topics, he measured electronically their psysiological responses (heart rate, blood-flow rate, perspiration, and the presence of stress-related hormones in the urine and blood). Then, he followed up these interviews with questionnaires and conversations to determine what the spouses were thinking and feeling during the interviews and what they imagine their partners were thinking and feeling. He also used questionnaires and conducted an oral history about the state of their marriage through the years.

Gottman discovered that "human relationships, like other natural processes, are not random and unknowable, but appear to obey certain laws." In the face of popular misconceptions about what undermines relationships, he argues that there are four variables that, by themselves, do not lead to the failure of relationships and predict divorce. First, couples who create a volatile relationship characterized by a lot of conflict and anger do not necessarily end up divorced. Indeed, constructive anger focused on a particular issue and expressed without contempt or criticism is healthy, perhaps even necessary. It acts a lot like "spice that keeps the relationship from going flat." Gottman maintains that "blunt, straightforward anger seems to immunize marriages against deterioration."

Second, the other side of this coin is equally true. Couples who tend to minimize or avoid conflict at all costs do not face the inevitable breakdown of their marriages.

Third, couple incompatibility regarding central issues such as religion, politics, and the use of money does not lead to marital dissolution either. What is crucial is the way in which the spouses manage their incompatibilities.

Finally, sexual differences do not in themselves unravel marriages. Gottman found out that, in satisfying marriages, there are virtually no gender differences in the expression of emotions and that men who do housework are more likely "to be more happily engaged and involved in their marriages than men who did not, and less lonely, less stressed, and less likely to be sick four years" after his initial interviews of them.

What does lead to the dissolution of relationships and predicts divorce are what he calls the "Four Horsemen of the Apocalypse," a set of behaviors which attack and destroy the bonds of affection, trust, and commitment. These enemies are excessive criticism of the partner, defensiveness in the face of the partner's dissatisfactions and complaints, emotionally withdrawing and isolating oneself from one's partner (stonewalling), and contempt expressed verbally and nonverbally.

What is indispensable for the well-being of a couple's relationship and a lasting marriage is an "emotional ecological balance" that includes five positive emotional interactions to every one negative interchange. If a couple can create this sort of balance between their positive and negative interactions, they can weather conflict, anger, boredom, incompatibilities, and sexual problems.

From a different perspective, Scheff and Retzinger have come up with a remarkably

4. RELATING TO OTHERS

similar conclusion. Their method was to videotape interviews with couples and subject these interviews to a sequential analysis of the spouses' discourse. The couple was asked to discuss three topics, each for 15 minutes: something neutral like the events of the day; an issue about which they frequently argue; and activities they enjoy doing as a couple. Using verbal, nonverbal, and visual cues, the researchers sought to infer the emotions communicated by the couple.

Scheff and Retzinger contend that the strength and vitality of the social bond between persons in an intimate relationship depends upon the extent of healthy or genuine pride awakened in the relationship. The opposite of genuine pride is shame (Gottman's "contempt"). Attention to the condition of the social bond can not be optional, for the social bond is being strengthened, maintained, repaired, or weakened in every transaction. The emotions of genuine pride or shame are triggered in every interaction and signal the state of the social bond.

Partners communicate something about the other's worth by means of every word, gesture, facial expression, and action. When partners understand and acknowledge each other's "thoughts, feelings, and actions" as well as their "intentions and character," they increase healthy pride in each other and build secure bonds. When spouses misunderstand, fail to "ratify," and reject each other, they awaken shame in each other and damage their social bond.

Positive emotional messages strengthen the couple's solidarity, increase cooperation between them, and make for clear and unambiguous communication. In sharp contrast, critical, judgmental, and humiliating interactions lead to unremitting conflict, distorted, confused communication, and alienation.

Scheff and Retzinger agree with Gottman that anger and conflict in and of themselves are not injurious to lasting marriages. They go one step beyond him with their assertion that anger usually is the way people defend themselves against the shame activated by the interaction. Shame and anger go hand in hand. What leads to alienation and often domestic violence is that the shame is not acknowledged and the consequent alienation is not dealt with.

Couples frequently get swept up in shame-rage spirals that can escalate to physical violence. What causes marital breakdown is the couple's unwillingness or inability to address their shame and alienation and repair their damaged or severed emotional bond. The viability and permanence of a committed relationship hinges upon whether persons can acknowledge and resolve humiliating interactions.

Criticism, defensiveness, stonewalling, and contemptuous or shaming encounters attack the bonds of marriage and leave attachments fractured or broken. What is common to the first three of those negative behaviors is that they trigger shame. Of the "Four Horsemen," shame is the most deadly.

Shame is the most hurtful and debilitating of all emotions, "an inner torment" and "sickness of the soul," according to psychologist Silvan Tomkins. When people feel terrible about themselves in America's culture of narcissism, they are more likely to experience shame, not guilt. Shame is the companion to narcissistic injury. Exposing the self to itself, shame illuminates our profound alienation from ourselves and others. What this emotion discloses to us is our defectiveness, deficiency, inadequacy, unworthiness, weakness, and sense of failure. In addition, shame involves not only sobering self-exposure, but exposure of the self to others. Shame is a negative evaluation of the self from the perspective of others, "a vicarious experience of the other's scorn." No wonder this "affect of inferiority" is so corrosive to marriages.

> *"Criticism, defensiveness, stonewalling, and contemptuous or shaming encounters attack the bonds of marriage and leave attachments fractured or broken."*

Not all shame erodes intimate social bonds; only unacknowledged shame does. Indeed, a certain amount of shame is inevitable in close relationships. Marriages fail when couples can not identify their own shame reactions, do not recognize or admit that they are humiliating each other, and do not communicate about it. In turn, unacknowledged shame triggers rage, leading to intractable conflict and, all too often, domestic violence.

What can repair and renew damaged social bonds? What can revitalize intimate relationships when the partners have become estranged, embittered, and hopeless? What can restore respect, trust, and affection after alienation has set in? What is powerful enough to heal the wounds of shame? The answer is forgiveness.

This claim is not accepted universally. Psychologists Michael McCullough and Everett Worthington, Jr., argue convincingly that, despite extensive research, there is insufficient empirical data "to conclude that forgiving has any clear physical or psychological benefits." Nor is the weight of therapeutic practice on the side of endorsing the value or utility of forgiveness in therapy. Neither secular nor religious counselors make extensive use of forgiveness techniques in their work. There is scant social scientific evidence that forgiveness actually reduces negative effects and none that it enhances a sense of well-being, leaving a dilemma wherein it is known what leads to social alienation and relationship failure, but not what transforms estranged relationships.

For their part, Gottman, Retzinger, and Scheff neither rule out forgiveness as an answer to marital breakdown nor make any claims for it. Yet, most individuals can attest from experience to the power of an apology and the offer of forgiveness to heal interpersonal injuries and repair fractured social bonds. Until more empirical research is done on forgiveness, it will be necessary to trust the wisdom that comes from religious traditions, clinical insights, and personal experiences informed by reason, intuition, and common sense.

What is forgiveness? The dictionary defines it as giving up resentment, vengeful feelings, and all claims to punishment. How do people forgive when the natural thing to do when they have been hurt and humiliated is to retaliate and settle the score? Can forgiveness really transform estranged relationships? Is it always safe to forgive? At the heart of the Judaeo-Christian tradition is the belief that God is a god of forgiveness who requires believers to forgive those who have betrayed, rejected, injured, and therefore shamed them. This tradition claims that forgiveness can resolve anger, resentment, and shame and reconcile damaged relationships. Of course, this is a value commitment and has not yet been *proven* by social scientific research.

From a psychological perspective, the most compelling and cogent expositions of forgiveness have been to approach it in terms of a series of stages. A case in point is the work of family therapist Terry Hargrave. He asserts that forgiveness is an arduous process that incorporates two stages: exoneration and overt forgiveness. Exoneration—setting someone free from the blame of wrongdoing—involves insight and understanding.

Insight identifies what concrete behaviors actually caused the injury, the extent of the damage, and who is responsible. It clarifies the bases of powerful emotional reactions of fear, shame, and anger when someone has been harmed, and it aids in protecting oneself by setting limits to further injury at the hands of the perpetrator of the hurt. Insight also can function as an effective restraint against retaliation and inflicting injury upon someone else.

Understanding opens the door to a greater

comprehension of the offender's position, limitations, development, efforts, and intent. Individuals are able to comprehend better what led the offender to injure and humiliate them. The work of exoneration empowers people to hold the offender responsible and accountable for his or her actions while enabling them to identify with the offender's flawed humanity since they, too, have been or could be the inflictor of injury upon others. Hargrave claims that understanding can lessen the tendency to blame either the offender or ourselves, and therefore can dilute pain and shame.

Not everyone will move to the next phase of overt forgiveness. For whatever reasons, some will conclude that the broken relationship is not worth repairing or can not be restored. The injured individual could conclude that the offender is unable or unwilling to make amends and change his or her ways; therefore, it is not safe to move to the next phase. In this case, the person offended could decide that he or she is unwilling to make himself or herself vulnerable even in small, measured ways to the offender.

Overt forgiveness has two parts. In the first, the injured person offers the offender opportunities to prove gradually that he or she can be trusted. The offender has to acknowledge his or her wrongdoing and take responsibility for it in a way that is congruent with the offended one's understanding of the injury. This surely will involve an apology by the wrongdoer and acceptance of it by the hurt one. The apology functions as a method or promise of restitution for the injustices of the past. This move is risky and could lead to more hurt and deeper alienation.

In part two, the one offended has to extend overt forgiveness to the person who has hurt him or her. The offended one, in effect, gives up any claim to injustice and moves beyond resentment and the desire to punish. For this to happen, both individuals have to want to overcome their alienation and restore a relationship of love, trust, and fairness.

Forgiveness is not the only force that can dilute or dissolve shame and repair and renew the "interpersonal bridge," but I believe it is the most powerful and effective means. Much more empirical research is needed to test this proposition, though. The way of forgiveness is not easy or likely to become popular and widespread. It requires a disciplined commitment to the value and belief that the most meaningful and enduring relationships thrive in this way of life.

Shame is a painful part of close relationships and can shatter intimate bonds if it is not acknowledged and processed. The most effective way to cope with shame and undercut its corrosive consequences is with disciplined forgiveness.

Patterns of Abuse

Two million women are beaten every year, one every 16 seconds. Who's at risk, why does violence escalate—and when should a woman fear for her life?

THE STORIES SPILL OUT FROM BEhind bedroom walls and onto the front pages. Back in 1983, before talk shows dissolved into daily confessionals, actor David Soul offered up the stunning admission that he'd abused his wife, Patti. Two years later, John Fedders, the chief regulator of the Securities and Exchange Commission, resigned after he acknowledged that he'd broken his wife's eardrum, wrenched her neck and left her with black eyes and bruises. In 1988, the nation sat mesmerized by Hedda Nussbaum and her testimony about being systematically beaten by her companion, a brooding New York lawyer named Joel Steinberg, who also struck the blows that killed their adopted daughter, Lisa. Now America is riveted again, this time by the accumulating evidence of O. J. Simpson's brutality against his wife, Nicole. Yet, for all the horror, there is a measure of futility in these tales: one moment, they ignite mass outrage; then the topic fades from the screen.

Americans often shrug off domestic violence as if it were no more harmful than Ralph Kramden hoisting a fist and threatening: "One of these days, Alice . . . Pow! Right in the kisser!" But there's nothing funny about it—and the phenomenon of abuse is just as complicated as it is common. About 1,400 women are killed by their husbands, ex-husbands and boyfriends each year and about 2 million are beaten—on average, one every 16 seconds. Although some research shows women are just as likely as men to start a fight, Justice Department figures released last February reveal that women are the victims 11 times more often than men. Battering is also a problem among gay couples: the National Coalition on Domestic Violence estimates that almost one in three same-sex relationships are abusive, seemingly more than among heterosexual couples. But violence against women is so entrenched that in 1992 the U.S. Surgeon General ranked abuse by husbands and partners as the leading cause of injuries to women aged 15 to 44. Despite more hot lines and shelters and heightened awareness, the number of assaults against women has remained about the same over the last decade.

A disturbing double standard also remains. "If O. J. Simpson had assaulted Al Cowlings nine times and if A.C. called the police, O.J. couldn't have told them, 'This is a family matter'," says Mariah Burton Nelson, author of the book "The Stronger Women Get the More Men Love Football." "Hertz and NBC would have dropped him and said, 'This man has a terrible problem.' But family violence is accepted as no big deal." New York University law professor Holly Maguigan says wife-beating was actually once sanctioned by the so-called Rule of Thumb—English common law, first cited in America in an 1824 Mississippi Supreme Court decision, that said a man could physically chastise his wife as long as the stick he used was no wider than his thumb. Even now, Maguigan says, "we're not very far removed from a time when the criminal-justice system saw its task as setting limits on the amount of force a man could use, instead of saying that using force against your wife is a crime."

Changing attitudes is difficult. Although advocacy groups are already claiming that Nicole Simpson's case can do for spousal abuse what Rock Hudson did for AIDS and Anita Hill did for sexual harassment, that may be more rhetoric than reality; there is great ambivalence about family violence. Americans cling to a "zone of privacy"—the unwritten code that a man's home is his castle and what happens inside should stay there. It helps explain why, in some states, a man who strikes his wife is guilty only of a misdemeanor, but if he attacks a stranger, it's a felony. It helps explain why a woman can walk away from a friend who says she got her black eye walking into a door. And it helps explain why men retreat when a buddy dismisses brutality as the ups and downs that "all" marriages go through.

So many look away because they don't know what constitutes domestic violence. Who's a victim? Who's an abuser? Most people believe that, unless a woman looks as pathetic as Hedda Nussbaum did—her nose flattened, her face swollen—she couldn't possibly be a victim. And despite highly publicized cases of abuse, celebrity still bestows credibility. What's more, it's hard for many to comprehend how anything short of daily brutality can be wife-beating. Even Nicole's sister fell into the trap. "My definition of a battered woman is somebody who gets beat up all the time," Denise Brown told The New York Times last week. "I don't want people to think it was like that. I know Nicole. She was a very strong-willed person. If she was beaten up, she wouldn't have stayed with him. That wasn't her." Or was it? The patterns of abuse—who's likely to be at risk, why women take action and when battering turns deadly—can often be surprising, as paradoxical as the fact that love can coexist with violence.

MICHELE INGRASSIA AND MELINDA BECK, WITH REPORTING BY GINNY CARROLL, NINA ARCHER BIDDLE, KAREN SPRINGEN, PATRICK ROGERS, JOHN MCCORMICK, JEANNE GORDON, ALLISON SAMUELS AND MARY HAGER.

WHO IS MOST AT RISK

EXPERTS USED TO THINK THAT BATTERED WOMEN WERE "asking for it"—somehow masochistically provoking abuse from their men. Mercifully, that idea has now been discredited. But researchers do say that women who are less educated, unemployed, young and poor may be more likely to have abusive relationships than others. Pregnant women seem to make particular targets: according to one survey, approximately one in six is abused; another survey cites one in three. There are other common characteristics: "Look for low self-esteem, a background in an abusive family, alcohol and drug abuse, passivity in relationships, dependency, isolation and a high need for approval, attention and affection," says psychologist Robert Geffner, president of the Family Violence and Sexual Assault Institute in Tyler, Texas. "The more risk factors a woman has, the more likely she is to become a candidate."

But not all women fit that profile: statistically, one woman in four will be physically assaulted by a partner or ex-partner during her lifetime, so it's not surprising that abuse cuts across racial, ethnic, religious and socioeconomic lines. "I'm treating physicians, attorneys, a judge and professors who are, or were, battered women," says Geffner. "Intelligent people let this happen, too. What goes on inside the home does not relate to what's outside."

And what's outside is often deceiving. Dazzling blond Nicole Simpson didn't look like someone who could have low self-esteem. But she met O.J. when she was just 18, and devoted herself to being his wife. In her 1992 divorce papers, she claimed that O.J. forced her to quit junior college and be with him all the time. She

Ten Risk Factors
Previous domestic violence is the highest risk factor for future abuse. Homes with two of these others show twice as much violence as those with none. In those with seven or more factors, the violence rate is 40 times higher.

- Male unemployed
- Male uses illicit drugs at least once each year
- Male and female have different religious backgrounds
- Male saw father hit mother
- Male and female cohabit and are not married
- Male has blue-collar occupation, if employed
- Male did not graduate from high school
- Male is between 18 and 30 years of age
- Male or female use severe violence toward children in home
- Total family income is below the poverty line

SOURCE: RISK-MARKERS OF MEN WHO BATTER, A 1994 ANALYSIS BY RICHARD J. GELLES, REGINA LACKNER AND GLENN D. WOLFNER

Striking a wife can be a misdemeanor while hitting a stranger is a felony

said she'd do anything to keep him from being angry: "I've always told O.J. what he wants to hear. I've always let him . . . it's hard to explain." For all their jet-setting, she was isolated—and reluctant to discuss what was happening at home, even though some friends say they had known. "She would wear unsuitable clothing to cover the bruises, or sunglasses to hide another shiner," says one. "She was trapped. She didn't have any training to do anything, and he knew that and he used it."

But even feisty women with their own careers can get involved with violent men. Earlier this month, Lisa (Left Eye) Lopes, a singer with the hip-hop group TLC, allegedly burned down the $800,000 home of her boyfriend, Atlanta Falcons' wide receiver Andre Rison. Police say the barely 5-foot, 100-pound Lopes appeared bruised and beaten when they arrived on the scene; friends say it was an open secret that she was abused. (Rison denies the allegations.) Curiously, the lyrics of Lopes's debut album are peppered with references about standing up to men: "I have my own control/I can't be bought or sold/ And I never have to do what I'm told . . ." Was that just a tough act to mask insecurity? Jacquelyn Campbell, a researcher in domestic violence at Johns Hopkins University, concludes that a woman's risk of being battered "has little to do with her and everything to do with who she marries or dates."

WHO BECOMES AN ABUSER

WHAT KIND OF MAN HEAPS PHYSICAL AND EMOTIONAL abuse on his wife? It's only in the last decade that researchers have begun asking. But one thing they agree on is the abuser's need to control. "There is no better way of making people compliant than beating them up on an intermittent basis," says Richard Gelles, director of the Family Violence Research Program at the University of Rhode Island. Although Gelles says men who have less education and are living close to the poverty line are more likely to be abusers, many white-collar men—doctors, lawyers and accountants—also beat their partners.

"Amy," a 50-year-old Colorado woman, spent 23 years married to one of them. Her husband was an attorney, well heeled, well groomed, a pillar of the community. She says he hit her, threw her down the stairs, tried to run her over. "One night in Vail, when he had one of his insane fits, the police came and put him in handcuffs," says Amy, who asked that her real name not be used. "My arms were still red from where he'd trapped them in the car window, but somehow, he talked his way out of it." Lenore Walker, director of the Domestic Violence Institute in Denver, sees the pattern all the time. "It's like Jekyll and Hyde—wonderful one minute, dark and terrifying the next."

Indiana University psychologist Amy Holtzworth-Munroe divides abusers into three behavioral types. The majority of men who hit their wives do so infrequently and their violence doesn't escalate. They look ordinary, and they're most likely to feel remorse after an attack. "When they use violence, it reflects some lack of communication skills, combined with a dependence on the wife," she says.

A second group of men are intensely jealous of their wives and fear abandonment. Most likely, they grew up with psychological and

4. RELATING TO OTHERS

sexual abuse. Like those in the first group, these men's dependence on their wives is as important as their need to control them—if she even talks to another man, "he thinks she's leaving or sleeping around," says Holtzworth-Munroe. The smallest—and most dangerous—group encompasses men with an antisocial personality disorder. Their battering fits into a larger pattern of violence and getting in trouble with the law. Neil S. Jacobson, a marital therapist at the University of Washington, likens such men to serial murderers. Rather than becoming more agitated during an attack, he says, they become calmer, their heart rates drop. "They're like cobras. They're just like criminals who beat up anybody else when they're not getting what they want."

For women aged 15 to 44, domestic abuse is the leading cause of injury

Men who batter share something else: they deny what they've done, minimize their attacks and always blame the victims. Evan Stark, codirector of the Domestic Violence Training Project in New Haven, Conn., was intrigued by Simpson's so-called suicide note. "He never takes responsibility for the abuse. These are just marital squabbles. Then he blames her—'I felt like a battered husband'." Twenty-nine-year-old "Fidel" once felt the same way. When he began getting counseling in Houston's Pivot Project, he blamed everyone else for his violence—especially his new wife, who, he discovered, was pregnant by another man. "When I came here, I couldn't believe I had a problem," he says. "I always thought of myself as a well-mannered person."

Avoiding Abuse

Battered women use a range of desperate methods to discourage partners from injuring them, from running away to fighting back.

STRATEGIES USED BY WOMEN TO END SEVERE SPOUSAL VIOLENCE

Avoid him or avoid certain topics	69%
Talking him out of it	59
Get him to promise no more violence	57
Threaten to get a divorce	54
Physically fight back	52
Hide or go away	37
Threaten to call the police	36
Leave home for two or more days	32

SOURCE: INTIMATE VIOLENCE, BY RICHARD J. GELLES AND MURRAY A. STRAUS (DATA FROM A 1985 STUDY)

STOPPING ABUSE: WHAT WORKS

Can a man who batters his partner learn to stop? Can psychotherapy turn an abuser into a respectful companion? Specialized treatment programs have proliferated in recent years, most of them aimed at teaching wife-beaters to manage their anger. But abusive men tend to resist treatment, and there are no proven formulas for reforming them. "We don't have any research that tells us any particular intervention is effective in a particular situation," says Eve Lipchik, a private therapist in Milwaukee. "We have nothing to go on."

Some abusers are less treatable than others. Researchers have identified a hard core, perhaps 10 to 20 percent, who seem beyond the reach of therapy. Experts differ on how best to handle the rest, but they agree that abusers shouldn't be coddled, even if they have grown up as victims themselves. "These men need to be confronted," says New York psychologist Matthew Campbell, who runs a treatment program in Suffolk County. "Giving them TLC just endangers women. The man has to take full responsibility. He has to learn to say, 'I can leave. I can express upset. But I cannot be abusive'."

Some therapists favor counseling abusers and victims as couples provided the beating has stopped and the relationship has a healthy dimension to build on. But couples therapy is controversial, especially among feminists. In fact, several states have outlawed it. "Couples therapy says to the victim, 'If you change, this won't happen'," says Campbell. "That's dangerous."

To avoid that message, most clinics deal exclusively with abusers, often having them confront each other in groups. During a typical session at Houston's Pivot Project, a private, not-for-profit counseling agency, batterers take

WHY WOMEN STAY

IT LOOKS SO SIMPLE FROM THE OUTSIDE. MANY WOMEN THINK that if a mate ever hit them, they'd pack up and leave immediately. But women who have been in abusive relationships say it isn't that easy. The violence starts slowly, doesn't happen every day and by the time a pattern has emerged there may be children, and financial and emotional bonds that are difficult to break. "I know when I took my marriage vows, I meant 'for better or for worse'," G. L. Bundow, a South Carolina physician, wrote in The Journal of the American Medical Association, describing her own abusive relationship. "But when 'until death do us part' suddenly became a frightening reality, I was faced with some terrifying decisions."

With more women working and greater availability of shelters, financial dependence is less of a factor than it used to be. The emotional dependence is often stronger. "Women are trained to think that we can save these men, that they can change," says Angela Caputi, a professor of American Studies at the University of New Mexico. That mythology, she notes, is on full display in "Beauty and the Beast": the monster smashing furniture will turn into a prince if only the woman he's trapped will love him.

Many abusers *can* be charming—and abused women often fall for their softer side. Denver's Lenore Walker says there are three parts to the abuse cycle that are repeat over and over—a phase where tension is building and the woman tries desperately to keep the man calm; an explosion with acute battering, and then a period where the batterer is loving and contrite. "During this last phase, they listen to the woman, pay attention, buy her flowers—they become the ideal guy," Walker says. Geffner adds that in this part of the relationship, "they make love, the sex is good. And that also keeps them going."

Eventually, however, the repeated cycles wear women down until some are so physically and mentally exhausted that leaving is almost impossible. The man gradually takes control of the woman's psyche and destroys her ability to think clearly. Even the memory of past

34. Patterns of Abuse

turns recounting the past week's conflicts. (As a reminder that women aren't property, the participants must refer to their partners by name. Anyone using the phrase "my wife" has to hold a stuffed donkey.) As each man testifies, his peers offer criticism. Therapist Toby Myers says one client recently boasted that he had avoided punching his wife by ramming his fist through a wall. Instead of praising him, a counselor asked the other participants what message the gesture had sent to the man's wife. A group member's reply: "It says she better be careful or she's next."

There's no question that such exercises can change men's behavior. At the Domestic Abuse Project in Minneapolis, follow-up studies suggest that two out of three clients haven't battered their partners 18 months after finishing treatment. Unfortunately, few abusers get that far. Only half of the men who register at the Abuse Project show up, even though most are under court orders. And only half of those who start treatment see it through.

Drug treatment may someday provide another tool. Preliminary findings suggest that Prozac-style antidepressants, which enhance a brain chemical called serotonin, help curb some men's aggressiveness. Neither counseling nor drug treatment is a cure-all. "We need psychological services," says Campbell, the New York psychologist. "But services mean nothing without sanctions. Men need to know that if they don't change, they'll go to jail."

Not every abuser is sensitive to that threat. Dr. Roland Maiuro, director of the Harborview Anger Management and Domestic Violence Program in Seattle, notes that some men simply become more bitter—and more dangerous—after they're arrested. But until treatment becomes a surer science, keeping those men behind bars may be the best way to keep their victims alive.

GEOFFREY COWLEY with GINNY CARROLL in Houston and bureau reports

abuse keeps the woman in fear and in check. "You can't underestimate the terror and brainwashing that takes place in battering relationships," says psychiatrist Elaine Carmen of the Solomon Carter Fuller Mental Health Center in Boston. "She really comes to believe that she deserves the abuse and is incompetent."

WHEN WOMEN TAKE ACTION

THE TURNING POINT MAY COME WHEN A WOMAN CAN NO longer hide the scars and bruises. Or when her own financial resources improve, when the kids grow up—or when she begins to fear for their safety. Sometimes, neighbors hear screaming and call police—or a doctor challenges a woman's made-up story about how she got those broken ribs. "There are different moments of truth," says psychiatrist Carmen. "Acting on them partly depends on how safe it is to get up and leave." Walker says that women decide to get help when the pain of staying in a relationship outweighs the emotional, sexual or financial benefits.

For "Emma," a bank teller, the final straw came the day she returned from work to find that her husband hadn't mowed the lawn as she asked. "You promised me you'd mow the lawn," she said, then dropped the issue. Later they were seated calmly on the couch, when suddenly he was standing on the coffee table, coming down on her with his fists. He beat her into the wall until plaster fell down. "I was dragged through the house by my hair. At some point I began thinking I don't want to live anymore. If it hadn't been for this tiny voice in the background saying, 'Mama, please don't die,' I would have surrendered." Emma finally crawled to the car but couldn't see to drive, so her grandmother took her to the emergency room, where the doctor didn't believe her story about being mugged. "He said, 'You're not fine. You're bleeding internally. You've got a concussion.' He got a mirror and showed me my face. I looked like a monster in a horror movie. It was the first time I recognized how bad things had gotten." For a while, though, life got even harder. "When I arrived in Chicago, I had two children, two suitcases and $1,500 in my pocket to start a new life." She found it running a coalition that provides shelter for more than 700 battered women.

When women do take action, it can run the gamut from calling a hot line, seeking counseling, filing for divorce or seeking a court order of protection. Often those measures soothe the abuser—but only temporarily. "They think he's changed. Then it starts three months later," says Chicago divorce attorney David Mattenson. Some women weaken, too: they may lock the doors, check the shadows—but still let him have the keys to the house. Emma herself briefly returned to her husband when he begged and pleaded. "The same week I went back, he was beating me again."

WHEN COPS AND COURTS STEP IN

BLUNTLY PUT, COPS HATE DOMESTIC CALLS—IN PART because they are so unpredictable. A neighbor may simply report a disturbance and cops have no idea what they will find on the scene. The parties may have cooled down and be sitting in stony silence. Or one may be holding the other hostage, or the kids. Sometimes, warring spouses even turn on cops—which is why many police forces send them in pairs and tell them to maintain eye contact with each other at all times. But dangerous as family combat is, many cops still don't see such calls as real police work, says Jerome Storch, a professor of law and police science at John Jay College of Criminal Justice in New York. "There's this thing in the back of the [cops'] mind that it's a domestic matter, not criminal activity."

Many cities have started training programs to make police take domestic-violence calls more sensitively—and seriously. For several years, the San Diego Police Department has even used details of O. J. Simpson's 1989 arrest for spousal battery as an example to recruits not to be intimidated by a famous name or face. Laws requiring police to make arrests in domestic cases are on the books in 15 states. But compliance is another matter. Since 1979, New York City has had a mandatory-arrest law, which also requires cops to report every domestic call. Yet a 1993 study found that reports were filed in only 30 percent of approximately 200,000 annual domestic-violence calls, and arrests were made in only 7 percent of the cases. Many cops insist they need to be able to use their own judgment. "If there's a minor assault, are you going to make an arrest just because it's 'a domestic crime'?" asks Storch. "Then if you take it to court and the judge says, 'This is minor,' it's dismissed. If you place mandates on the police, you must place them on the courts."

Prosecutors are just as frustrated. Testimony is often his word against hers; defense attorneys scare off victims with repeated delays and many victims decline to cooperate or press charges. "When women call the police, they don't call because they want to prosecute," says Mimi Rose, chief of the Family Violence and Assault Unit at the Philadelphia District Attorney's Office. "They are scared and want the violence to stop. Ten days later when they get the subpoena to appear in court, the situation has changed. The idea of putting someone you live with in jail becomes impossible." Pressing charges is just the first step. The victim is faced with a range of potential legal remedies: orders of protection, criminal prosecution, family-court prosecution, divorce, a child-custody agreement. Each step is complex and time-consuming, requiring frequent court appearances by the victim—and the abuser, if he'll show up.

Courts around the country have made an effort to streamline the procedures; more than 500 bills on domestic violence were introduced in state legislatures last year, and 100 of them became law. In California alone, new bills are pending that would impose mandatory minimum jail sentences and long-term counseling for abusers, set up computer registries for restraining orders, ban abusers from carrying firearms, mandate training for judges—and even raise the "domestic-violence surcharge" on marriage licenses by $4 to be used for shelter services. On the national level, women's groups are pushing for the $1.8 million Violence Against Women act that would

4. RELATING TO OTHERS

set up a national hot line, provide police training, toughen penalties and aid shelters and prevention programs. But those in the field say the question is whether the justice system can solve a highly complex social problem. "We need to rethink what we're doing," says Rose. "Prosecution isn't a panacea. It's like a tourniquet. We put it on when there is an emergency and we keep it on as long as necessary. But the question is, then what?"

WHEN ABUSE TURNS DEADLY

AFTER YEARS OF ABUSE, LEAVING IS OFTEN THE MOST dangerous thing a woman can do. Probably the first thing a battered wife learns in counseling is that orders of protection aren't bulletproof. Severing ties signals the abuser that he's no longer in control, and he often responds in the only way he knows how—by escalating the violence. Husbands threaten to "hunt them down and kill them," says Margaret Byrne, who directs the Illinois Clemency Project for Battered Women. One man, she recalled, told his wife he would find her shelter and burn it down, with her in it. "It's this male sense of entitlement—'If I can't have her,

One third of women in prison for homicide have killed an intimate

no one can'," says University of Illinois sociologist Pauline Bart. Friends claim O.J. made similar threats to Nicole.

Although conventional wisdom has it that women are most vulnerable in the first two years after they separate, researcher Campbell is suspicious of limiting danger to a particular time. Typically, she says, women report they're harassed for about a year after a breakup, "but we think the really obsessed guys remain that way much longer." In the last 16 years, the rate of homicides in domestic-abuse cases has actually gone down slightly—particularly for black women—according to an analysis of FBI data by James Fox, dean of the College of Criminal Justice at Northeastern University. Fox is not certain why. "More and more women are apparently getting out of a relationship before it's too late."

Or perhaps women are getting to the family gun first. While studying some 22,000 Chicago murders since 1965, researcher Carolyn Block of the Illinois Criminal Justice Information Authority discovered that among black couples, women were more likely to kill men in domestic-abuse situations than the other way round. In white relationships, by contrast, only about 25 percent of the victims were male. Nationwide, about one third of the women in prison for homicide have killed an intimate, according to the Bureau of Justice Statistics. While judges and juries are increasingly sympathetic to "Burning Bed" tales of longtime abuse, the vast majority don't get off.

Whatever the numbers, men and women kill their partners for very different reasons. For men, it's usually an escalation of violence. For women, killing is often the last resort. "The woman who is feisty and strong would have left," says Geffner. "The one who murders her husband is squashed, terrified by, 'You're never going to get away from me, I'm going to take the kids.' There's nothing left for her. To protect herself or her kids, she ends up killing the batterer."

Getting Help

These national information and referral centers handle domestic-violence calls from male and female victims as well as abusers, whether gay or straight. Or contact local mental-health organizations.

- **National Victim Center**
  1-800-FYI-CALL
- **National Coalition Against Domestic Violence**
  303-839-1852

WHAT HAPPENS TO THE KIDS

THE CHILDREN OF O.J. AND NICOLE SIMPSON WERE REPORTEDLY with their maternal grandparents in Orange County, Calif., last week, riding their bikes and playing with cousins on the beach. Sydney, 9, and Justin, 5, know their mother is dead, but they reportedly have not been told that their father has been charged in her murder. Even if their family unplugs the TV and hides the newspapers, the scars may already be too deep.

"The worst thing that can happen to kids is to grow up in an abusive family," says Gelles. Research has shown that children reared amid violence risk more problems in school and an increased likelihood of drug and alcohol abuse. And, of course, they risk repeating the pattern when they become parents. Former surgeon general C. Everett Koop says domestic violence is often three-generational: in families in which a grandparent is abused, the most likely assailant is the daughter—who's likely to be married to a man who abuses her. Together, they abuse their children. "If you are going to break the chain," Koop says, "you have to break it at the child level."

The effects of violence can play out in many ways. Some boys get angry when they watch their father beat their mother, as Bill Clinton did as a teenager. Other children rebel and withdraw from attachment. All of them, says Northwestern University child psychiatrist David Zinn, suffer by trying to hide their family's dirty little secret. As a result, they feel isolated and unlike other kids. Sadly, it's a good bet the Simpsons' children will never again feel like everyone else. "The worst of all tragedies is to become social orphans—they lost their mother through a horrific crime and now their father has been turned into Mephistopheles," says Gelles. It's difficult enough for any child to overcome the legacy of domestic violence; having it play out on a national stage may make it all but impossible.

The Secret World of Siblings

Emotional ambivalence often marks the most enduring relationship in life

They have not been together like this for years, the three of them standing on the close-cropped grass, New England lawns and steeples spread out below the golf course. He is glad to see his older brothers, has always been glad to have "someone to look up to, to do things with." Yet he also knows the silences between them, the places he dares not step, even though they are all grown men now. They move across the greens, trading small talk, joking. But at the 13th hole, he swings at the ball, duffs it and his brothers begin to needle him. "I should be better than this," he thinks. Impatiently, he swings again, misses, then angrily grabs the club and breaks it in half across his knee. Recalling this outburst later, he explains, simply: "They were beating me again."

As an old man, Leo Tolstoy once opined that the simplest relationships in life are those between brother and sister. He must have been delirious at the time. Even lesser mortals, lacking Tolstoy's acute eye and literary skill, recognize the power of the word *sibling* to reduce normally competent, rational human beings to raw bundles of anger, love, hurt, longing and disappointment— often in a matter of minutes. Perhaps they have heard two elderly sisters dig at each other's sore spots with astounding accuracy, much as they did in junior high. Or have seen a woman corner her older brother at a family reunion, finally venting 30 years of pent-up resentment. Or watched remorse and yearning play across a man's face as he speaks of the older brother whose friendship was chased away long ago, amid dinner table taunts of "Porky Pig, Porky Pig, oink, oink, oink!"

Sibling relationships—and 80 percent of Americans have at least one—outlast marriages, survive the death of parents, resurface after quarrels that would sink any friendship. They flourish in a thousand incarnations of closeness and distance, warmth, loyalty and distrust. Asked to describe them, more than a few people stammer and hesitate, tripped up by memory and sudden bursts of unexpected emotion.

Traditionally, experts have viewed siblings as "very minor actors on the stage of human development," says Stephen Bank, Wesleyan University psychologist and coauthor of *The Sibling Bond*. But a rapidly expanding body of research is showing that what goes on in the playroom or in the kitchen while dinner is being cooked exerts a profound influence on how children grow, a contribution that approaches, if it may not quite equal, that of parenting. Sibling relationships shape how people feel about themselves, how they understand and feel about others, even how much they achieve. And more often than not, such ties represent the lingering thumbprint of childhood upon adult life, affecting the way people interact with those closest to them, with friends and coworkers, neighbors and spouses—a topic explored by an increasing number of popular books, including *Mom Loved You Best*, the most recent offering by Dr. William and Mada Hapworth and Joan Heilman.

Shifting landscape. In a 1990s world of shifting social realities, of working couples, disintegrating marriages, "blended" households, disappearing grandparents and families spread across a continent, this belated validation of the importance of sibling influences probably comes none too soon. More and more children are stepping in to change diapers, cook meals and help with younger siblings' homework in the hours when parents are still at the office. Baby boomers, edging into middle age, find themselves squaring off once again with brothers and sisters over the care of dying parents or the division of inheritance. And in a generation where late marriages and fewer children are the norm, old age may become for many a time when siblings—not devoted sons and daughters—sit by the bedside.

It is something that happened so long ago, so silly and unimportant now that she is 26 and a researcher at a large, downtown office and her younger brother is her best friend, really, so close that she talks to him at least once a week. Yet as she begins to speak she is suddenly a 5-year-old again on

4. RELATING TO OTHERS

Christmas morning, running into the living room in her red flannel pajamas, her straight blond hair in a ponytail. He hasn't even wrapped it, the little, yellow-flowered plastic purse. Racing to the tree, he brings it to her, thrusts it at her—"Here's your present, Jenny!"—smiling that stupid, adoring, little brother smile. She takes the purse and hurls it across the room. "I don't want your stupid present," she yells. A small crime, long ago forgiven. Yet she says: "I still feel tremendously guilty about it."

Sigmund Freud, perhaps guided by his own childhood feelings of rivalry, conceived of siblingship as a story of unremitting jealousy and competition. Yet, observational studies of young children, many of them the groundbreaking work of Pennsylvania State University psychologist Judy Dunn and her colleagues, suggest that while rivalry between brothers and sisters is common, to see only hostility in sibling relations is to miss the main show. The arrival of a younger sibling may cause distress to an older child accustomed to parents' exclusive attention, but it also stirs enormous interest, presenting both children with the opportunity to learn crucial social and cognitive skills: how to comfort and empathize with another person, how to make jokes, resolve arguments, even how to irritate.

The lessons in this life tutorial take as many forms as there are children and parents. In some families, a natural attachment seems to form early between older and younger children. Toddlers as young as 14 months miss older siblings when they are absent, and babies separated briefly from their mothers will often accept comfort from an older sibling and go back to playing happily. As the younger child grows, becoming a potential playmate, confidant and sparring partner, older children begin to pay more attention. But even young children monitor their siblings' behavior closely, showing a surprisingly sophisticated grasp of their actions and emotional states.

Parental signals. To some extent, parents set the emotional tone of early sibling interactions. Dunn's work indicates, for example, that children whose mothers encourage them to view a newborn brother or sister as a human being, with needs, wants and feelings, are friendlier to the new arrival over the next year, an affection that is later reciprocated by the younger child. The quality of parents' established relationships with older siblings can also influence how a new younger brother or sister is received. In another of Dunn's studies, first-born daughters who enjoyed a playful, intense relationship with their mothers treated newborn siblings with more hostility, and a year later the younger children were more hostile in return. In contrast, older daughters with more contentious relationships with their mothers greeted the newcomer enthusiastically—perhaps relieved to have an ally. Fourteen months later, these older sisters were more likely to imitate and play with their younger siblings and less apt to hit them or steal their toys.

In troubled homes, where a parent is seriously ill, depressed or emotionally unavailable, siblings often grow closer than they might in a happier environment, offering each other solace and protection. This is not always the case, however. When parents are on the brink of separation or have already divorced and remarried, says University of Virginia psychologist E. Mavis Hetherington, rivalry between brothers and sisters frequently increases, as they struggle to hold on to their parents' affection in the face of the breakup. If anything, it is sisters who are likely to draw together in a divorcing family, while brothers resist forming tighter bonds. Says Hetherington: "Males tend to go it alone and not to use support very well."

Pretend play is never wasted. Toddlers who engage regularly in make-believe activity with older siblings later show a precocious grasp of others' behavior.

Much of what transpires between brothers and sisters, of course, takes place when parents are not around. "Very often the parent doesn't see the subtlety or the full cycle of siblings' interactions," says University of Hartford psychologist Michael Kahn. Left to their own devices, children tease, wrestle and play make-believe. They are the ones eager to help pilot the pirate ship or play storekeeper to their sibling's impatient customer. And none of this pretend play, researchers find, is wasted. Toddlers who engage regularly in make-believe with older siblings later show a precocious grasp of others' behavior. Says Dunn: "They turn out to be the real stars at understanding people."

Obviously, some degree of rivalry and squabbling between siblings is natural. Yet in extreme cases, verbal or physical abuse at the hands of an older brother or sister can leave scars that last well into adulthood. Experts like Wesleyan University's Bank distinguish between hostility that takes the form of humiliation or betrayal and more benign forms of conflict. From the child's perspective, the impact of even normal sibling antagonism may depend in part on who's coming out ahead. In one study, for example, children showed higher self-esteem when they "delivered" more teasing, insults and other negative behaviors to their siblings than they received. Nor is even intense rivalry necessarily destructive. Says University of Texas psychologist Duane Buhrmester: "You may not be happy about a brother or sister who is kind of pushing you along, but you may also get somewhere in life."

They are two sides of an equation written 30 years ago: Michèle, with her raven-black hair, precisely made-up lips, restrained smile; Arin, two years older, her easy laugh filling the restaurant, the sleeves of her gray turtleneck pulled over her hands.

This is what Arin thinks about Michèle: "I have always resented her, and she has always looked up to me. When we were younger, she used to copy me, which would drive me crazy. We have nothing in common except our family history—isn't that terrible? I like her spirit of generosity, her direction and ambition. I dislike her vapid conversation and her idiotic friends. But the reality is that we are very close, and we always will be."

This is what Michèle sees: "Arin was my ideal. I wanted to be like her, to look like her. I think I drove her crazy. Once, I gave her a necklace I thought was very beautiful. I never saw her wear it. I think it wasn't good enough, precious enough. We are so different—I wish that we could be more like friends. But as we get older, we accept each other more."

It is something every brother or sister eventually marvels at, a conundrum that novelists have played upon in a thousand different ways: There are two children. They grow up in the same house, share the same parents, experience many of the same events. Yet they are stubbornly, astonishingly different.

A growing number of studies in the relatively new field of behavioral genetics are finding confirmation for this popular observation. Children raised in the same family, such studies find, are only very slightly more similar to each other on a variety of personality dimensions than they are, say, to Bill Clinton or to the neighbor's son. In cognitive abilities, too, siblings appear more different than alike. And the extent to which siblings *do* resemble one another in these traits is largely the result of the genes they share—a conclusion drawn from twin studies, comparisons of biological siblings raised apart and biological children and adopted siblings raised together.

Contrasts. Heredity also contributes to the *differences* between siblings. About 30 percent of the dissimilarity between brothers and sisters on many personality dimensions can be accounted for by differing genetic endowments from parents. But that still leaves 70 percent that *cannot* be attributed to genetic causes, and it is this unexplained portion of contrasting traits that scientists find so intriguing. If two children who grow up in the same family are vastly different, and genetics accounts for only a minor part of these differences, what else is going on?

The answer may be that brothers and sisters don't really share the same family at all. Rather, each child grows up in a unique family, one shaped by the way he perceives other people and events, by the chance happenings he alone experiences, and by how other people—parents, siblings and teachers—perceive and act toward him. And while for decades experts in child development have focused on the things that children in the same family share—social class, child-rearing attitudes and parents' marital satisfaction, for example—what really seem to matter are those things that are not shared. As Judy Dunn and Pennsylvania State behavioral geneticist Robert Plomin write in *Separate Lives: Why Siblings Are So Different*, "Environmental factors important to development are those that two children in the same family experience differently."

Asked to account for children's disparate experiences, most people invoke the age-old logic of birth order. "I'm the middle child, so I'm cooler headed," they will say, or "Firstborns are high achievers." Scientists, too, beginning with Sir Francis Galton in the 19th century, have sought in birth order a way to characterize how children diverge in personality, IQ or life success. But in recent years, many researchers have backed away from this notion, asserting that when family size, number of siblings and social class are taken into account, the explanatory power of birth ranking becomes negligible. Says one psychologist: "You wouldn't want to make a decision about your child based on it."

At least one researcher, however, argues that birth order does exert a strong influence on development, particularly on attitudes toward authority. Massachusetts Institute of Technology historian Frank Sulloway, who has just completed a 20-year analysis of 4,000 scientists from Copernicus through the 20th century, finds that those with older siblings were significantly more likely to have contributed to or supported radical scientific revolutions, such as Darwin's theory of evolution. Firstborn scientists, in contrast, were more apt to champion conservative scientific ideas. "Later-borns are consistently more open-minded, more intellectually flexible and therefore more radical," says Sulloway, adding that later-borns also tend to be more agreeable and less competitive.

Hearthside inequities. Perhaps most compelling for scientists who study sibling relationships are the ways in which parents treat their children differently and the inequalities children perceive in their parents' behavior. Research suggests that disparate treatment by parents can have a lasting effect, even into adulthood. Children who receive more affection from fathers than their siblings do, for example, appear to aim their sights higher in terms of education and professional goals, according to a study by University of Southern California psychologist Laura Baker. Seven year-olds treated by their mothers in a less affectionate, more controlling way than their brothers or sisters are apt to be more anxious and depressed. And adolescents who say their parents favor a sibling over themselves are more likely to report angry and depressed feelings.

Parental favoritism spills into sibling relationships, too, sometimes breeding the hostility made famous by the Smothers Brothers in their classic 1960s routine, "Mom always loved you best." In families where parents are more punitive and restrictive toward one child, for instance that child is more likely to act in an aggressive, rivalrous and unfriendly manner toward a brother or sister, according to work by Hetherington. Surprisingly, it may not matter who is favored. Children in one study were more antagonistic toward siblings even when *they* were the ones receiving preferential treatment.

Many parents, of course, go to great lengths to distribute their love and attention equally. Yet even the most

4. RELATING TO OTHERS

consciously egalitarian parenting may be seen as unequal by children of different ages. A mother may treat her 4-year-old boy with the same care and attention she lavished on her older son when he was 4. But from the 7-year-old's perspective, it may look like his younger brother is getting a better deal. Nor is there much agreement among family members on how evenhandedly love is apportioned: Adolescents report favoritism when their mothers and fathers insist that none exists. Some parents express surprise that their children feel unequally treated, while at the same time they describe how one child is more demanding, another needs more discipline. And siblings almost never agree in their assessments of who, exactly, Mom loves best.

Nature vs. nurture. Further complicating the equation is the contribution of heredity to temperament, each child presenting a different challenge from the moment of birth. Plomin, part of a research team led by George Washington University psychiatrist David Reiss that is studying sibling pairs in 700 families nationwide, views the differences between siblings as emerging from a complex interaction of nature and nurture. In this scheme, a more aggressive and active child, for example, might engage in more conflict with parents and later become a problem child at school. A quieter, more timid child might receive gentler parenting and later be deemed an easy student.

In China, long ago, it was just the two of them, making dolls out of straw together in the internment camp, putting on their Sunday clothes to go to church with their mother. She mostly ignored her younger sister, or goaded her relentlessly for being so quiet. By the time they were separated—her sister sailing alone at 13 for the United States—there was already a wall between them, a prelude to the stiff Christmas cards they exchange, the rebuffed phone calls, the impersonal gifts that arrive in the mail.

Now, when the phone rings, she is wishing hard for a guardian angel, for someone to take away the pain that throbs beneath the surgical bandage on her chest, keeping her curled under the blue and white cotton coverlet. She picks up the receiver, recognizes her sister's voice instantly, is surprised, grateful, cautious all at once. How could it be otherwise after so many years? It is the longest they have spoken in 50 years. And across the telephone wire, something is shifting, melting in the small talk about children, the wishes for speedy recovery. "I think we both realized that life can be very short," she says. Her pain, too, is dulling now, moving away as she listens to her sister's voice. She begins to say a small prayer of thanks.

For a period that seems to stretch forever in the timelessness of childhood, there is only the family, only the others who are unchosen partners, their affection, confidences, attacks and betrayals defining the circumference of a limited world. But eventually, the boundaries expand, friends and schoolmates taking the place of brothers and sisters, highways and airports leading to other lives, to office parties and neighborhood meetings, to other, newer families.

Adult bonds. Rivalry between siblings wanes after adolescence, or at least adults are less apt to admit competitive feelings. Strong friendships also become less intense, diluted by geography, by marriage, by the concerns of raising children and pursuing independent careers. In national polls, 65 percent of Americans say they would like to see their siblings more often than the typical "two or three times a year." And University of Indianapolis psychologist Victoria Bedford finds, in her work, that men and women of child-rearing age often show longing toward siblings, especially those close in age and of the same sex. Yet for some people, the detachment of adulthood brings relief, an escape from bonds that are largely unwanted but never entirely go away. Says one woman about her brothers and sisters: "Our values are different, our politics diametrically opposed. I don't feel very connected, but there's still a pressure to keep up the tie, a kind of guilt that I don't have a deeper sense of kinship."

How closely sibling ties are maintained and nurtured varies with cultural and ethnic expectations. In one survey, for example, 54 percent of low-income blacks reported receiving help from a brother or sister, in comparison with 44 percent of low-income Hispanics and 36 percent of low-income whites. Siblings in large families are also more likely to give and receive support, as are those who live in close geographical proximity to one another. Sex differences are also substantial. In middle and later life, sisters are much more likely than brothers to keep up close relationships.

So important, in fact, is the role that sisters play in cementing family ties that some families all but fall apart without them. They are the ones who often play the major role in caring for aging parents and who make sure family members stay in touch after parents die. And in later life, says Purdue University psychologist Victor Cicirelli, sisters can provide a crucial source of reassurance and emotional security for their male counterparts. In one study, elderly men with sisters reported greater feelings of happiness and less worry about their life circumstances.

Warmth or tolerance? Given the mixed emotions many adults express about sibling ties, it is striking that in national surveys the vast majority—more than 80 percent—deem their relationships with siblings to be "warm and affectionate." Yet this statistic may simply reflect the fact that ambivalence is tolerated more easily at a distance, warmth and affection less difficult to muster for a few days a year than on a daily basis. Nor are drastic breaches between siblings—months or years of silence, with no attempt at rapprochement—unheard of. One man, asked by a researcher about his brother, shouted, "Don't mention that son of a bitch to me!" and slammed the door in the psychologist's face.

Sibling feuds often echo much earlier squabbles and are sparked by similar collisions over shared responsibility or resources—who is doing more for an ailing

ONLY CHILDREN
Cracking the myth of the pampered, lonely misfit

Child-rearing experts may have neglected the psychology of sibling ties, but they have never been hesitant to warn parents about the perils of siring a single child. Children unlucky enough to grow up without brothers or sisters, the professional wisdom held, were bound to be self-centered, unhappy, anxious, demanding, pampered and generally maladjusted to the larger social world. "Being an only child is a disease in itself," psychologist G. Stanley Hall concluded at the turn of the century.

Recent research paints a kinder picture of the only child—a welcome revision at a time when single-child families are increasing. The absence of siblings, psychologists find, does not doom children to a life of neurosis or social handicap. Day care, preschool and other modern child-care solutions go far in combatting an only child's isolation and in mitigating the willfulness and self-absorption that might come from being the sole focus of parental attention. And while only children may miss out on some positive aspects of growing up around brothers and sisters, they also escape potentially negative experiences, such as unequal parenting or severe aggression by an older sibling. Says University of Texas at Austin social psychologist Toni Falbo: "The view of only children as selfish and lonely is a gross exaggeration of reality."

Indeed, Falbo goes so far as to argue that only children are often better off—at least in some respects—than those with brothers and sisters. Reviewing over 200 studies conducted since 1925, she and her colleague Denise Polit conclude that only children equal firstborns in intelligence and achievement, and score higher than both firstborns and later-borns with siblings on measures of maturity and leadership. Other researchers dispute these findings, however. Comparing only children with firstborns over their life span, for example, University of California at Berkeley psychologist B. G. Rosenberg found that only children—particularly females—scored lower on intelligence tests than did firstborns with a sibling.

Rosenberg distinguishes between three types of only children. "Normal, well-adjusted" onlies, he says, are assertive, poised and gregarious. "Impulsive, acting out" only children adhere more to the old stereotype, their scores on personality tests indicating they are thin-skinned, self-indulgent and self-dramatizing. The third group resembles the firstborn children of larger families, scoring as dependable, productive and fastidious.

Perhaps the only real disadvantage to being an only child comes not in childhood but much later in life. Faced with the emotional and financial burdens of caring for aging parents, those without siblings have no one to help out. But as Falbo points out, even in large families such burdens are rarely distributed equally.

parent, how inheritance should be divided. Few are long lasting, and those that are probably reflect more severe emotional disturbance. Yet harmonious or antagonistic patterns established in childhood make themselves felt in many adults' lives. Says psychologist Kahn: "This is not just kid stuff that people outgrow." One woman, for example, competes bitterly with a slightly older co-worker, just as she did with an older brother growing up. Another suspects that her sister married a particular man in part to impress her. A scientist realizes that he argues with his wife in exactly the same way he used to spar with an older brother.

For most people, a time comes when it makes sense to rework and reshape such "frozen images" of childhood—to borrow psychologist Bank's term—into designs more accommodating to adult reality, letting go of ancient injuries, repairing damaged fences. In a world of increasingly tenuous family connections, such renegotiation may be well worth the effort. Says author Judith Viorst, who has written of sibling ties: "There is no one else on Earth with whom you share so much personal history."

ERICA E. GOODE

Dynamics of Personal Adjustment: The Individual and Society

The passing of each decade brings changes to society. Some historians have suggested that changes are occurring more rapidly now than in the past. In other words, history appears to take less time to occur. How has American society changed historically? The inventory is long. Technological advances can be found everywhere. A decade ago, few people knew what "user-friendly" or "16MB RAM" signified. Today these terms are readily identified with the quickly expanding computer industry. Fifteen years ago, Americans felt fortunate to own a 13-inch television that received three local stations. Now people feel deprived if they cannot select from 100 different worldwide channels on their big, rear-screen sets. Today we can fax a message to the other side of the world faster than we can propel a missile to the same place.

In the Middle Ages, Londoners worried about the bubonic plague. Before vaccines were available, people feared polio and other diseases. Today much concern is focused on the transmission and cure of AIDS, the discovery of more carcinogenic substances, and the greenhouse effect. In terms of mental health, psychologists see few hysterics, the type of patient seen by Sigmund Freud in the 1800s. Psychosomatic ulcers and alcohol and drug addiction are more common today. In other words, lifestyle, more than disease, is killing Americans. Similarly, issues concerning the changing American family continue to grab headlines. Nearly every popular magazine carries a story or two bemoaning the passing of the traditional, nuclear family and the decline in "family values." And as if these spontaneous or unplanned changes are not enough to cope with, some individuals are intentionally trying to change the world. Witness the continuing dramatic changes in Eastern Europe and the Middle East, for example.

This list of societal transformations, while not exhaustive, reflects society's continual demand for adaptation by each of its members. However, it is not just society at large that places stress on us. Smaller units within society, such as our work group, demand constant adaptation by individuals. Work groups expand and contract with every economic fluctuation. Even when group size remains stable, new members come and go as turnover takes place; hence, changes in the dynamics of the group occur in response to the new personalities. Each of these changes, welcome or not, probably places less strain on society as a whole and more stress on the individual, who then needs to adjust or cope with the change.

This unit addresses the interplay between the individual and society in producing the problems each creates for the other.

The first three essays feature ideas about societal problems such as violence and racism. Both are pervasive problems in our society. The murder rate continues to climb in American cities. In the initial article, Patrick Fagan blames the disintegration of the nuclear family. He supports his arguments by looking at declines in both white and black families. He says that to reduce street violence, we need to reevaluate and revive the role of the family. In "Mixed Blood," racism is discussed by Jefferson Fish, who believes that our use of the word "race" and our categories for race in the United States are contrived and are unlike any others found in the rest of the world. If Fish is correct, our research into race differences, for example, differences in intelligence, are misguided. In the third article, Ray Surette blames the media for encouraging our violent behavior. He examines research into media violence. These writers seem to tell us that violence and racism are rising in American society, and the causes might be multiple. Approaches to decreasing them, then, might also have to be multipronged.

While on the topic of media violence, it might also serve us well to investigate the effects of other media on us. Robert Wright, in the next selection for this unit, suggests that the introduction of technology, such as computers, into our lives is antithetical to our very being. Humans, he claims, were meant to be social creatures, and technology isolates us.

UNIT 5

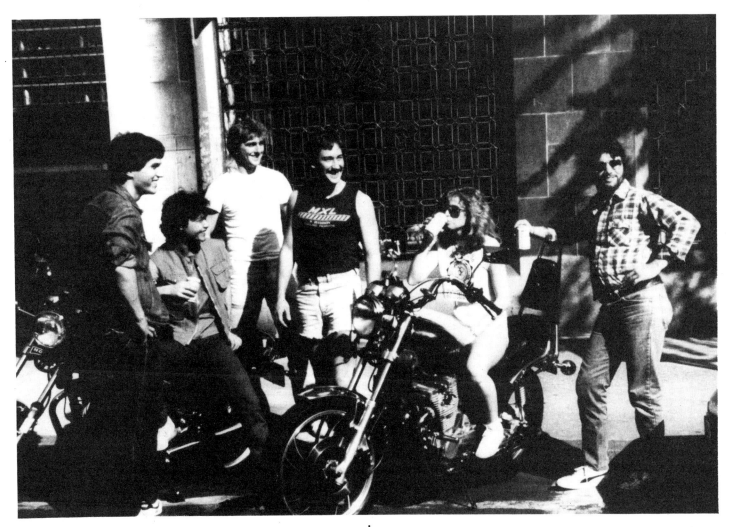

The last article of this unit, "Psychotrends: Taking Stock of Tomorrow's Family and Sexuality," discusses developments in human sexuality. As the AIDS epidemic continues, laypersons and researchers alike are interested in human sexuality and changes in sex behaviors and attitudes. Shervert Frazier tracks recent changes.

Looking Ahead: Challenge Questions

What is the definition of race in American society? Do other cultures use this same definition? If not, why not? What is it about our society that perpetuates the "isms" (racism, sexism and other prejudices)? How can we eliminate or overcome racism, sexism, and sexual harassment?

What do you think has caused the epidemic of violence on American streets? Discuss whether or not televised violence has encouraged this epidemic. Is the decline of the family an important ingredient? If so, what can we do to reduce violence? If not, what else has caused violence to increase over the last decade? To what positive uses can television be put? For what negative uses has television been developed? Should we censor or restrict certain types of television? Why, and for whom? Do you agree that networks should voluntarily make programming changes or that such changes should be legislated? Why or why not? If families are important, how can true family values be revived?

Besides television, what other modern technologies are available to us? How do these technologies enhance the human experience? How might they be detrimental to it?

What has spawned the renewed interest in the sexual revolution? What changes have recently occurred in sexual behavior and attitudes? How do these changes relate to American families? To each gender?

Disintegration of the Family VIOLENT

"... The popular assumption that there is an association between race and crime is false. Illegitimacy, not race, is the key factor. It is the absence of marriage and the failure to maintain intact families that explain the incidence of crime among whites as well as blacks."

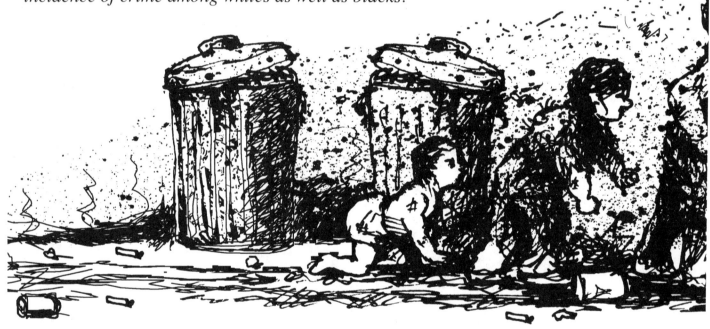

Patrick F. Fagan

SOCIAL SCIENTISTS, criminologists, and many other observers at long last are coming to recognize the connection between the breakdown of families and various social problems that have plagued American society. In the debate over welfare reform, for instance, it now is a widely accepted premise that children born into single-parent families are much more likely than those in intact families to fall into poverty and welfare dependency.

While the link between the family and chronic welfare dependency is understood much better these days, there is another link—between the family and crime—that deserves more attention. Entire communities, particularly in urban areas, are being torn apart by crime. We desperately need to uncover the real root cause of criminal behavior and learn how criminals are formed in order to be able to fight this situation.

There is a wealth of evidence in the professional literature of criminology and sociology to suggest that the breakdown of family is the real root cause of crime in the U.S. Yet, the orthodox thinking in official Washington assumes that it is caused by material conditions, such as poor employment opportunities and a shortage of adequately funded state and Federal social programs.

The Violent Crime Control and Law Enforcement Act of 1994, supported by the Clinton Administration, perfectly embodies Washington's view of crime. It provides for

Mr. Fagan is William H.G. Fitzgerald Fellow for Family and Cultural Studies, Heritage Foundation, Washington, D.C. This article is based on a Hillsdale (Mich.) College Center for Constructive Alternatives seminar on "Crime in America: Fighting Back with Moral and Market Virtues."

36. Disintegration of the Family Is the Real Root Cause of CRIME

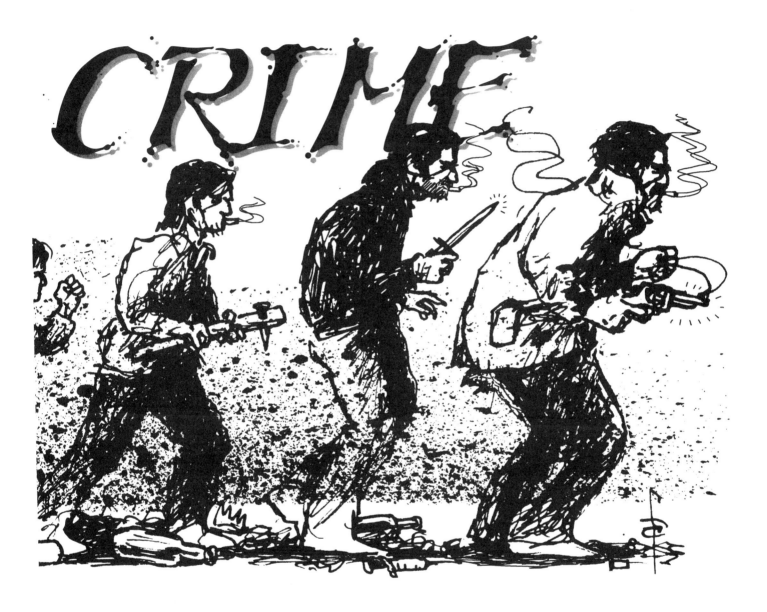

billions of dollars in new spending, adding 15 social programs on top of a welfare system that has cost taxpayers five trillion dollars since the War on Poverty was declared in 1965. There is no reason to suppose that increased spending and new programs will have any significant positive impact. Since 1965, welfare spending has grown 800% in real terms, while the number of major felonies per capita today is roughly three times the rate prior to 1960. As Sen. Phil Gramm (R.-Tex.) rightly observes, "If social spending stopped crime, America would be the safest country in the world."

Still, Federal bureaucrats and lawmakers persist in arguing that poverty is the primary cause of crime. In its simplest form, this contention is absurd; if it were true, there would have been more crime in the past, when more people were poorer. Moreover, in less-developed nations, the crime rates would be higher than in the U.S. History defies the assumption that deteriorating economic circumstances breed crime and improving conditions reduce it. America's crime rate actually rose during the long period of economic growth in the early 20th century. As the Great Depression set in and incomes dropped, the crime rate also fell. It went up again between 1965 and 1974, when incomes rose. Most recently, during the recession of 1982, there was a slight dip in crime, not an increase.

Washington also believes that race is the second most important cause of crime. The large disparity in crime rates between whites and blacks often is cited as proof. However, a closer look at the data shows that the real variable is not race, but family structure and all that it implies in terms of commitment and love between adults and children.

A 1988 study of 11,000 individuals found

5. DYNAMICS OF PERSONAL ADJUSTMENT: THE INDIVIDUAL AND SOCIETY

that "the percentage of single-parent households with children between the ages of 12 and 20 is significantly associated with rates of violent crime and burglary." The same study makes it clear that the popular assumption that there is an association between race and crime is false. Illegitimacy, not race, is the key factor. It is the absence of marriage and the failure to form and maintain intact families that explains the incidence of crime among whites as well as blacks.

There is a strong, well-documented pattern of circumstances and social evolution in the life of a future violent criminal. The pattern may be summarized in five basic stages:

Stage one: Parental neglect and abandonment of the child in early home life. When the future violent criminal is born, his father already has abandoned the mother. If his parents are married, they are likely to divorce by the third year of his life. He is raised in a neighborhood with a high concentration of single-parent families. He does not become securely attached to his mother during the critical early years. His child care frequently changes.

The adults in his life often quarrel and vent their frustrations physically. He, or a member of his family, may suffer one or more forms of abuse, including sexual. There is much harshness in his home, and he is deprived of affection.

He becomes hostile, anxious, and hyperactive. He is difficult to manage at age three and is labeled a "behavior problem." Lacking his father's presence and attention, he becomes increasingly aggressive.

Stage two: The embryonic gang becomes a place for him to belong. His behavior continues to deteriorate at a rapid rate. He satisfies his needs by exploiting others. At age five or six, he hits his mother. In first grade, his aggressive behavior causes problems for other children. He is difficult for school officials to handle.

He is rejected socially at school by "normal" children. He searches for and finds acceptance among similarly aggressive and hostile youngsters. He and his friends are slower at school. They fail at verbal tasks that demand abstract thinking and at learning social and moral concepts. His reading scores trail behind the rest of his class. He has lessening interest in school, teachers, and learning.

By now, he and his friends have low educational and life expectations for themselves. These are reinforced by teachers and family members. Poor supervision at home continues. His father, or father substitute, still is absent. His life primarily is characterized by aggressive behavior by himself and his peers and a hostile home life.

Stage three: He joins a delinquent gang. At age 11, his bad habits and attitudes are well-established. By age 15, he engages in criminal behavior. The earlier he commits his first delinquent act, the longer he will be likely to lead a life of crime.

His companions are the main source of his personal identity and his sense of belonging. Life with his delinquent friends is hidden from adults. The number of delinquent acts increases in the year before he and his friends drop out of school.

His delinquent girlfriends have poor relationships with their mothers, as well as with "normal" girls in school. A number of his peers use drugs. Many, especially the girls, run away from home or just drift away.

Stage four: He commits violent crime and the full-fledged criminal gang emerges. High violence grows in his community with the increase in the number of single-parent families. He purchases a gun, at first mainly for self-defense. He and his peers begin to use violence for exploitation. The violent young men in his delinquent peer group are arrested more than the nonviolent criminals, but most of them do not get caught at all.

Gradually, different friends specialize in different types of crime—violence or theft. Some are more versatile than others. The girls are involved in prostitution, while he and the other boys are members of criminal gangs.

Stage five: A new child—and a new generation of criminals—is born. His 16-year-old girlfriend is pregnant. He has no thought of marrying her; among his peers this simply isn't done. They stay together for awhile until the shouting and hitting start. He leaves her and does not see the baby anymore.

One or two of his criminal friends are experts in their field. Only a few members of the group to which he now belongs—career criminals—are caught. They commit hundreds of crimes per year. Most of those he and his friends commit are in their own neighborhood.

For the future violent criminal, each of these five stages is characterized by the absence of the love, affection, and dedication of his parents. The ordinary tasks of growing up are a series of perverse exercises, frustrating his needs, stunting his capacity for empathy as well as his ability to belong, and increasing the risk of his becoming a twisted young adult. This experience is in stark contrast to the investment of love and dedication by two parents normally needed to make compassionate, competent adults out of their offspring.

The impact of violent crime

When one considers some of the alarming statistics that make headlines today, the future of our society appears bleak. In the mid 1980s, the chancellor of the New York City school system warned: "We are in a situation now where 12,000 of our 60,000 kindergartners have mothers who are still in their teenage years and where 40% of our students come from single-parent households."

Today, this crisis is not confined to New York; it afflicts even small, rural communities. Worse yet, the national illegitimacy rate is predicted to reach 50% within the next 12-20 years. As a result, violence in school is becoming worse. The Centers for Disease Control recently reported that more than four percent of high school students surveyed had brought a firearm at least once to school. Many of them, in fact, were regular gun carriers.

The old injunction clearly is true—violence begets violence. Violent families are producing violent youths, and violent youths are producing violent communities. The future violent criminal is likely to have witnessed numerous conflicts between his parents. He may have been physically or sexually abused. His parents, brothers, and sisters also may be criminals, and thus his family may have a disproportionate negative impact on the community. Moreover, British and American studies show that fewer than five percent of all criminals account for 50% of all criminal convictions. Over all, there has been an extraordinary increase in community violence in most major American cities.

Government agencies are powerless to make men and women marry or stay wed. They are powerless to guarantee that parents will love and care for their children. They are powerless to persuade anyone to make and keep promises. In fact, government agencies often do more harm than good by enforcing policies that undermine stable families and by misdiagnosing the real root cause of such social problems as violent crime.

Nevertheless, ordinary American are not powerless. They know full well how to fight crime effectively. They do not need to survey the current social science literature to know that a family life of affection, cohesion, and parental involvement prevents delinquency. They instinctively realize that paternal and maternal affection and the father's presence in the home are among the critical elements in raising well-balanced children. They acknowledge that parents should encourage the moral development of their offspring—an act that best is accomplished within the context of religious belief and practice.

None of this is to say that fighting crime or rebuilding stable families and communities will be easy. What *is* easy is deciding what we must do at the outset. Begin by affirming four simple principles: First, marriage is vital. Second, parents must love and nurture their children in spiritual as well as physical ways. Third, children must be taught how to relate to and empathize with others. Finally, the backbone of strong neighborhoods and communities is friendship and cooperation among families.

These principles constitute the real root solution to the problem of violent crime. We should do everything in our power to apply them in our own lives and the life of the nation, not just for our sake, but for that of our children.

Mixed Blood

Race is an immutable biological given, right? So how come the author's daughter can change her race just by getting on a plane? Because race is a social classification, not a biological one. We might just have categorized people according to body type rather than skin color. As for all those behavioral differences attributed to race, like I.Q.—don't even ask.

Jefferson M. Fish, Ph.D.

Jefferson M. Fish, Ph.D., is a professor of psychology at St. John's University, in New York.

Last year my daughter, who had been living in Rio de Janeiro, and her Brazilian boyfriend paid a visit to my cross-cultural psychology class. They had agreed to be interviewed about Brazilian culture. At one point in the interview I asked her, "Are you black?" She said, "Yes." I then asked him the question, and he said "No."

"How can that be?" I asked. "He's darker than she is."

Psychologists have begun talking about race again. They think that it may be useful in explaining the biological bases of behavior. For example, following publication of *The Bell Curve,* there has been renewed debate about whether black-white group differences in scores on IQ tests reflect racial differences in intelligence. (Because this article is about race it will mainly use racial terms, like black and white, rather than cultural terms, like African-American and European-American.)

The problem with debates like the on[e] over race and IQ is that psychologists on both sides of the controversy make a totally unwarranted assumption: that there is a biological entity called "race." If there were such an entity, then it would at least be possible that differences in behavior between "races" might be biologically based.

Before considering the controversy, however, it is reasonable to step back and ask ourselves "What is race?" If, as happens to be the case, race is not a biologically meaningful concept, then looking for biologically based racial differences in behavior is simply a waste of time.

The question "What is race?" can be divided into two more limited ones. The answers to both questions have long been known by anthropologists, but seem not to have reached other social or behavioral scientists, let alone the public at large. And both answers differ strikingly from what we Americans think of as race.

The first question is "How can we understand the variation in physical appearance among human beings?" It is interesting to discover that Americans (including researchers, who should know better) view only a part of the variation as "racial," while other equally evident variability is not so viewed.

The second question is "How can we understand the kinds of racial classifications applied to differences in physical appearance among human beings?" Surprisingly, different cultures label these physical differences in different ways. Far from describing biological entities, American racial categories are merely one of numerous, very culture-specific schemes for reducing uncertainty about how people should respond to other people. The fact that Americans believe that Asians, blacks, Hispanics, and whites constitute biological entities called races is a matter of cultural interest rather than scientific substance. It tells us something about American culture—but nothing at all about the human species.

The short answer to the question "What is race?" is: There is no such thing. Race is a myth. And our racial classification scheme is loaded with pure fantasy.

Let's start with human physical variation. Human beings are a species, which means that people from anywhere on the planet can mate with others from anywhere else and produce fertile offspring. (Horses and donkeys are two different species because, even though they can mate with each other, their offspring—mules—are sterile.)

Our species evolved in Africa from earlier forms and eventually spread out around the planet. Over time, human populations that were geographically separated from

The American concept of race does not correspond to the ways physical appearance varies.

one another came to differ in physical appearance. They came by these differences through three major pathways: mutation, natural selection, and genetic drift. Since genetic mutations occur randomly, different mutations occur and accumulate over time in geographically separated populations. Also, as we have known since Darwin, different geographical environments select for different physical traits that confer a survival advantage. But the largest proportion of variability among populations may well result from purely random factors; this random change in the frequencies of already existing genes is known as genetic drift.

If an earthquake or disease kills off a large segment of a population, those who

5. DYNAMICS OF PERSONAL ADJUSTMENT: THE INDIVIDUAL AND SOCIETY

survive to reproduce are likely to differ from the original population in many ways. Similarly, if a group divides and a subgroup moves away, the two groups will, by chance, differ in the frequency of various genes. Even the mere fact of physical separation will, over time, lead two equivalent populations to differ in the frequency of genes. These randomly acquired population differences will accumulate over successive generations along with any others due to mutation or natural selection.

A number of the differences in physical appearance among populations around the globe appear to have adaptive value. For example, people in the tropics of Africa and South America came to have dark skins, presumably, through natural selection, as protection against the sun. In cold areas, like northern Europe or northern North America, which are dark for long periods of time, and where people covered their bodies for warmth, people came to have light skins—light skins make maximum use of sunlight to produce vitamin D.

The indigenous peoples of the New World arrived about 15,000 years ago, during the last ice age, following game across the Bering Strait. (The sea level was low enough to create a land bridge because so much water was in the form of ice.) Thus, the dark-skinned Indians of the South American tropics are descended from light-skinned ancestors, similar in appearance to the Eskimo. In other words, even though skin color is the most salient feature thought by Americans to be an indicator of race—and race is assumed to have great time depth—it is subject to relatively rapid evolutionary change.

Meanwhile, the extra ("epicanthic") fold of eyelid skin, which Americans also view as racial, and which evolved in Asian populations to protect the eye against the cold, continues to exist among South American native peoples because its presence (unlike a light skin) offers no reproductive disadvantage. Hence, skin color and eyelid form, which Americans think of as traits of different races, occur together or separately in different populations.

Like skin color, there are other physical differences that also appear to have evolved through natural selection—but which Americans do not think of as racial. Take, for example, body shape. Some populations in very cold climates, like the Eskimo, developed rounded bodies. This is because the more spherical an object is, the less surface area it has to radiate heat. In contrast, some populations in very hot climates, like the Masai, developed lanky bodies. Like the tubular pipes of an old-fashioned radiator, the high ratio of surface area to volume allows people to radiate a lot of heat.

In terms of Americans' way of thinking about race, lanky people and rounded people are simply two kinds of whites or blacks. But it is equally reasonable to view light-skinned people and dark-skinned people as two kinds of "lankys" or "roundeds." In other words, our categories for the racial classification of people arbitrarily include certain dimensions (light versus dark skin) and exclude others (rounded versus elongated bodies).

There is no biological basis for classifying race according to skin color instead of body form—or according to any other variable, for that matter. All that exists is variability in what people look like—and the arbitrary and culturally specific ways different societies classify that variability. There is noting left over that can be called race. This is why race is a myth.

Skin color and body form do not vary together: Not all dark-skinned people are lanky; similarly, light-skinned people may be lanky or rounded. The same can

Race is just one culture-specific scheme for reducing uncertainty about how people should respond.

be said of the facial features Americans think of as racial—eye color, nose width (actually, the ratio of width to length), lip thickness ("evertedness"), hair form, and hair color. They do not vary together either. If they did, then a "totally white" person would have very light skin color, straight blond hair, blue eyes, a narrow nose, and thin lips; a "totally black" person would have very dark skin color, black tight curly hair, dark brown eyes, a broad nose, and thick lips; those in between would have—to a correlated degree—wavy light brown hair, light brown eyes, and intermediate nose and lip forms.

While people of mixed European and African ancestry who look like this do exist, they are the exception rather than the rule. Anyone who wants to can make up a chart of facial features (choose a location with a diverse population, say, the New York City subway) and verify that there are people with all possible admixtures of facial features. One might see someone with tight curly blond hair, light skin, blue eyes, broad nose, and thick lips—whose features are half "black" and half "white." That is, each of the person's facial features occupies one end or the other of a supposedly racial continuum, with no intermediary forms (like wavy light brown hair). Such people are living proof that supposedly racial features do not vary together.

Since the human species has spent most of its existence in Africa, different populations in Africa have been separated from each other longer than East Asians or Northern Europeans have been separated from each other or from Africans. As a result, there is remarkable physical variation among the peoples of Africa, which goes unrecognized by Americans who view then all as belonging to the same race.

In contrast to the very tall Masai, the diminutive stature of the very short Pygmies may have evolved as an advantage in moving rapidly through tangled forest vegetation. The Bushmen of the Kalahari desert have very large ("steatopygous") buttocks, presumably to store body fat in one place for times of food scarcity, while leaving the rest of the body uninsulated to radiate heat. They also have "peppercorn" hair. Hair in separated tufts, like tight curly hair, leaves space to radiate the heat that rises through the body to the scalp; straight hair lies flat and holds in body heat, like a cap. By viewing Africans as constituting a single race, Americans ignore their greater physical variability, while assigning racial significance to lesser differences between them.

Although it is true that most inhabitants of northern Europe, east Asia, and central Africa look like Americans' conceptions of one or another of the three purported races, most inhabitants of south Asia, southwest Asia, north Africa, and the Pacific islands do not. Thus, the 19th century view of the human species as comprised of Caucasoid, Mongoloid, and Negroid races, still held by many Americans, is based on a partial and unrepresentative view of human variability. In other words, what is now known about human physical variation does not correspond to what Americans think of as race.

In contrast to the question of the actual physical variation among human beings, there is the question of how people classify that variation. Scientists classify things in scientific taxonomies—chemists' periodic table of the elements, biologists' classification of life forms into kingdoms, phyla, and so forth.

In every culture, people also classify things along culture-specific dimensions of meaning. For example, paper clips and staples are understood by Americans as paper fasteners, and nails are not, even though, in terms of their physical properties, all three consist of differently shaped pieces of metal wire. The physical variation in pieces of metal wire can be seen as analogous to human physical variation; and the categories of cultural meaning, like paper fasteners vs. wood fasteners, can be seen as analogous to races. Anthropologists refer to these kinds of classifications as folk taxonomies.

Consider the avocado—is it a fruit or a vegetable? Americans insist it is a vegetable. We eat it in salads with oil and vinegar. Brazilians, on the other hand, would say it is a fruit. They eat it for dessert with lemon juice and sugar.

How can we explain this difference in classification?

The avocado is an edible plant, and the American and Brazilian folk taxonomies, while containing cognate terms, classify some edible plants differently. The avocado

Americans believe in 'blood,' a folk term for the quality presumed carried by members of 'races.'

does not change. It is the same biological entity; but its folk classification changes, depending on who's doing the classifying.

Human beings are also biological entities. Just as we can ask if an avocado is a fruit or a vegetable, we can ask if a person is white or black. And when we ask race questions, the answers we get come from folk taxonomies, not scientific ones. Terms like "white" or "black" applied to people—or "vegetable" or "fruit" applied to avocados—do not give us biological information about people or avocados. Rather, they exemplify how cultural groups (Brazilians or Americans) classify people and avocados.

Americans believe in "blood," a folk term for the quality presumed to be carried by members of so-called races. And the way offspring—regardless of their physical appearance—always inherit the less prestigious racial category of mixed parentage is called "hypo-descent" by anthropologists. A sentence thoroughly intelligible to most Americans might be, "Since Mary's father is white and her mother is black, Mary is black because she has black 'blood.'" American researchers who think they are studying racial differences in behavior would, like other Americans, classify Mary as black—although she has just as much white "blood."

According to hypo-descent, the various purported racial categories are arranged in a hierarchy along a single dimension, from the most prestigious ("white"), through intermediary forms ("Asian"), to the least prestigious ("black"). And when a couple come from two different categories, all their children (the "descent" in "hypo-descent") are classified as belonging to the less prestigious category (thus, the "hypo"). Hence, all the offspring of one "white" parent and one "black" parent—regardless of the children's physical appearance—are called "black" in the United States.

The American folk concept of "blood" does not behave like genes. Genes are units which cannot be subdivided. When several genes jointly determine a trait, chance decides which ones come from each parent. For example, if eight genes determine a trait, a child gets four from each parent. If a mother and a father each have the hypothetical genes BBBBWWWW, then a child could be born with any combination of B and W genes, from BBBBBBBB to WWWWWWWW. In contrast, the folk concept "blood" behaves like a uniform and continuous entity. It can be divided in two indefinitely—for example, quadroons and octoroons are said to be people who have one-quarter and one-eighth black "blood," respectively. Oddly, because of hypo-descent, Americans consider people with one-eighth black "blood" to be black rather than white, despite their having seven eighths white "blood."

Hypo-descent, or "blood," is not informative about the physical appearance of people. For example, when two parents called black in the United States have a number of children, the children are likely to vary in physical appearance. In the case of skin color, they might vary from lighter than the lighter parent to darker than the darker parent. However, they would all receive the same racial classification—black—regardless of their skin color.

All that hypo-descent tells you is that, when someone is classified as something other than white (e.g., Asian), at least one of his or her parents is classified in the same way, and that neither parent has a less prestigious classification (e.g., black). That is, hypo-descent is informative about ancestry—specifically, parental classification—rather than physical appearance.

There are many strange consequences of our folk taxonomy. For example, someone who inherited no genes that produce "African"-appearing physical features would still be considered black if he or she has a parent classified as black. The category "passing for white" includes many such people. Americans have the curious belief that people who look white but have a parent classified as black are "really" black in some biological sense, and are being deceptive if they present themselves as white. Such examples make it clear that race is a social rather than a physical classification.

From infancy, human beings learn to recognize very subtle differences in the faces of those around them. Black babies see a wider variety of black faces than white faces, and white babies see a wider variety of white faces than black faces. Because they are exposed only to a limited range of human variation, adult members of each "race" come to see their own group as containing much wider variation than others. Thus, because of this perceptual learning, blacks see greater physical variation among themselves than among whites, while whites see the opposite. In this case, however, there is a clear answer to the question of which group contains greater physical variability. Blacks are correct.

Why is this the case?

Take a moment. Think of yourself as an amateur anthropologist and try to step out of American culture, however briefly.

It is often difficult to get white people to accept what at first appears to contradict the evidence they can see clearly with their own eyes—but which is really the result of a history of perceptual learning. However, the reason that blacks view themselves as more varied is not that their vision is more accurate. Rather, it is that blacks too have a long—but different—history of perceptual learning from that of whites (and also that they have been observers of a larger range of human variation).

The fact of greater physical variation among blacks than whites in America goes back to the principle of hypo-descent, which classifies all people with one black parent and one white parent as black. If they were all considered white, then there would be more physical variation among whites.

5. DYNAMICS OF PERSONAL ADJUSTMENT: THE INDIVIDUAL AND SOCIETY

Someone with one-eighth white "blood" and seven-eighths black "blood" would be considered white; anyone with *any* white ancestry would be considered white. In other words, what appears to be a difference in biological variability is really a difference in cultural classification.

Perhaps the clearest way to understand that the American folk taxonomy of race is merely one of many—arbitrary and unscientific like all the others—is to contrast it with a very different one, that of Brazil. The Portuguese word that in the Brazilian folk taxonomy corresponds to the American "race" is "*tipo*." *Tipo*, a cognate of the English word "type," is a descriptive term that serves as a kind of shorthand for a series of physical features. Because people's physical features vary separately from one another, there are an awful lot of tipos in Brazil.

Since tipos are descriptive terms, they vary regionally in Brazil—in part reflecting regional differences in the development of colloquial Portuguese, but in part because the physical variation they describe is different in different regions. The Brazilian situation is so complex I will limit my delineation of tipos to some of the main ones used in the city of Salvador, Bahia, to describe people whose physical appearance is understood to be made up of African and European features. (I will use the female terms throughout; in nearly all cases the male term simply changes the last letter from "a" to "o.")

Proceeding along a dimension from the "whitest" to the "blackest" tipos, a *loura* is whiter-than-white, with straight blond hair, blue or green eyes, light skin color, narrow nose, and thin lips. Brazilians who come to the United States think that a *loura* means a "blond," and are surprised to find that the American term refers to hair color only. A *branca* has light skin color, eyes of any color, hair of any color or form except tight curly, a nose that is not broad, and lips that are not thick. *Branca* translates as "white," though Brazilians of this tipo who come to the United States—especially those from elite families—are often dismayed to find that they are not considered white here, and, even worse, are viewed as Hispanic despite the fact that they speak Portuguese.

A *morena* has brown or black hair that is wavy or curly but not tight curly, tan skin, a nose that is not narrow, and lips that are not thin. Brazilians who come to the United States think that a *morena* is a "brunette," and are surprised to find that brunettes are considered white but *morenas* are not. Americans have difficulty classifying *morenas*, many of whom are of Latin American origin: Are they black or Hispanic? (One might also observe that *morenas* have trouble with Americans, for not just accepting their appearance as a given, but asking instead "Where do you come from?" "What language did you speak at home?" "What

> 'When researchers study racial differences in behavior in search of biological causes, they are wasting their time.'

was your maiden name?" or even, more crudely, "What *are* you?")

A *mulata* looks like a *morena*, except with tight curly hair and a slightly darker range of hair colors and skin colors. A *preta* looks like a *mulata*, except with dark brown skin, broad nose, and thick lips. To Americans, *mulatas* and *pretas* are both black, and if forced to distinguish between them would refer to them as light-skinned blacks and dark-skinned blacks, respectively.

If Brazilians were forced to divide the range of tipos, from *loura* to *preta*, into "kinds of whites" and "kinds of blacks" (a distinction they do not ordinarily make), they would draw the line between *morenas* and *mulatas*; whereas Americans, if offered only visual information, would draw the line between *brancas* and *morenas*.

The proliferation of tipos, and the difference in the white–black dividing line, do not, however, exhaust the differences between Brazilian and American folk taxonomies. There are tipos in the Afro-European domain that are considered to be neither black nor white—an idea that is difficult for Americans visiting Brazil to comprehend. A person with tight curly blond (or red) hair, light skin, blue (or green) eyes, broad nose, and thick lips, is a *sarará*. The opposite features—straight black hair, dark skin, brown eyes, narrow nose, and thin lips—are those of a *cabo verde*. *Sarará* and *cabo verde* are both tipos that are considered by Brazilians in Salvador, Bahia, to be neither black nor white.

When I interviewed my American daughter and her Brazilian boyfriend, she said she was black because her mother is black (even though I am white). That is, from her American perspective, she has "black blood"—though she is a *morena* in Brazil. Her boyfriend said that he was not black because, viewing himself in terms of Brazilian tipos, he is a *mulato* (not a *preto*).

There are many differences between the Brazilian and American folk taxonomies of race. The American system tells you about how people's parents are classified but not what they look like. The Brazilian system tells you what they look like but not about their parents. When two parents of intermediate appearance have many children in the United States, the children are all of one race; in Brazil they are of many tipos.

Americans believe that race is an immutable biological given, but people (like my daughter and her boyfriend) can change their race by getting on a plane and going from the United States to Brazil—just as, if they take an avocado with them, it changes from a vegetable into a fruit. In both cases, what changes is not the physical appearance of the person or avocado, but the way they are classified.

I have focused on the Brazilian system to make clear how profoundly folk taxonomies of race vary from one place to another. But the Brazilian system is just one of many. Haiti's folk taxonomy, for example, includes elements of both ancestry and physical appearance, and even includes the amazing term (for foreigners of African appearance) *un blanc noir*—literally, "a black white." In the classic study *Patterns of Race in the Americas*, anthropologist Marvin Harris gives a good introduction to the ways in which the conquests by differing European powers of differing New World peoples and ecologies combined with differing patterns of slavery to produce a variety of folk taxonomies. Folk taxonomies of race can be found in many—though by no means all—cultures in other parts of the world as well.

The American concept of race does not correspond to the ways in which human physical appearance varies. Further, the American view of race ("hypo-descent") is just one among many folk taxonomies, none of which correspond to the facts of human physical variation. This is why race is a myth and why races as conceived by Americans (and others) do not exist. It is also why differences in behavior between "races" cannot be explained by biological differences between them.

When examining the origins of IQ scores (or other behavior), psychologists sometimes use the term "heritability"—a statistical concept that is not based on observations of genes or chromosomes. It is important to understand that questions about the heritability of IQ have nothing to do with racial differences in IQ. "Heritability" refers only to the relative ranking of individuals *within* a population, under given environmental conditions, and not to differences *between* populations. Thus, among the population of American whites, it may be that those with high IQ's tend to have higher-IQ children than do those with low IQs. Similarly, among American blacks, it may be that those with high IQs also tend to have higher-IQ children.

In both cases, it is possible that the link between the IQs of parents and children may exist for reasons that are not entirely environmental. This heritability of IQ *within* the two populations, even if it exists, would in no way contradict the average social advantages of American whites as a group compared to the average social disadvantages of American blacks as a group. Such differences in social environments can easily account for any differences in the average test scores *between* the two groups. Thus, the heritability of IQ *within* each group is irrelevant to understanding differences *between* the groups.

Beyond this, though, studies of differences in behavior between "populations" of whites and blacks, which seek to find biological causes rather than only social ones, make a serious logical error. They assume that blacks and whites are populations in some biological sense, as sub-units of the human species. (Most likely, the researchers make this assumption because they are American and approach race in terms of the American folk taxonomy.)

In fact, though, the groups are sorted by a purely social rule for statistical purposes. This can easily be demonstrated by asking researchers how they know that the white subjects are really white and the black subjects are really black. There is no biological answer to this question, because race as a biological category does not exist. All that researchers can say is, "The tester classified them based on their physical appearance," or "Their school records listed their race," or otherwise give a social rather than biological answer.

So when American researchers study racial differences in behavior, in search of biological rather than social causes for differences between socially defined groups, they are wasting their time. Computers are wonderful machines, but we have learned about "garbage in/garbage out." Applying complex computations to bad data yields worthless results. In the same way, the most elegant experimental designs and statistical analyses, applied flawlessly to biologically meaningless racial categories, can only produce a very expensive waste of time.

As immigrants of varied physical appearance come to the United States from countries with racial folk taxonomies different from our own, they are often perplexed and dismayed to find that the ways they classify themselves and others are irrelevant to the American reality. Brazilians, Haitians, and others may find themselves labeled by strange, apparently inappropriate, even pejorative terms, and grouped together with people who are different from and unreceptive to them. This can cause psychological complications (a Brazilian immigrant—who views himself as white—being treated by an American therapist who assumes that he is not).

Immigration has increased, especially from geographical regions whose people do not resemble American images of blacks, whites, or Asians. Intermarriage is also increasing, as the stigma associated with it diminishes. These two trends are augmenting the physical diversity among those who marry each other—and, as a result, among their children. The American folk taxonomy of race (purportedly comprised of stable biological entities) is beginning to change to accommodate this new reality. After all, what race is someone whose four grandparents are black, white, Asian, and Hispanic?

Currently, the most rapidly growing census category is "Other," as increasing numbers of people fail to fit available options. Changes in the census categories every 10 years reflect the government's attempts to grapple with the changing self-identifications of Americans—even as statisticians try to maintain the same categories over time in order to make demographic comparisons. Perhaps they will invent one or more "multiracial" categories, to accommodate the wide range of people whose existence defies current classification. Perhaps they will drop the term "race" altogether. Already some institutions are including an option to "check as many as apply," when asking individuals to classify themselves on a list of racial and ethnic terms.

Thinking in terms of physical appearance and folk taxonomies helps to clarify the emotionally charged but confused topic of race. Understanding that different cultures have different folk taxonomies suggests that we respond to the question "What race is that person?" not by "Black" or "White," but by "Where?" and "When?"

MEDIA, VIOLENCE, YOUTH, AND SOCIETY

Ray Surette

Ray Surette is professor of criminal justice in the School of Public Affairs and Services, Florida International University, North Miami, and author of Media, Crime and Criminal Justice: Images and Realities.

It is guns, it is poverty, it is overcrowding, and it is the uniquely American problem of a culture that is infatuated with violence. We love it, we glamorize it, we teach it to our children.[1]

The above testimony by Dr. Deborah Prothrow-Stith on gangs and youth violence presented before the U.S. Senate contains two important points concerning the mass media and youth violence. First, it does not mention the media as a factor in violence, lending support to the view that the media are not crucial agents in youth violence. Second, it does cite an American culture that is infatuated with violence, and the glamorization and teaching of violence to our children, as problems. Culture, glamorization, and instruction, however, are areas where the media have been shown to play important social roles. The above statement simultaneously provides support for the position that the media are indeed important players in the production of youth violence and yet paradoxically also supports the position that they are not contributors. The relative validity of these two dichotomous positions, the media as unimportant and the media as central in fostering youth violence, has dominated the public discussion, resulting in much confusion about this issue and public posturing by various groups and individuals. The actual relationship of the media to youth violence lies somewhere between these two extremes.

Research interest in the relationship of the mass media to social violence has been elevated for most of this century. Over the twentieth century, the issue of the media as a source of violence has moved into and out of the public consciousness in predictable ten-to twenty-year cycles. If a consensus has emerged from the research and public interest, it is that the sources of violence are complex and tied to our most basic nature as well as the social world we have created and that the media's particular relationship to social violence is extremely complicated. (See the discussion in this author's *Media, Crime, and Criminal Justice* [1992] and in *Crime and Human Nature* [1985] by J. Wilson and R. Herrnstein.)

Therefore, when discussing the nature of the relationship between the media and violence, it is important not to be myopic. Social violence is embedded in historical, social forces and phenomena, while the media are components of a larger information system that creates and distributes knowledge about the world. The media and social violence must both be approached as parts of phenomena that have numerous interconnections and paths of influence between them. Too narrow a perspective on youth violence or the media's role in its generation oversimplifies both the problem and the solutions we pursue. Nowhere is this more apparent than in the current concern about media, youth, and violence.

STATISTICS ON YOUTH VIOLENCE

The source of this concern is revealed by a brief review of the statistics of youth violence.[2] Youth violence, and particularly violent crime committed by youth, has recently increased dramatically. Today about 5 out of every 20 robbery arrests and 3 of every 20 murder, rape, and aggravated assault arrests are of juveniles. In raw numbers, this translates into 3,000 murder, 6,000 forcible rape, 41,000 robbery, and 65,000 aggravated assault arrests of youths annually.

The surge in youth criminal violence is concentrated within the past five years. During the first part of the 1980s, there was a general decline in youth arrests for both violent and property crimes. In the latter half of the 1980s, however, youth arrests increased at a pace greater than that of adults for violent crimes. Youth arrests increased substantially between 1981 and 1990 for nonaggravated assault (72 percent), murder and nonnegligent manslaughter (60 percent), aggravated assault (57 percent), weapons violations (41 percent), and forcible rape (28 percent). Looking over a generational time span from 1965 to 1989, the arrest rate for violent crimes by youths grew between the mid-1960s and the mid-1970s but then leveled off and remained relatively constant until the late 1980s. At that time, the rate again began to increase, reaching its highest recorded level in the most recent years.

Thus, while the proportion of youth in the general population has declined as the baby-boom generation has aged, the rate of violence from our youth has increased significantly. We have fewer youth proportionately, but they are more violent and account for increased proportions of our violent crime. Attempts to comprehend and explain this change have led invariably to the mass media as prime suspects, but deciphering the media's role has not been a simple or straightforward task.

This difficulty in deciphering the media's role is due to the fact that the relationship of media to violence is complex, and the media's influence can be both direct and indirect. Research on their relationship (reported, for example, in George Comstock's 1980 study *Television in America*) has revealed that media effects that appear when large groups are examined are not predictable at the individual subject level. The media are also related to social violence in ways not usually considered in the public debate, such as their effects on public policies and general social attitudes toward violence.

Adding to the complexity of the media's relationship, there are many other sources of violence that either interact with the media or work alone to produce violence. These sources range from individual biology to characteristics of our history and culture. The importance of nonmedia factors such as neighborhood and family conditions, individual psychological and genetic traits, and our social structure, race relations, and economic conditions for the generation of violence are commonly acknowledged and analyzed, as in Jeffrey Goldstein's 1986 study *Aggression and Crimes of Violence*. The role of the mass media is confounded with these other sources, and its significance is often either lost or exaggerated. One task of this essay is thus to dispel the two popular but polarizing notions that have dominated the public debate. The first is that the media are the primary cause of violence in society. The second is that the media have no, or a very limited, effect on social violence.

The former view of the media as the source of primary effects is often advanced along with draconian policy demands such as extensive government intervention or direct censorship of the media. The counterargument to this position is supported by a number of points. The most basic is that we were a violent nation before we had mass media, and there is no evidence that the removal of violent media would make us nonviolent.[3] Some research into copy-cat crime additionally provides no evidence of a criminalization effect from the media as a cause.[4] The media alone cannot turn a law-abiding individual into a criminal one nor a nonviolent youth into a violent one. In sum, individual and national violence cannot be blamed primarily on the media, and violence-reducing policies directed only at the media will have little effect.

The latter argument, that the media have limited to no effect on levels of social violence, is structured both in posture and approach to the tobacco industry's response to research linking smoking to lung cancer and it rings just as hollow. The argument's basic approach is to expound inherent weaknesses in the various methodologies of the media-violence research and to trumpet the lack of evidence of strong, direct effects, while ignoring the persistent pattern of positive findings. Proponents of the nil effect point out that laboratory experiments are biased toward finding an effect. To isolate the effect of a single factor, in this case the media, and observe a rare social behavior, namely violence, experiments must exaggerate the link between media and aggression and create a setting that will elicit violent behavior. They therefore argue that all laboratory research on the issue is irrelevant. They continue, however, to dismiss the nonlaboratory research because of a lack of strict variable controls and designs that leave open noncausal interpretations of the results. "No effects" proponents lastly argue that while society reinforces some behaviors shown in the media such as that found in commercials, it does not condone or reinforce violence and, therefore, a violence-enhancing effect should not be expected (a view discussed in "Smoking Out the Critics," a 1984 *Society* article [21:36–40] by A. Wurtzel and G. Lometti).

In reality, the research shows persistent behavioral effects from violent media under diverse situations for differing groups.[5] Regarding the strong behavioral effects apparent in fashion and fad, effects that Madison Avenue touts, the argument of a behavioral effect only on sanctioned behavior but not on unsanctioned violence is specious. The media industry claim of

If a consensus has emerged from the research and public interest, it is that the media's particular relationship to social violence is extremely complicated.

having only positive behavioral effects is as valid as the tobacco industry claiming that their ads do not encourage new smokers but only persuade brand switching among established smokers. First, violence is sometimes socially sanctioned, particularly within the U.S. youth and hypermasculine culture that is the target audience of the most prominently violent media. And although the media cannot criminalize someone not having criminal predispositions, media-generated, copy-cat crime is a significant criminal phenomenon with ample anecdotal and case evidence providing a form for criminality to take.[6] The recurring mimicking of dangerous film stunts belies the argument of the media having only positive behavioral effects. It is apparent that while the media alone cannot make someone a criminal, it can change the criminal behavior of a predisposed offender.

CONFLICTING CAUSAL CLAIMS

The two arguments of primary cause and negligible cause compete for public support. These models not only posit differing causal relations between the media and violence but imply vastly different public policies regarding the media as well. The primary-cause model (fig. 1) is that of a significant, direct linear relationship between violent media and violent behavior. In this model, violent media, independent of other factors, directly cause violent behavior. If valid, it indicates that strong intervention is necessary in the content, distribution, and creation of violent media.

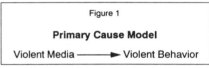

The negligible-cause model (fig. 2) concedes a statistical association between the media and violent behavior but poses the connection as due not to a causal relationship but to persons predisposed to violence simultaneously seeking out violent media and more often behaving violently. As the relationship is associative and not causal in this model, policies targeted at the media will have no effects on violent behavior and the media can be safely ignored.

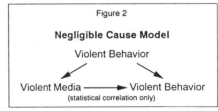

Both models inaccurately describe the media-violence relationship. The actual relationship between the factors is felt to be bidirectional and cyclical (fig. 3). In addition to violently predisposed people seeking out violent media and violent media causing violent behavior, violent media play a role in the generation of violently predisposed people through their effects on attitudes. And as the made-for-TV movie industry reflects, violent behavior sometimes results in the creation of more violent media. Finally, by providing live models of violence and creating community and home environments that are more inured to and tolerant of violence, violent behavior helps to create more violently predisposed youth in society. Therefore, while the direct effect of media on violence may not be initially large, its influence cycles through the model and accumulates.

The view of the media as the source of primary effects is often advanced along with draconian policy demands such as extensive government intervention or direct censorship of the media.

An area of research that provides an example of the bidirectional model is the relationship of pornography to sexual violence; a recent (1993) overview of such research can be found in *Pornography*, by D. Linz and N. Malamuth. On one hand, the research establishes that depictions of sexual violence, specifically those that link sex with physical violence toward women, foster antisocial attitudes toward women and lenient perceptions of the

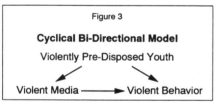
Figure 3
Cyclical Bi-Directional Model

crime of rape. Aberrant perceptions, such as increased belief in the "rape myth" (that women unconsciously want to be raped or somehow enjoy being raped), have been reported. Virtually none of the research, however, reveals strong direct effects from pornography, and even sexually violent media do not appear to negatively affect all male viewers. Many cultural and individual factors appear to mediate the effects and to foster the predisposition to sexually violent media and sexual violence. Researchers in this area have concluded that the media are one of many social forces that affect the development of intervening variables, such as thought patterns, sexual arousal patterns, motivations, and personality characteristics that are associated with tolerance for sexual violence and perhaps an increase in sexually violent behavior in society.[7] As in other areas of media-violence research, sexually violent media emerge as neither a primary engine nor an innocuous social factor.

THE KEY TO MEDIA EFFECTS

The key to media effects occurring in any particular instance, then, are the intermediate, interactive factors. In terms of the media, there are numerous interactive factors that have been identified as conducive to generating aggressive effects. Among the many delineated in the research, a sample includes: reward or lack of punishment for the perpetrator, portrayal of violence as justified, portrayal of the consequences of violence in a way that does not stir distaste, portrayal of violence without critical commentary, the presence of live peer models of violence, and the presence of sanctioning adults (all discussed in Comstock's *Television in America*). Only unambiguous linking of violent behavior with undesirable consequences or motives by the media appears capable of inhibiting subsequent aggression in groups of viewers.

A list of nonmedia factors deemed significant in the development of crime and the number of violently predisposed individuals can be culled from *Crime and Human Nature* by J. Wilson and R. Herrnstein. The authors list constitutional, developmental, and social-context factors including gender, age, intelligence, personality, psychopathology, broken and abusive families, schools, community, labor markets, alcohol and heroin, and finally history and culture. As can be seen, most aspects of modern life are implicated, and only tangential factors like diet and climate (which other researchers would have included) are left out. With such a large number of factors coming into play, the levels of interactions and complexity of relationships are obviously enormous.

The research on violence suggests that certain factors are basic to violent crime, as detailed by Wilson and Herrnstein. None of these factors dominates, but none are without significant effects.

Accordingly, the research (contained in this author's 1992 study *Media, Crime and Criminal Justice*) clearly signifies the media as only some of many factors in the generation of youth violence and that media depictions of violence do not affect all persons in the same way. The media contribute to violence in combination with other social and psychological factors. Whether or not a particular media depiction will cause a particular viewer to act more aggressively is not a straightforward issue. The emergence of an effect depends on the interaction between each individual viewer, the content of the portrayal, and the setting in which exposure to the media occurs. This gives the media significant aggregate effects but makes these effects difficult to predict for individuals. There is no doubt, however, that violent children, including those who come to have significant criminal records, spend more time exposed to violent media than do less violent children. The issue is not the existence of a media effect but the magnitude or importance of the effect.

Media violence correlates as strongly with and is as causally related to the magnitude of violent behavior as any other social behavioral variable that has been studied. This reflects both the media's impact and our lack of knowledge about the etiology of violence. Because of the many individual and social factors that come into play in producing any social behavior, one should not expect to find more than a modest direct relationship between the media and violence. Following their review of the research, Thomas Cook and his colleagues conclude:

No effects emerge that are so large as to hit one between the eyes, but early measure of viewing violence adds to the predictability of later aggression over and above the predictability afforded by earlier measures of aggression. These lagged effects are consistently positive, but not large, and they are rarely statistically significant, although no reliable lagged negative effects have been reported.... But is the association causal? If we were forced to render a judgment, probably yes.... There is strong evidence of causation in the wrong setting (the lab) with the right population (normal children) and in the right setting (outside the lab) with the wrong population (abnormal adults).[8]

MEDIA AMONG MANY FACTORS

In summation, despite the fact that the media are among many factors, they should not be ignored, regardless of the level of their direct impact. Because social violence is a pressing problem, even those factors that only modestly contribute to it are important. Small effects of the media accumulate and appear to have significant long-term social effects.[9] The research strongly indicates that we are a more violent society because of our mass media. Exactly how and to what extent the media cause long-term changes in violent behavior remains unknown, but the fact that it plays an important, but not independent, role is generally conceded.

What public policies are suggested by the knowledge we now possess about media and violence? Not all of the factors discussed above are good candidates for public intervention strategies, but there are three sources of youth violence that government policy can influence. In order of importance, they are: extreme differences in economic conditions and the concentration of wealth in America; the American gun culture; and, exacerbating the problems created by the first two, the media's violence-enhancing messages. Family, neighborhood, and personality factors may be more important for generating violence in absolute magnitude, but they are not easily influenced by public actions.

The magnitude of economic disparity and the concentration of wealth in the United States is greater than in comparable (and, not surprisingly, less violent) societies. Our richest citizens not only earn vastly more than our poorest, but, more important, the wealth in the country is increasingly concentrated in fewer and fewer hands. The trend during this century, which accelerated during the 1980s, is for an ever-shrinking percentage of the richest Americans to control greater proportions of the country's wealth, while the poorest have access to increasingly smaller proportions. The burden of this

The fear and loathing we feel toward criminals—youthful, violent, or not—is tied to our media-generated image of criminality.

economic disenfranchisement, both psychologically and fiscally, falls heavily on the young, and especially on the young who are urban poor minorities, as is shown in Elliott Currie's 1985 study *Confronting Crime*. In a consumerism-saturated society like the United States, hopelessness, bitterness, and disregard for moral values and law are heightened by this growing economic disparity.

And as the economic polarization and violent crime have grown, we also became nationally fixated on heightening and extending our punishment capacities in an attempt to suppress violent behavior, evidenced by Diana Gordon's 1991 study *The Justice Juggernaut*. Since 1975, we have increased the rate of juvenile incarceration steadily. Today we hold in custody approximately one hundred thousand juveniles every year. Despite our strengthened capacity to punish, however, youth violence has not abated.

This result should have been expected because two social mechanisms are needed to reduce violence—punishing violent criminal behavior and rewarding law-abiding, nonviolent behavior. Societies that are more successful in balancing the two mechanisms are less violent, as shown in *Crime and Control in Comparative Perspective*, by H. Heiland and L. Shelley (1992). While punishment of violent behavior is certainly necessary and justified, its emphasis, coupled with the concentration of wealth in America, has resulted in the degrading of the equally important social capacity to reward law-abiding behavior. By emphasizing one, we have lamed and discredited the other. Nonmaterial rewards like social status, an esteemed reputation, and a clear conscience have been losing their legitimacy with the young, while material rewards for law-abiding life-styles such as careers, comfortable incomes and affordable goods are less generally available to our poorest and, not surprisingly most crime-prone and violent citizens.

We have chosen to emphasize the mechanism, punishment, that is actually the weaker of the two in actually influencing behavior. As operant conditioning theory would predict, punishment, if severe enough, can suppress one type of violent crime. But the suppression of one behavior gives no push toward a desirable replacement activity, and a substitute violent crime will likely emerge. So "smash and grab" robberies give way to "bump and rob" holdups. Shaping behavior requires a credible reward system. In social terms, youth must see law-abiding behavior as credible and potentially rewarding as well as seeing violent behavior as potentially resulting in punishment.

The second area that government policy can immediately address is the gun culture in America. Our culture of violence, referred to in the opening quote, is made immeasurably more deadly by the enfolded gun culture. The availability of guns as cheap killing mechanisms is simply a national insanity. The mass production of these killing "toys" and the easy access to them must be addressed. The most recent statistics show that one out of every ten high school students report that they carry a handgun. Gun buy-back programs should be supported, and production and availability must be reduced if a positive net effect is to be expected. Irrespective of the difficulty of controlling the sources of individual violent behavior, the implements of fatal violence should not be ignored.

The third area of policy concern, the mass media, exacerbates the gun culture by portraying guns as glamorous, effective, omnipotent devices. The mass media also heighten the negative effects of economic disparities through their consumer messages in advertising and entertainment. Although both of these effects that add to the problem of youth violence are sometimes discussed, the debate about the media remains tightly focused on measuring and reviewing violent media content. Within this focus, the emphasis has been on counting violent acts rather than on exploring the context of its portrayal. Deciphering the media's moral and value messages about violence has been mostly ignored.

EFFECTS ON CRIMINAL JUSTICE

A closer examination of the context of violence in the media would tell us that we should not try to purge the media of violence, for violent media can be good when programs teach that violence is bad. Our goal should be to reduce graphic, gratuitous, and glorified violence; to portray it not as a problem solver but as a reluctant, distasteful, last resort with tragic, unanticipated consequences. Violence shown consistently as a generator of pain and suffering, not as a personal or social panacea, would be positive media violence. Too often, violence in the media is shown as an effective solution, and, too often, it is simply met by increased counterviolence. But, despite the recurring interest and current debate about media violence, there is little direction for the media industry regarding the context of violence and its effects. A goal should be to provide better information to the industry that details the various contexts and messages of violence and their effects.

Perhaps the most significant social effect of media violence is, however, not the direct generation of social violence but its

A Brief History of Television and Youth Violence Research

The logic of science requires that in order to establish the causal effect of a variable, one must be able to examine a situation without the variable's effect. In terms of television and violence, this requirement means that a group of subjects (a control group) who have not been exposed to violent television is necessary for comparison with a violent television-exposed group. Television, however, is ubiquitous and an integral part of a modern matrix of influences on social behaviors. Therefore, when the interest is in the effects of television on mainstream citizens in Western industrialized and urbanized nations, finding nontelevision-exposed controls is essentially impossible. In response, artificial laboratory situations are created, or statistical controls and large data sets are employed. Thus, while social sciences abound with research reporting variables that are correlated with one another, research firmly establishing causal relationships is rare. Unlike the content of television, there are few smoking guns in social science. Rather than conclusively proven, cause is more often inferred in a trial-like decision from the predominance of evidence. Such is the case with television and violence.

In a traditional laboratory experiment, two sets of matched, usually randomly assigned, subjects are placed in identical situations except for a single factor of interest. Early research in the television-violence quest were in this vein, with the seminal ones conducted in the 1960s by researchers Bandura, Ross, and Ross.[1] These laboratory studies basically consisted of exposing groups of young children to either a short film containing violence (frequently an adult beating up an inflated Bobo doll) or a similar but nonviolent film. The two groups of children were then placed in playrooms and observed. Children who watched the film where a doll was attacked would significantly more often attack a similar doll if given the opportunity shortly after viewing their film than children who had observed a nonviolent film. These and other studies established the existence of an "observational imitation" effect from visual violence; in short, children will imitate violence they see in the media. It was concluded by many that television violence must therefore be a cause of youth violence.

However, critics of this conclusion argued that because laboratory situations are purposely artificial and contrived to isolate the influence of a single variable, the social processes producing aggression in the laboratory are not equal to those found in the real world. In summary, one cannot assume that behavior and variable relationships observed in the lab are occurring in the home or street.

In addition to the laboratory studies, at about the same time a number of survey studies were reporting positive correlations between youth aggression and viewing violent television.[2] Efforts to extend the laboratory findings and determine if the correlational studies reflected real-world causal relationships led to two types of research: natural field experiments[3] and longitudinal panel studies.

The better known and most discussed research efforts came from longitudinal panel studies conducted in the 1970s and early '80s. Expensive and time consuming, in panel studies a large number of subjects are selected and followed for a number of years. Three such studies are particularly important due to their renown, similarities in approach, and differences in conclusions.

The first study (called the Rip van Winkle study) by L. Rowell Huesmann, Leonard Eron, and their colleagues used a cross-lag panel design (that is, comparison over time and with different populations) in which television habits at grade three (approximately age eight) were correlated with aggression in grade three and with television viewing and aggression ten years later for a sample of 211 boys.[4] The researchers collected their data in rural New York State from students in the third, eighth, and "thirteenth" grades (one year after graduation). Favorite television programs were rated based on their violent content, and frequency of viewing was obtained from the children's mothers in grade three and from the subjects in grades eight and thirteen. The measure of aggression was a peer-nominated rating obtained from responses to questions such as, "Who starts fights over nothing?" The most significant finding

---

1. See, for example, A. Bandura, D. Ross, and S. A. Ross, "Transmission of Aggression through Imitation of Aggressive Models," *Journal of Abnormal and Social Psychology* 63 (1961), 575-82; and "Imitation of film-mediated aggressive models" *Journal of Abnormal and Social Psychology* 66 (1963), 3-11.

2. See G. Comstock, et al., *Television and Human Behavior* (New York: Columbia University Press, 1978) for a review.

3. Natural field experiments typically take advantage of a planned introduction of television to a previously unexposed population. This allows both a pretelevision and posttelevision comparison of the new television group and comparisons with similar but still unexposed other groups. Although rare because of the unique circumstances necessary and by definition confined to non-mainstream populations, these studies report significant increases in aggressive behavior for children who watched a lot of television in the new-television populations. See, for example, G. Granzberg, "The Introduction of Television into a Northern Manitoba Cree Community" in G. Granzberg and J. Steinberg, eds. *Television and the Canadian Indian* (Winnipeg, Manitoba; University of Winnipeg Press, 1980); and T. Williams, ed., *The Impact of Television: A Natural Experiment in Three Communities* (New York: Academic Press, 1985).

4. M. Lefkowitz, et al., "Television Violence and Child Aggression: A Follow-up Study" in G. A. Comstock and E. A. Rubinstein, eds. *Television and Social Behavior*, vol 3 *Television and Adolescent Aggressiveness* (Washington, D.C.: U.S. Government Printing Office, 1971).

reported was a strong, positive association between violent television viewing at grade three and aggression at grade thirteen. However, this study was criticized for a number of reasons. For example, the measure of aggression used in grade thirteen was poorly worded and phrased in the past tense (i.e., "Who started fights over nothing?") and thus the answers were ambiguous in that the grade thirteen subjects may have been referring to general reputations rather than current behaviors. In addition, cross-lagged correlation analysis has a built-in bias toward finding relationships where none exist. Despite the study's weaknesses, Huesmann and Eron concluded that a causal relationship between television violence and aggression existed. This study had a strong public impact.

A second longitudinal panel study was conducted by Ronald Milavsky and his colleagues in the early 1970s that had an opposite conclusion. This study was based on surveys of about 2,400 elementary students age seven to twelve, and 403 male teenagers age twelve to sixteen in Minneapolis, Minnesota, and Fort Worth, Texas.[5] The subjects were surveyed five to six times over nineteen months. This study also used peer-nominated aggression measures for the younger group and four self-reported measures of aggression for the teenagers.[6] Unlike the "van Winkle" study, which used the children's mothers' selection of favorite programs, this study measured exposure to violent programming based on the subjects' own reports. Their analysis further controlled for earlier levels of aggression and exposure to television violence, in effect searching for evidence of significant incremental increases in youth aggression that could be attributed to past exposure to television violence after taking into account past levels of aggressive behavior.

Huesmann and Eron report meaningful lagged associations between later aggression and a number of prior conditions such as earlier aggression in a child's classroom, father's use of physical punishment, family conflict, and violent environments—but not for prior exposure to violent television. Although some significant positive relationships were found between exposure to television violence and later aggression, the overall pattern and number of findings regarding television were interpreted as inconsistent. These researchers conclude that chance, not cause, is the best explanation for their findings regarding television and aggression.

Partly in response to the Milavsky study and criticisms of their earlier methodology, Huesmann, Eron, and their colleagues conducted a third panel study (the Chicago Circle study) in the late 1970s using first and third graders in Chicago public and parochial schools as subjects.[7] Six hundred seventy-two students were initially sampled and tested for three consecutive years in two groups. One group was followed from first through third grades, the second from third through fifth grades. Aggression was measured once more by a peer-generated scale in which each child designated other children on fifteen descriptive statements, ten of which dealt with aggression. (An example is, "Who pushes and shoves other children?") Exposure to violent television was measured by asking each child to select the show most often watched and frequency of watching from eight different ten-program lists. Each list contained a mix of violent and nonviolent programs.

The study was simultaneously conducted in the United States, Australia, Finland, Israel, the Netherlands, and Poland. Their analysis of the U.S. data showed a significant general effect for television violence on girls but not for boys. However, the interaction of viewing violent television and identification with aggressive television characters was a significant predictor of male aggression. Huesmann and Eron conclude that the relationship between television violence and viewer aggression is causal and significant but bidirectional.

At this time, most reviewers of these studies and the subsequent research that followed conclude that a modest but genuine causal association does exist between media violence and aggression.[8] The fact is that, once introduced, the effect of television on a society or an individual can never be fully extricated from all the other forces that may contribute to violence. Television's influence is so intertwined with these parallel forces that searches for strong direct causal effects are not likely to be fruitful. But similar to smoking/lung cancer research, evidence of a real causal connection of some sort has been established beyond a reasonable doubt for most people.

—*R.S.*

---

5. J. Milavsky, et al., *Television and Aggression: A Panel Study* (New York: Academic Press, 1982).

6. Personal aggression toward others, aggression against a teacher (rudeness or unruliness), property aggression (theft and vandalism), and delinquency (serious or criminal behaviors).

7. See Rowell Huesmann and Leonard Eron, "Television Violence and Aggressive Behavior" in D. Pearl, L. Bouthilet, and J. Lazar, eds. *Television and Behavior: Ten Years of Scientific Progress and Implications for the 80's* (Washington, D.C., 1982); and "Factors Influencing the Effect of Television Violence on Children" in Michael Howe, ed., *Learning from Television: Psychological and Educational Research* (New York: Academic Press, 1983).

8. See, for example, L. Heath, L. Bresolin, and R. Rinaldi, "Effects of Media Violence on Children: A Review of the Literature," *Archives of General Psychiatry* 46 (1989), 376–79.

impact on our criminal justice policy. The fear and loathing we feel toward criminals—youthful, violent, or not—is tied to our media-generated image of criminality. The media portray criminals as typically animalistic, vicious predators. This media image translates into a more violent society by influencing the way we react to all crime in America. We imprison at a much greater rate and make reentry into law-abiding society, even for our nonviolent offenders, more difficult than other advanced (and, not coincidentally, less violent) nations. The predator-criminal image results in policy based on the worst-case criminal and a constant ratcheting up of punishments for all offenders. In its cumulative effect, the media both provide violent models for our youth to emulate and justify a myopic, harshly punitive public reaction to all offenders.

Currently, the debate concerning both the media and youth violence has evolved into "circles of blame" in which one group ascribes blame for the problem to someone else in the circle. Thus, in the media circle, the public blames the networks and studios, which blame the producers and writers, who blame the advertisers, who blame the public. In the violence circle, the government blames the youth, who blame the community, which blames the schools, which blame the parents, who blame the government. A more sensible, productive process would be a shift to a "ring of responsibility," with the groups addressing their individual contributions to the problem and arriving at cooperative policies. We can't selectively reduce one aspect of violence in a violent society and expect real results. Youth violence will not be seriously reduced without violence in other aspects of our culture being addressed. In the same vein, modifying media violence alone will not have much effect but to ignore it will make efforts on other fronts less successful. Ironically, despite the fact that the media have limited independent effects on youth violence, we need to expand the focus on them. This should incorporate other social institutions, such as the media industry itself, and the social norms and

Youth violence will not be seriously reduced without violence in other aspects of our culture being addressed.

values reflected in the media. We could then derive more general models of media effects and social violence.

Violence is a cultural product. The media are reflections of the culture and engines in the production process. Although they are not the only or even the most powerful causes, they are tied into the other violence-generating engines, and youth pay particular attention to them. The aggregate result of all of these forces in the United States is a national character that is individualistic, materialistic, and violence prone. If we wish to change our national character regarding violence, we cannot take on only some aspects of its genesis. We must address everything we can, such as economic inequities, the gun culture, and the glamorization of violence. And, by a slow, painful, generational process of moral leadership and example, we must work to modify the individual, family, and neighborhood factors that violently predispose youth.

In conclusion, our youth will be violent as long as our culture is violent. The local social conditions in which they are raised and the larger cultural and economic environments that they will enter generate great numbers of violently predisposed individuals. As we have experienced, violently predisposed youth, particularly among our poor, will fully develop their potential and come to prey upon us. Faced with frightful predators, we subsequently and justly punish them, but the use of punishment alone will not solve the problem. The role that the media play in the above scenario versus their potential role in deglorifying violence and showing our youth that armed aggression is not an American cultural right, will determine the media's ultimate relationship to youthful violence in society.

NOTES

1. Dr. Deborah Prothrow-Stith testifying before the Senate Subcommittee on Juvenile Justice, November 26, 1991.

2. Sources of the statistics cited in this essay are drawn from "Arrests of Youth 1990," January 1992, *Office of Juvenile Justice and Delinquency Prevention Update on Statistics; and Sourcebook of Criminal Justice Statistics—1992*, Bureau of Justice Statistics, U.S. Department of Justice, 1993.

3. Hugh Davis Graham and Ted Robert Gurr, eds., *Violence in America* (Beverly Hills, CA: Sage, 1979).

4. See S. Milgram and R. Shotland, *Television and Antisocial Behavior: Field Experiments* (New York: Academic Press, 1973) and A. Schmid and J. de Graaf, *Violence as Communication* (Newbury Park, CA: Sage, 1982).

5. T. Cook, D. Kendzierski, and S. Thomas, "The Implicit Assumptions of Television Research," *Public Opinion Quarterly* 47: 161-201.

6. For a listing of examples see S. Pease and C. Love, "The Copy-Cat Crime Phenomenon," in *Justice and the Media* by R. Surette (Springfield IL: Charles C. Thomas, 1984), 199-211; and A. Schmid and J. de Graaf, *Violence as Communication* (Newbury Park, CA: Sage, 1982).

7. N. Malamuth and J. Briere (1986), "Sexual Violence in the Media: Indirect Effects on Aggression against Women," *Journal of Social Issues* 42, 89.

8. T. Cook, D. Kendzierski, and S. Thomas (1993), "The Implicit Assumptions of Television Research," *Public Opinion Quarterly* 47: 191-92.

9. R. Rosenthal (1986), "Media Violence, Anti-Social Behavior, and the Social Consequences of Small Effects," *Journal of Social Issues* 42: 141-54.

ADDITIONAL READING

George Comstock, *Television in America*, Sage, Newbury Park, Calif., 1980.
Elliott Currie, *Confronting Crime*, Pantheon, New York, 1985.
Jeffrey Goldstein, *Aggression and Crimes of Violence*, Oxford University Press, New York, 1986.
Diana Gordon, *The Justice Juggernaut*, Rutgers University Press, New Brunswick, N.J., 1991.
Joshua Meyrowitz, *No Sense of Place*, Oxford University Press, New York, 1985.
Ray Surette, *Media, Crime, and Criminal Justice*, Brooks/Cole, Pacific Grove, Calif., 1992.
James Q. Wilson and Richard Herrnstein, *Crime and Human Nature*, Simon & Schuster, New York, 1985.

The Evolution of Despair

A new field of science examines the mismatch between our genetic makeup and the modern world, looking for the source of our pervasive sense of discontent

ROBERT WRIGHT

"[I] attribute the social and psychological problems of modern society to the fact that society requires people to live under conditions radically different from those under which the human race evolved..." —THE UNABOMBER

THERE'S A LITTLE BIT OF THE UNABOMBER IN MOST OF us. We may not share his approach to airing a grievance, but the grievance itself feels familiar. In the recently released excerpts of his still unpublished 35,000-word essay, the serial bomber complains that the modern world, for all its technological marvels, can be an uncomfortable, "unfulfilling" place to live. It makes us behave in ways "remote from the natural pattern of human behavior." Amen. VCRs and microwave ovens have their virtues, but in the everyday course of our highly efficient lives, there are times when something seems deeply amiss. Whether burdened by an overwhelming flurry of daily commitments or stifled by a sense of social isolation (or, oddly, both); whether mired for hours in a sense of life's pointlessness or beset for days by unresolved anxiety; whether deprived by long workweeks from quality time with offspring or drowning in quantity time with them—whatever the source of stress, we at times get the feeling that modern life isn't what we were designed for.

And it isn't. The human mind—our emotions, our wants, our needs—evolved in an environment lacking, for example, cellular phones. And, for that matter, regular phones, telegraphs and even hieroglyphs—and cars, railroads and chariots. This much is fairly obvious and, indeed, is a theme going back at least to Freud's *Civilization and Its Discontents*. But the analysis rarely gets past the obvious; when it does, it sometimes veers toward the dubious. Freud's ideas about the evolutionary history of our species are now considered—to put it charitably—dated. He hypothesized, for example, that our ancestors lived in a "primal horde" run by an autocratic male until one day a bunch of his sons rose up, murdered him and ate his flesh—a rebellion that not only miraculously inaugurated religion but somehow left a residue of guilt in all subsequent descendants, including us. Any questions?

A small but growing group of scholars—evolutionary psychologists—are trying to do better. With a method less fanciful than Freud's, they're beginning to sketch the contours of the human mind as designed by natural selection. Some of them even anticipate the coming of a field called "mismatch theory," which would study maladies resulting from contrasts between the modern environment and the "ancestral environment," the one we were designed for. There's no shortage of such maladies to study. Rates of depression have been doubling in some industrial countries roughly every 10 years. Suicide is the third most common cause of death among young adults in North America, after car wrecks and homicides. Fifteen percent of Americans have had a clinical anxiety disorder. And, pathological, even murderous alienation is a hallmark of our time. In that sense, the Unabomber is Exhibit A in his own argument.

Evolutionary psychology is a long way from explaining all this with precision, but it is already shedding enough light to challenge some conventional wisdom. It suggests, for example, that the conservative nostalgia for the nuclear family of the 1950s is in some ways misguided—that the household of Ozzie and Harriet is hardly a "natural" and healthful living arrangement, especially for wives. Moreover, the bygone American life-styles that do look fairly natural in light of evolutionary psychology appear to have been eroded largely by capitalism—another challenge to conservative orthodoxy. Perhaps the biggest surprise from evolutionary psychology is its depiction of the "animal" in us. Freud, and various thinkers since, saw "civilization" as an oppressive force that thwarts basic animal urges such as lust and aggression, transmuting them into psychopathology. But evolutionary psychology suggests that a larger threat to mental health may be the way civilization thwarts civility. There is a kinder, gentler side of human nature, and it seems increasingly to be a victim of repression.

THE EXACT SERIES OF SOCIAL CONTEXTS THAT SHAPED the human mind over the past couple of million years is, of course, lost in the mists of prehistory. In trying to reconstruct the "ancestral environment," evolutionary psychologists analyze the nearest approximations available—the sort of technologically primitive societies that the Unabomber extols. The most prized examples are the various hunter-gatherer societies that anthropologists have studied this century, such as the Ainu of Japan, the !Kung San of southern Africa and the Ache of South America. Also valuable are societies with primitive agriculture in the few cases where—as with some Yanomamo villages in Venezuela—they lack the contaminating contact with moderners that reduces the anthropological value of some hunter-gatherer societies.

None of these societies is Nirvana. Indeed, the anthropological record provides little support for Jean-Jacques Rousseau's notion of the "noble savage" and rather more for Thomas Hobbes' assertion that life for our distant ancestors was "nasty, brutish, and short." The anthropologist Napoleon Chagnon has written of his first encounter with the Yanomamo: "The excitement of meeting my first Indians was almost unbearable as I duck-waddled through the low passage into the village clearing." Then "I looked up and gasped when I saw a dozen burly, naked, filthy, hideous men staring at us down the shafts of their drawn arrows!" It turned out that Chagnon "had arrived just after a serious fight. Seven women had been abducted the day before by a neighboring group, and the local men and their guests has just that morning recovered five of them in a brutal club fight." The men were vigilantly awaiting retaliation when Chagnon popped in for a chat.

5. DYNAMICS OF PERSONAL ADJUSTMENT: THE INDIVIDUAL AND SOCIETY

In addition to the unsettling threat of *mano-à-mano* violence, the ancestral environment featured periodic starvation, incurable disease and the prospect of being eaten by a beast. Such inconveniences of primitive life have recently been used to dismiss the Unabomber's agenda. The historian of science Daniel Kevles, writing in the *New Yorker*, observes how coarse the "preindustrial past" looks, once "stripped of the gauzy romanticism of myth." Regarding the Unabomber's apparent aim of reversing technological history and somehow transporting our species back toward a more primitive age, Kevles declares, "Most of us don't want to live in a society like that."

Quite so. Though evolutionary psychologists would love somehow to visit the ancestral environment, few would buy a one-way ticket. Still, to say we wouldn't want to live in our primitive past isn't to say we can't learn from it. It is, after all, the world in which our currently malfunctioning minds were designed to work like a Swiss watch. And to say we'll decline the Unabomber's invitation somehow to turn the tide of technological history isn't to say technology doesn't have its dark side. We don't have to slavishly emulate, say, the Old Order Amish, who use no cars, electricity or alcohol; but we can profitably ask why it is that they suffer depres-

---

The problem is that too little of our "social" contact is social in the natural, intimate sense of the word.

---

sion at less than one-fifth the rate of people in nearby Baltimore.

The barbaric violence Chagnon documented is in some ways misleading. Though strife does pervade primitive societies, much of the striving is subtler than a club fight. Our ancestors, it seems, competed for mates with guile and hard work. They competed for social status with combative wordplay and social politicking. And this competition, however subtle, had Darwinian consequences. Anthropologists have shown, for example, that hunter-gatherer males successful in status competition have better luck in mating and thus getting genes into the next generation.

And getting genes into the next generation was, for better or worse, the criterion by which the human mind was designed. Mental traits conducive to genetic proliferation are the traits that survived. They are what constitute our minds today; they are us, we are designed to steer genes through a technologically primitive social structure. The good news is that doing this job entailed some quite pleasant feelings. Because social cooperation improves the chances of survival, natural selection imbued our minds with an infrastructure for friendship, including affection, gratitude and trust. (In technical terms, this is the machinery for "reciprocal altruism.") And the fact that offspring carry our genes into posterity accounts for the immense joy of parental love.

Still, there is always a flip side. People have enemies—social rivals—as well as friends, feel resentful as well as grateful, feel nervously suspicious as well as trusting. Their children, being genetic conduits, can make them inordinately proud but also inordinately disappointed, angry or anxious. People feel the thrill of victory but also the agony of defeat, not to mention pregame jitters. According to evolutionary psychology, such unpleasant feelings are with us today because they helped our ancestors get genes into the next generation. Anxiety goaded them into keeping their children out of harm's way or adding to food stocks even amid plenty. Sadness or dejection—after a high-profile social failure, say—led to soul-searching that might discourage repeating the behavior that led to the failure. ("Maybe flirting with the wives of men larger than me isn't a good idea.") The past usefulness of unpleasant feelings is the reason periodic unhappiness is a natural condition, found in every culture, impossible to escape.

What isn't natural is going crazy—for sadness to linger on into debilitating depression, for anxiety to grow chronic and paralyzing. These are largely diseases of modernity. When researchers examined rural villagers in Samoa, they discovered what were by Western standards extraordinarily low levels of cortisol, a biochemical by-product of anxiety. And when a Western anthropologist tried to study depression among the Kaluli of New Guinea, he couldn't find any.

One thing that helps turn the perfectly natural feeling of sadness or dejection into the pathology known as depression is social isolation. Today one-fourth of American households consist of a single person. That's up from 8% in 1940—and, apparently, from roughly zero percent in the ancestral environment. Hunter-gatherer societies, for all their diversity, typically feature intimacy and stability: people live in close contact with roughly the same array of several dozen friends and relatives for decades. They may move to another village, but usually either to join a new family network (as upon marriage) or to return to an old one (as upon separation). The evolutionary psychologists John Tooby and Leda Cosmides see in the mammoth popularity of the TV show *Cheers* during the 1980s a visceral yearning for the world of our ancestors—a place where life brought regular, random encounters with friends, and not just occasional, carefully scheduled lunches with them; where there were spats and rivalries, yes, but where grievances were usually heard in short order and tensions thus resolved.

As anyone who has lived in a small town can attest, social intimacy comes at the price of privacy: everybody knows your business. And that's true in spades when next-door neighbors live not in Norman Rockwell clapboard homes but in thatched huts.

Still, social transparency has its virtues. The anthropologist Phillip Walker has studied the bones of more than 5,000 children from hundreds of preindustrial cultures, dating back to 4,000 B.C. He has yet to find the scattered bone bruises that are the skeletal hallmark of "battered-child syndrome." In some modern societies, Walker estimates, such bruises would be found on more than 1 in 20 children who die between the ages of one and four. Walker accounts for this contrast with several factors, including a grim reminder of Hobbesian barbarism: unwanted children in primitive societies were often killed at birth, rather than resented and brutalized for years. But another factor, he believes, is the public nature of primitive child rearing, notably the watchful eye of a child's aunts, uncles, grandparents or friends. In the ancestral environment, there was little mystery about what went on behind closed doors, because there weren't any.

In that sense, Tooby and Cosmides have noted, nostalgia for the suburban nuclear family of the 1950s—which often accompanies current enthusiasm for "family values"—is ironic. The insular coziness of Ozzie and Harriet's home is less like our natural habitat than, say, the more diffuse social integration of Andy Griffith's Mayberry. Andy's son Opie is motherless, but he has a dutiful great-aunt to watch over him—and, anyway, can barely sit on the front porch without seeing a family friend.

To be sure, keeping nuclear families intact has virtues that are underscored by evolutionary psychology, notably in keeping children away from stepfathers, who, as the evolutionary psychologists Martin Daly and Margo Wilson predicted and then documented, are much more prone to child abuse than biological fathers. But to worship the suburban household of the 1950s is to miss much of the trouble with contemporary life.

Though people talk about "urbanization" as the process that ushered in modern ills, many urban neighborhoods at mid-century were in fact fairly communal; it's hard to walk into a Brooklyn brownstone day after day without bumping into neighbors. It was suburbanization that brought the combination of transience and residential isolation that leaves many people feeling a bit alone in their own neighborhoods. (These days, thanks to electric garage-door openers, you can drive straight into your house, never risking contact with a neighbor.)

The suburbs have been particularly hard on women with

young children. In the typical hunter-gatherer village, mothers can reconcile a homelife with a work life fairly gracefully, and in a richly social context. When they gather food, their children stay either with them or with aunts, uncles, grandparents, cousins or lifelong friends. When they're back at the village, child care is a mostly public task—extensively social, even communal. The anthropologist Marjorie Shostak wrote of life in an African hunter-gatherer village, "The isolated mother burdened with bored small children is not a scene that has parallels in !Kung daily life."

Evolutionary psychology thus helps explain why modern feminism got its start after the suburbanization of the 1950s. The landmark 1963 book *The Feminine Mystique* by Betty Friedan grew out of her 1959 conversation with a suburban mother who spoke with "quiet desperation" about the anger and despair that Friedan came to call "the problem with no name" and a doctor dubbed "the housewife's syndrome." It is only natural that modern mothers rearing children at home are more prone to depression than working mothers, and that they should rebel.

But even working mothers suffer depression more often than

The suburbs have been particularly hard on women.

---

working men. And that shouldn't shock us either. To judge by hunter-gatherer societies, it is unnatural for a mother to get up each day, hand her child over to someone she barely knows and then head off for 10 hours of work—not as unnatural as staying home alone with a child, maybe, but still a likely source of guilt and anxiety. Finding a middle ground, enabling women to be workers and mothers, is one of the great social challenges of our day.

Much of this trouble, as the Unabomber argues, stems from technology. Suburbs are largely products of the automobile. (In the forthcoming book *The Lost City*, Alan Ehrenhalt notes the irony of Henry Ford, in his 60s, building a replica of his hometown—gravel roads, gas lamps—to recapture the "saner and sweeter idea of life" he had helped destroy.) And in a thousand little ways—from the telephone to the refrigerator to ready-made microwavable meals—technology has eroded the bonds of neighborly interdependence. Among the Aranda Aborigines of Australia, the anthropologist George Peter Murdock noted early this century, it was common for a woman to breast-feed her neighbor's child while the neighbor gathered food. Today in America it's no longer common for a neighbor to borrow a cup of sugar.

Of course, intensive interdependence also has its downside. The good news for our ancestors was that collectively fending off starvation or saber-toothed tigers forged bonds of a depth moderners can barely imagine. The bad news was that the tigers and the starvation sometimes won. Technology is not without its rewards.

Perhaps the ultimate in isolating technologies is television, especially when linked to a VCR and a coaxial cable. Harvard professor Robert Putnam, in a recent and much noted essay titled "Bowling Alone," takes the demise of bowling leagues as a metaphor for the larger trend of asocial entertainment. "Electronic technology enables individual tastes to be satisfied more fully," he concedes, but at the cost of the social gratification "associated with more primitive forms of entertainment." When you're watching TV 28 hours a week—as the average American does—that's a lot of bonding you're not out doing.

As the evolutionary psychiatrist Randolph Nesse has noted, television can also distort our self-perception. Being a socially competitive species, we naturally compare ourselves with people we see, which meant, in the ancestral environment, measuring ourselves against fellow villagers and usually finding at least one facet of life where we excel. But now we compare our lives with "the fantasy lives we see on television," Nesse writes in the recent book *Why We Get Sick: The New Science of Darwinian Medicine,* written with the eminent evolutionary biologist George Williams. "Our own wives and husbands, fathers and mothers, sons and daughters can seem profoundly inadequate by comparison. So we are dissatisfied with them and even more dissatisfied with ourselves." (And, apparently, with our standard of living. During the 1950s, various American cities saw theft rates jump in the particular years that broadcast television was introduced.)

Relief from TV's isolating and at times depressing effects may come from more communal technologies. The inchoate Internet is already famous for knitting congenial souls together. And as the capacity of phone lines expands, the Net may allow us to, say, play virtual racketball with a sibling or childhood friend in a distant city. But at least in its current form, the Net brings no visual (much less tactile) contact, and so doesn't fully gratify the social machinery in our minds. More generally the Net adds to the information overload, whose psychological effects are still unknown but certainly aren't wholly benign.

This idea that modern society is dangerously asocial would surprise Freud. In *Civilization and Its Discontents,* he lamented the tension between crude animal impulses and the dictates of society. Society, he said, tells us to cooperate with one another, indeed, even to "love they neighbor as thyself"; yet by our nature, we are tempted to exploit our neighbor, "to humiliate him, to cause him pain, to torture and to kill him. *Homo homini lupus* [Man is a wolf to man.]" The Unabomber, too, in his mode as armchair psychologist, celebrates our "WILD nature" and complains that in modern society "we are not supposed to hate anyone, yet almost everyone hates somebody at some time or other." This sort of cramping of our natural selves, he opines, creates "oversocialized" people. He seems to agree with Freud's claim that "primitive man was better off in knowing no restrictions of instinct."

Yet evolutionary psychology suggests that primitive man knew plenty of "restrictions of instinct." True, hatred is part of our innate social repertoire, and in other ways as well we are naturally crude. But the restraint of crude impulses is also part of our nature. Indeed, the "guilt" that Freud never satisfactorily explained is one built-in restrainer. By design, it discourages us from, say, neglecting kin through unbridled egoism, or imperiling friendships in the heat of anger—or, at the very least, it goads us to make amends after such imperiling, once we've cooled down. Certainly modern society may burden us unduly with guilt. After erupting in anger toward an acquaintance, we may not see him or her for

---

The ultimate in isolating technologies is television.

---

weeks, whereas in the ancestral environment we might have reconciled in short order. Still, feeling guilty about spasms of malice is no invention of modern civilization.

This points to the most ironic of evolutionary psychology's implications: many of the impulses created by natural selection's ruthless imperative of genetic self-interest aren't selfish in any straightforward way. Love, pity, generosity, remorse, friendly affection and enduring trust, for example, are part of our genetic heritage. And, oddly, some of these affiliative impulses are frustrated by the structure of modern society at least as much as the more obviously "animal" impulses. The problem with modern life, increasingly, is less that we're "oversocialized" than that we're undersocialized—or, that too little of our "social" contact is social in the natural, intimate sense of the word.

Various intellectual currents reflect this shortage of civility in modern civilization. The "communitarian" movement, lately championed by Democratic and Republican leaders alike, aims to restore a sense of social kinship, and thus of moral responsibility. And various scholars and politicians (including Putnam) are now

5. DYNAMICS OF PERSONAL ADJUSTMENT: THE INDIVIDUAL AND SOCIETY

bemoaning the shrinkage of civil society, that realm of community groups, from the Boy Scouts to the Rotary Club, that once not only kept America shipshape but met deep social needs.

The latest tribute to civil society comes in Francis Fukuyama's book *Trust*, whose title captures a primary missing ingredient in modern life. As of 1993, 37% of Americans felt they could trust most people, down from 58% in 1960. This hurts; according to evolutionary psychology, we are designed to seek trusting relationships and to feel uncomfortable in their absence. Yet the trend is hardly surprising in a modern, technology-intensive economy, where so much leisure time is spent electronically and so much "social" time is spent nurturing not friendships but professional contacts.

As scholars and public figures try to resurrect community, they might profitably draw on evolutionary psychology. Prominent communitarian Amitai Etzioni, in highlighting the shortcomings of most institutionalized child care, has duly stressed the virtues of parents' "co-oping," working part time at day-care centers. Still, the stark declaration in his book *The Spirit of Community* that "infants are better off at home" gives short shrift to the innately social nature of infants and mothers. That women naturally have a vocational calling as well as a maternal one suggests that workplace-based, co-operative day-care centers may deserve more attention.

Residential planners have begun to account implicitly for human nature. They're designing neighborhoods that foster affiliation—large common recreational spaces, extensive pedestrian thoroughfares and even, in some cases, parking spaces that make it hard to hop from car to living room without traversing some turf in between. In effect: drive-in, hunter-gatherer villages.

Still, many nice features of the ancestral environment can't be revived with bricks and mortar. Building physically intimate towns won't bring back the extended kin networks that enmeshed our ancestors and, among other benefits, made child rearing a much simpler task than it is for many parents today. Besides, most adults, given a cozy community, will still spend much of the day miles away, at work. And even if telecommuting increasingly allows them to work at home, they won't be out bonding with neighbors in the course of their vocations, as our ancestors were.

One reason the sinews of community are so hard to restore is that they are at odds with free markets. Capitalism not only spews out cars, TVs and other antisocial technologies; it also sorts people into little vocational boxes and scatters the boxes far and wide. Economic opportunity is what drew farm boys into cities, and it has been fragmenting families ever since. There is thus a tension within conservative ideology between laissez-faire economics and family values, as various people have noted. (The Unabomber complains that conservatives "whine about the decay of traditional values," yet "enthusiastically support technological progress and economic growth.")

That much modern psychopathology grows out of the dynamics of economic freedom suggests a dearth of miracle cures; Utopian alternatives to capitalism have a history of not working out. Even the more modest reforms that are imaginable—reforms that somewhat blunt modernization's antisocial effects—will hardly be easy or cheap. Workplace-based day care costs money. Ample and inviting public parks cost money. And it costs money to create good public schools—which by diverting enrollment from private schools offer the large communal virtue of making a child's neighborhood peers and schoolyard friends one and the same. Yikes: taxes! Taxes, as Newt Gingrich and others have patiently explained, slow economic growth. True enough. But if economic growth places such a strain on community to begin with—a fact that Gingrich seems to grasp—what's so bad about a marginally subdued rate of growth?

Besides, how large is the psychological toll? Evolutionary psychology suggests that we're designed to compare our material well-being not so much with some absolute standard but with that of our neighbors. So if our neighbors don't get richer—and if the people on *Lifestyles of the Rich and Famous* don't get richer—then we shouldn't, in theory, get less happy than we already are. Between 1957 and 1990, per capita income in America more than doubled in real terms. Yet, as the psychologist David Myers notes in *The Pursuit of Happiness*, the number of Americans who reported being "very happy" remained constant, at one-third. Plainly, more gross domestic product isn't the answer to our deepest needs. (And that's especially true when growth only widens the gap between richest and poorest, as has done lately.)

There is a lesson here not just for policymakers but also for the rest of us. "It is human nature always to want a little more," writes the psychologist Timothy Miller in the recent book *How to Want What You Have*, perhaps the first self-help book based explicitly on evolutionary psychology. "People spend their lives honestly believing that they have almost enough of whatever they want. Just a little more will put them over the top; then they will be contented forever." This is a built-in illusion, Miller notes, engrained in our minds by natural selection.

We are designed to seek trusting relationships.

The illusion was designed to keep us constantly striving, adding tiny increments to the chances that our genes would get into the next generation. Yet in a modern environment—which, unlike the ancestral environment, features contraception—our obsession with material gain rarely has that effect. Besides, why should any of us choose to pursue maximum genetic proliferation—or relentless material gain, or anything else—just because that is high on the agenda of the process that designed the human mind? Natural selection, for better or worse, is our creator, but it isn't God; the impulses it implanted into our minds aren't necessarily good, and they aren't wholly beyond resisting.

Part of Miller's point is that the instinctive but ultimately fruitless pursuit of More—the 60-hour workweeks, the hour a month spent perusing the Sharper Image catalog—keeps us from indulging what Darwin called "the social instincts." The pursuit of More can keep us from better knowing our neighbors, better loving our kin—in general, from cultivating the warm, affiliative side of human nature whose roots science is just now starting to fathom.

PSYCHOTRENDS

Taking Stock of Tomorrow's Family and Sexuality

Where are we going and what kind of people are we becoming? Herewith, a road map to the defining trends in sexuality, family, and relationships for the coming millenium as charted by the former chair of Harvard's psychiatry department. From the still-rollicking sexual revolution to the painful battle for sexual equality to the reorganization of the family, America is in for some rather interesting times ahead.

Shervert H. Frazier, M.D.

Has the sexual revolution been sidetracked by AIDS, and the return to traditional values we keep hearing about? In a word, no. The forces that originally fueled the revolution are all still in place and, if anything, are intensifying: mobility, democratization, urbanization, women in the workplace, birth control, abortion and other reproductive interventions, and media proliferation of sexual images, ideas, and variation.

Sexuality has moved for many citizens from church- and state-regulated behavior to a medical and self-regulated behavior. Population pressures and other economic factors continue to diminish the size of the American family. Marriage is in sharp decline, cohabitation is growing, traditional families are on the endangered list, and the single-person household is a wave of the future.

AIDS has generated a great deal of heat in the media but appears to have done little, so far, to turn down the heat in the bedroom. It is true that in some surveys people *claimed* to have made drastic changes in behavior—but most telling are the statistics relating to marriage, divorce, cohabitation, teen sex, out-of-wedlock births, sexually transmitted diseases (STDs), contraception, and adultery. These are far more revealing of what we *do* than what we *say* we do. And those tell a tale of what has been called a "postmarital society" in continued pursuit of sexual individuality and freedom.

Studies reveal women are more sexual now than at any time in the century.

Arguably there are, due to AIDS, fewer visible sexual "excesses" today than there were in the late 1960s and into the 1970s, but those excesses (such as sex clubs, bathhouses, backrooms, swinging singles, group sex, public sex acts, etc.) were never truly reflective of norms and were, in any case, greatly inflated in the media. Meanwhile, quietly and without fanfare, the public, even in the face of the AIDS threat, has continued to expand its interest in sex and in *increased,* rather than decreased, sexual expression.

Numerous studies reveal that women are more sexual now than at any time in the century. Whereas sex counselors used to deal with men's complaints about their wives' lack of "receptivity," it is now more often the women complaining about the men. And women, in this "postfeminist" era, are doing things they never used to believe were "proper." Fellatio, for example, was seldom practiced (or admitted to) when Kinsey conducted his famous sex research several decades ago. Since that time, according to studies at UCLA and elsewhere, this activity has gained acceptance among women, with some researchers reporting that nearly all young women now practice fellatio.

Women's images of themselves have also changed dramatically in the past two decades, due, in large part, to their movement into the workplace and roles previously filled exclusively by men. As Lilian Rubin, psychologist at the University of California Institute for the Study of Social Change and author of *Intimate Strangers,* puts it, "Women feel empowered sexually in a way they never did in the past."

Meanwhile, the singles scene, far from fading away (the media just lost its fixation on this subject), continues to grow. James Bennett, writing in *The New Republic,* characterizes this growing population of no-reproducers thusly: "Single adults in America display a remarkable tendency to multiply without being fruitful."

Their libidos are the target of million-dollar advertising budgets and entrepreneurial pursuits that seek to put those sex drives on line in the information age. From video dating to computer coupling to erotic faxing, it's now "love at first

5. DYNAMICS OF PERSONAL ADJUSTMENT: THE INDIVIDUAL AND SOCIETY

byte," as one commentator put it. One thing is certain: the computer is doing as much today to promote the sexual revolution as the automobile did at the dawn of that revolution.

Political ideologies, buttressed by economic adversities, *can* temporarily retard the sexual revolution, as can sexually transmitted diseases. But ultimately the forces propelling this revolution are unstoppable. And ironically, AIDS itself is probably doing more to promote than impede this movement. It has forced the nation to confront a number of sexual issues with greater frankness than ever before. While some conservatives and many religious groups have argued for abstinence as the only moral response to AIDS, others have lobbied for wider dissemination of sexual information, beginning in grade schools. A number of school districts are now making condoms available to students—a development that would have been unthinkable before the outbreak of AIDS.

Despite all these gains (or losses, depending upon your outlook) the revolution is far from over. The openness that it has fostered is healthy, but Americans are still ignorant about many aspects of human sexuality. Sexual research is needed to help us deal with teen sexuality and pregnancies, AIDS, and a number of emotional issues related to sexuality. Suffice it to say for now that there is still plenty of room for the sexual revolution to proceed—and its greatest benefits have yet to be realized.

THE REVOLUTION AND RELATIONSHIPS

The idea that the Sexual Revolution is at odds with romance (not to mention tradition) is one that is widely held, even by some of those who endorse many of the revolution's apparent objectives. But there is nothing in our findings to indicate that romance and the sexual revolution are inimical—unless one's defense of romance disguises an agenda of traditional male dominance and the courtly illusion of intimacy and communication between the sexes.

The trend now, as we shall see, is away from illusion and toward—in transition, at least—a sometimes painful reality in which the sexes are finally making an honest effort to *understand* one another.

But to some, it may seem that the sexes are farther apart today than they ever have been. The real gender gap, they say, is a communications gap so cavernous that only the most intrepid or foolhardy dare try to bridge it. Many look back at the Anita Hill affair and say that was the open declaration of war between the sexes.

The mistake many make, however, is saying that there has been a *recent* breakdown in those communications, hence all this new discontent. This conclusion usually goes unchallenged, but there is nothing in the data we have seen from past decades to indicate that sexual- and gender-related communication were ever better than they are today. On the contrary, a more thoughtful analysis makes it very clear they have always been *worse*.

What has changed is our *consciousness* about this issue. Problems in communication between the sexes have been masked for decades by a rigid social code that strictly prescribes other behavior. Communication between the sexes has long been preprogrammed by this code to produce an exchange that has been as superficial as it is oppressive. As this process begins to be exposed by its own inadequacies in a rapidly changing world, we suddenly discover that we have a problem. But, of course, that problem was there for a long time, and the discovery does not mean a decline in communication between the sexes but, rather, provides us with the potential for better relationships in the long run.

Thus what we call a "breakdown" in communications might more aptly be called a *breakthrough*.

Seymour Parker, of the University of Utah, demonstrated that men who are the most mannerly with women, those who adhere most strictly to the "code" discussed above, are those who most firmly believe, consciously or unconsciously, that women are "both physically and psychologically weaker (i.e., less capable) than men." What has long passed for male "respect" toward women in our society is, arguably, *disrespect*.

Yet what has been learned can be unlearned—especially if women force the issue, which is precisely what is happening now. Women's views of themselves are changing and that, more than anything, is working to eliminate many of the stereotypes that supported the image of women as weak and inferior. Women, far from letting men continue to dictate to them, are making it clear they want more *real* respect from men and will accept nothing less. They want a genuine dialogue; they want men to recognize that they speak with a distinct and equal voice, not one that is merely ancillary to the male voice.

The sexual revolution made possible a serious inquiry into the ways that men and women are alike and the ways that each is unique. This revolutionary development promises to narrow the gender gap as nothing else can, for only by understanding the differences that make communication so complex do we stand any chance of mastering those complexities.

SUBTRENDS

Greater Equality Between the Sexes

Despite talk in the late 1980s and early 1990s of the decline of feminism and declarations that women, as a social and political force, are waning, equality between the sexes is closer to becoming a reality than ever before. Women command a greater workforce and wield greater political power than they have ever done. They are assuming positions in both public and private sectors that their mothers and grandmothers believed were unattainable (and their fathers and grandfathers thought were inappropriate) for women. Nonetheless, much remains to be achieved before women attain complete equality—but movement in that direction will continue at a pace that will surprise many over the next two decades.

Women voters, for example, who have long outnumbered male voters, are collectively a sleeping giant whose slumber many say was abruptly interrupted during the Clarence Thomas–Anita Hill hearings in 1991. The spectacle of a political "boy's club" raking the dignified Hill over the coals of sexual harassment galvanized the entire nation for days.

On another front, even though women have a long way to go to match men in terms of equal pay for equal work, as well as in equal opportunity, there is a definite *research* trend that shows women can match men in the skills needed to succeed in business. This growing body of data will make it more difficult for businesses to check the rise of women into the upper echelons of management and gradually help to change the corporate consciousness that still heavily favors male employees.

As for feminism, many a conservative wrote its obituary in the 1980s, only to find it risen from the dead in the 1990s. Actually, its demise was always imaginary. Movements make headway only in a context of dissatisfaction. And, clearly, there is still plenty for women to be dissatisfied about, particularly in the wake of a decade that tried to stifle meaningful change.

The "new feminism," as some call it, is less doctrinaire than the old, less extreme in the sense that it no longer has to be outrageous in order to call attention to itself. The movement today is less introspective, more goal oriented and pragmatic. Demands for liberation are superseded—and subsumed—by a well-organized quest for power. Women no longer want to burn bras, they want to manufacture and market them.

The New Masculinity

To say that the men's movement today is confused is to understate mercifully. Many men say they want to be more "sensitive" but also "less emasculated," "more open," yet "less vulnerable." While the early flux of this movement is often so extreme that it cannot but evoke guffaws, there is, nonetheless, something in it that commands some respect—for, in contrast with earlier generations of males, this one is making a real effort to examine and redefine itself. The movement, in a word, is *real*.

Innumerable studies and surveys find men dissatisfied with themselves and their roles in society. Part of this, undoubtedly, is the result of the displacement men are experiencing in a culture where *women* are so successfully transforming themselves. There is evidence, too, that men are dissatisfied because their own fathers were so unsuccessful in their emotional lives and were thus unable to impart to their sons a sense of love, belonging, and security that an increasing number of men say they sorely miss.

The trend has nothing to do with beating drums or becoming a "warrior." It relates to the human desire for connection, and this, in the long run, can only bode well for communications between humans in general and between the sexes in particular. Many psychologists believe men, in the next two decades, will be less emotionally closed than at any time in American history.

More (and Better) Senior Sex

People used to talk about sex after 40 as if it were some kind of novelty. Now it's sex after 60 and it's considered not only commonplace but healthy.

Some fear that expectations among the aged may outrun physiological ability and that exaggerated hopes, in some cases, will lead to new frustrations—or that improved health into old age will put pressure on seniors to remain sexually active beyond any "decent" desire to do so.

But most seem to welcome the trend toward extended sexuality. In fact, the desire for sex in later decades of life is *heightened*, studies suggest, by society's growing awareness and acceptance of sexual activity in later life.

Diversity of Sexual Expression

As sex shifts from its traditional reproductive role to one that is psychological, it increasingly serves the needs of the individual. In this context, forms of sexual expression that were previously proscribed are now tolerated and are, in some cases increasingly viewed as no more nor less healthy than long-accepted forms of sexual behavior. Homosexuality, for example, has attained a level of acceptance unprecedented in our national history.

More Contraception, Less Abortion

Though abortion will remain legal under varying conditions in most, if not all, states, its use will continue to decline over the next two decades as more—and better—contraceptives become available After a period of more than two decades in which drug companies shied away from contraceptive research, interest in this field is again growing. AIDS, a changed political climate, and renewed fears about the population explosion are all contributing to this change.

Additionally, scientific advances now point the way to safer, more effective, more convenient contraceptives. A male contraceptive that will be relatively side-effect free is finally within reach and should be achieved within the next decade, certainly the next two decades. Even more revolutionary in concept and probable impact is a vaccine, already tested in animals, that some predict will be available within 10 years—a vaccine that safely stops ovum maturation and thus makes conception impossible.

Religion and Sex: A More Forgiving Attitude

Just a couple of decades ago mainstream religion was monolithic in its condemnation of sex outside of marriage. Today the situation is quite different as major denominations across the land struggle with issues they previously wouldn't have touched, issues related to adultery, premarital sex, homosexuality, and so on.

A Special Committee on Human Sexuality, convened by the General Assembly of the Presbyterian Church (USA), for example, surprised many when it issued a report highly critical of the traditional "patriarchal structure of sexual relations," a structure the committee believes contributes, because of its repressiveness, to the proliferation of pornography and sexual violence.

All this will surely pale alongside the brave new world of virtual reality.

The same sort of thing has been happening in most other major denominations. It is safe to say that major changes are coming. Mainstream religion is beginning to perceive that the sexual revolution must be acknowledged and, to a significant degree, accommodated with new policies if these denominations are to remain in touch with present-day realities.

Expanding Sexual Entertainment

The use of sex to sell products, as well as to entertain, is increasing and can be expected to do so. The concept that "sex sells" is so well established that we need not belabor the point here. The explicitness of sexual advertising, however, may be curbed by recent research finding that highly explicit sexual content is so diverting that the viewer or reader tends to overlook the product entirely.

Sexual stereotyping will also be less prevalent in advertising in years to come. All this means, however, is that women will not be singled out as sex objects; they'll have plenty of male company, as is already the case. The female "bimbo" is now joined by the male "himbo" in ever-increasing numbers. Sexist advertising is still prevalent (e.g., male-oriented beer commercials) but should diminish as women gain in social and political power.

There's no doubt that films and TV have become more sexually permissive in the last two decades and are likely to continue in that direction for some time to come. But all this will surely pale alongside the brave (or brazen) new world of "cybersex" and virtual reality, the first erotic emanations of which may well be experienced by Americans in the coming two decades. Virtual reality aims to be just that—artificial, electronically induced experiences that are virtually indistinguishable from the real thing.

The sexual revolution, far from over, is in for some new, high-tech curves.

FROM BIOLOGY TO PSYCHOLOGY: THE NEW FAMILY OF THE MIND

Despite recent pronouncements that the traditional family is making a comeback, the evidence suggests that over the next two decades the nuclear family will share the same future as nuclear arms: there will be fewer of them, but those that remain will be better cared for.

Our longing for sources of nurturance has led us to redefine the family.

Demographers now believe that the number of families consisting of married couples with children will dwindle by yet another 12 percent by the year 2000. Meanwhile, single-parent households will continue to increase (up 41 percent over the past decade.) And household size will continue to decline (2.63 people in 1990 versus 3.14 in 1970). The number of households maintained by women, with no males present, has increased 300 percent since 1950 and will continue to rise into the 21st century.

Particularly alarming to some is the fact that an increasing number of people are choosing *never* to marry. And, throughout the developed world, the one-person household is now the fastest growing household category. To the traditionalists, this trend seems insidious—more than 25 percent of all households in the United States now consist of just one person.

There can be no doubt: the nuclear family has been vastly diminished, and it will continue to decline for some years, but at a more gradual pace. Indeed, there is a good chance that it will enjoy more stability in the next two decades than it did in the last two. Many of the very forces that were said to be weakening the traditional family may now make it stronger, though not more prevalent. Developing social changes have made traditional marriage more elective today, so that those who choose it may, increasingly, some psychologists believe, represent a subpopulation better suited to the situation and thus more likely to make a go of it.

As we try to understand new forms of family, we need to realize that the "traditional" family is not particularly traditional. Neither is it necessarily the healthiest form of family. The nuclear family has existed for only a brief moment in human history. Moreover, most people don't realize that no sooner had the nuclear family form peaked around the turn of the last century than erosion set in, which has continued ever since. For the past hundred years, reality has chipped away at this social icon, with increasing divorce and the movement of more women into the labor force. Yet our need for nurturance, security, and connectedness continues and, if anything, grows more acute as our illusions about the traditional family dissipate.

Our longing for more satisfying sources of nurturance has led us to virtually redefine the family, in terms of behavior, language, and law. These dramatic changes will intensify over the next two decades. The politics of family will be entirely transformed in that period. The process will not be without interruptions or setbacks. Some lower-court rulings may be overturned by a conservative U.S. Supreme Court, the traditional family will be revived in the headline from time to time, but the economic and psychological forces that for decades have been shaping these changes toward a more diverse family will continue to do so.

SUBTRENDS

Deceptively Declining Divorce Rate

The "good news" is largely illusory. Our prodigious national divorce rate, which more than doubled in one recent 10-year period, now shows signs of stabilization or even decline. Still, 50 percent of all marriages will break up in the next several years. And the leveling of the divorce rate is not due to stronger marriage but to *less* marriage. More people are skipping marriage altogether and are cohabiting instead.

The slight dip in the divorce rate in recent years has caused some prognosticators to predict that younger people, particularly those who've experienced the pain of growing up in broken homes, are increasingly committed to making marriage stick. Others, more persuasively, predict the opposite, that the present lull precedes a storm in which the divorce rate will soar to 60 percent or higher.

Increasing Cohabitation

The rate of cohabitation—living together without legal marriage—has been growing since 1970 and will accelerate in the next two decades. There were under half a million cohabiting couples in 1970; today there are more than 2.5. The trend for the postindustrial world is very clear: less marriage, more cohabitation, easier and—if Sweden is any indication—less stressful separation. Those who divorce will be less likely to remarry, more likely to cohabit. And in the United States, cohabitation will increasingly gather about it both the cultural acceptance and the legal protection now afforded marriage.

We need to realize the "traditional family" is not particularly traditional.

More Single-Parent Families and Planned Single Parenthood

The United States has one of the highest proportions of children growing up in single-parent families. More than one in five births in the United States is outside of marriage—and three quarters of those births are to women who are not in consensual unions.

What is significant about the single-parent trend is the finding that many single women with children now *prefer* to remain single. The rush to the altar of unwed mothers, so much a part of American life in earlier decades, is now, if anything, a slow and grudging shuffle. The stigma of single parenthood is largely a thing of the past—and the economic realities, unsatisfactory though they are, sometimes favor single parenthood. In any case, women have more choices today than they had even 10 years ago; they are choosing the psychological freedom of single parenthood over the financial security (increasingly illusory, in any event) of marriage.

More Couples Childless by Choice

In the topsy-turvy 1990s, with more single people wanting children, it shouldn't surprise us that more married couples *don't* want children. What the trend really comes down to is increased freedom of choice. One reason for increasing childlessness among couples has to do with the aging of the population, but many of the reasons are more purely psychological.

With a strong trend toward later marriage, many couples feel they are "too old" to have children. Others admit they like the economic advantages and relative freedom of being childless. Often both have careers they do not want to jeopardize by having children. In addition, a growing number of couples cite the need for lower population density, crime rates, and environmental concerns as reasons for not wanting children. The old idea that "there must be something wrong with them" if a couple does not reproduce is fast waning.

The One-Person Household

This is the fastest growing household category in the Western world. It has grown in the United States from about 10 percent in the 1950s to more than 25 percent of all households today. This is a trend that still has a long way to go. In Sweden, nearly *40 percent* of all households are now single person.

"Mr. Mom" a Reality at Last?

When women began pouring into the work force in the late 1970s, expectations were high that a real equality of the sexes was at hand and that men, at last, would begin to shoulder more of the household duties, including spending more time at home taking care of the kids. Many women now regard the concept of "Mr. Mom" as a cruel hoax; but, in fact, Mr. Mom *is* slowly emerging.

Men *are* showing more interest in the home and in parenting. Surveys make clear there is a continuing trend in that direction. Granted, part of the impetus for this is not so much a love of domestic work as it is a distaste for work outside the home. But there is also, among many men, a genuine desire to play a larger role in the lives of their children. These men say they feel "cheated" by having to work outside the home so much, cheated of the experience of seeing their children grow up.

As the trend toward more equal pay for women creeps along, gender roles in the home can be expected to undergo further change. Men will feel less pressure to take on more work and will feel more freedom to spend increased time with their families.

More Interracial Families

There are now about 600,000 interracial marriages annually in the United States, a third of these are black-white, nearly triple the number in 1970, when 40 percent of the white population was of the opinion that such marriages should be illegal. Today 20 percent hold that belief. There is every reason to expect that both the acceptance of and the number of interracial unions will continue to increase into the foreseeable future.

Recognition of Same-Sex Families

Family formation by gay and lesbian couples, with or without children, is often referenced by the media as a leading-edge signifier of just how far society has moved in the direction of diversity and individual choice in the family realm. The number of same-sex couples has steadily increased and now stands at 1.6 million such couples. There are an estimated 2 million gay parents in the United States.

And while most of these children were had in heterosexual relationships or marriages prior to "coming out," a significant number of gay and lesbian couples are having children through adoption, cooperative parenting arrangements, and artificial insemination. Within the next two decades, gays and lesbians will not only win the right to marry but will, like newly arrived immigrants, be some of the strongest proponents of traditional family values.

The Rise of Fictive Kinships

Multiadult households, typically consisting of unrelated singles, have been increasing in number for some years and are expected to continue to do so in coming years. For many, "roommates" are increasingly permanent fixtures in daily life.

In fact housemates are becoming what some sociologists and psychologists call "fictive kin." Whole "fictive families" are being generated in many of these situations, with some housemates even assigning roles ("brother," "sister," "cousin," "aunt," "mom," "dad," and so on) to one another. Fictive families are springing up among young people, old people, disabled people, homeless people, and may well define one of the ultimate evolutions of the family concept, maximizing, as they do, the opportunities for fulfillment of specific social and economic needs outside the constraints of biological relatedness.

THE BREAKUP OF THE NUCLEAR FAMILY

It's hard to tell how many times we've heard even well-informed health professionals blithely opine that "the breakup of the family is at the root of most of our problems." The *facts* disagree with this conclusion. Most of the social problems attributed to the dissolution of the "traditional" family (which, in reality, is *not* so traditional) are the product of other forces. Indeed, as we have seen, the nuclear family has itself created a number of economic, social, and psychological problems. To try to perpetuate a manifestly transient social institution beyond its usefulness is folly.

What *can* we do to save the nuclear family? Very little.

What *should* we do? Very little. Our concern should not be the maintenance of the nuclear family as a *moral* unit (which seems to be one of the priorities of the more ardent conservative "family values" forces), encompassing the special interests and values of a minority, but, rather, the strengthening of those social contracts that ensure the health, well-being, and freedom of individuals.

Enhancing Human Adjustment: Learning to Cope Effectively

On each college and university campus a handful of students experiences overwhelming stress and life-shattering crises. One student learns that her mother, living in a distant city, has terminal cancer and 2 months to live. Another receives the sad news that his parents are divorcing; he descends into a deep depression that lowers his grades. A sorority blackballs a young woman who was determined to become their sister; she commits suicide. The sorority sisters now experience the weighty sense of responsibility and guilt.

Fortunately, almost every campus houses a counseling center for students; some universities also offer assistance to employees. At the counseling service, trained professionals such as psychologists are available to offer aid and therapy to troubled members of the campus community.

On the other hand, many individuals are able to cope on their own. They are able to adapt to life's vagaries, even to life's disasters. Other individuals flounder. They simply do not know how to adjust to change and cope with negative and sometimes positive life events. These individuals sometimes seek temporary professional assistance from a therapist or counselor. For these professionals, the difficulty may be *how* to intervene as well as *when* to intervene. Very few individuals, fortunately, require long-term care or institutionalization in our society.

There are as many definitions of *maladjustment* as there are mental health professionals. Some practitioners define maladjustment or mental illness as "whatever society cannot tolerate." Others define maladjustment in terms of statistics: "If a majority do not behave that way, then the behavior signals maladjustment." Some professionals suggest that an inadequate self-concept is the cause of maladjustment. Others cite a lack of contact with reality as an indicator of mental illness. A few psychologists claim that mental disorder is a fiction: to call one individual ill suggests that the rest are healthy by contrast, when, in fact, there may be few real distinctions among people.

Because maladjustment is difficult to define, it is sometimes difficult to treat. For each definition, a theorist develops a different treatment strategy. Psychoanalysts press clients to recall their dreams, their childhoods, and their intrapsychic conflicts in order to empty and analyze the contents of the unconscious. Humanists encourage clients to explore all of the facets of their lives in order to become less defensive and more open to experience. Behaviorists are usually not concerned with the psyche but rather with observable and therefore treatable symptoms or behaviors. For behaviorists, no underlying causes such as intrapsychic conflict are postulated to be the roots of adjustment problems. Other therapists, namely psychiatrists who are physicians by training, may utilize these therapies and add somatotherapies, such as drugs and psychosurgery.

This brief list of interventions raises further questions. For instance, is one form of therapy more effective, less expensive, or longer lasting than another? Should a particular diagnosis be treated by one form of therapy while another diagnosis is more amenable to another treatment? Who should make the diagnosis? If two experts disagree on the diagnosis and treatment, which one is correct? Should psychologists be allowed to prescribe psychoactive drugs? These questions are being debated now.

Some psychologists question whether professional intervention is necessary at all. In one well-publicized but highly criticized study, researcher Hans Eysenck was able to show that spontaneous remission rates were as high as therapeutic "cure" rates. You, yourself, may be wondering whether professional help is always necessary. Can people be their own healers? Is support from friends as productive as professional treatment?

The first three readings offer general information to individuals who are having difficulty adjusting and coping. They pertain to three common forms of intervention. In "What You Can Change and What You Cannot Change," noted psychologist Martin Seligman discusses what can be realistically managed in terms of self-improvement. He emphasizes diets and various psychological disorders. In "Frontiers of Psychotherapy," Saúl Fuks discusses psychotherapy as widely available in the United States. Interestingly, there is now a wealth of research on whether psychotherapy works.

Because health insurance companies are reluctant to pay for years of counseling, and because Americans are more sophisticated in their knowledge of psychotherapy, therapists have had to change the way they deliver assistance. Besides being more short-term, therapy today is

UNIT 6

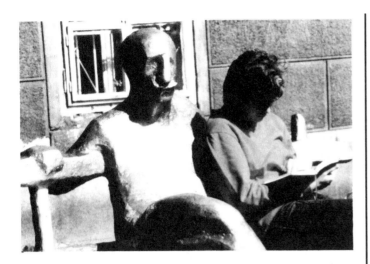

more empowering. These and other changes in how psychotherapy is practiced are detailed here.

Another form of treatment is medication. Many drugs are available to treat mental disorders. In "Prescriptions for Happiness," Seymour Fisher and Roger Greenberg review information on psychopharmacology, the study of drugs that affect the mind. Many medications today can alter the personality. Here the authors look at these medications and critique the research that establishes the effectiveness of such drugs and encourages faith in them.

In "Upset? Try Cybertherapy," Kerry Hannon takes a brief look at computerized psychological consultation. Because this form of therapy is new, practice standards, including ethical standards, have lagged. Caution is therefore needed.

We next look at various adjustment disorders. In "Defeating Depression," Nancy Wartik describes the complex relationship between heredity, personality, and life events that can trigger depression, a common disorder. Included are a self-assessment quiz and a discussion of various forms of treatment for depression.

Two other adjustment problems are discussed. One is addiction. Addictions to various substances have plagued humans for centuries. We are just now beginning to understand what causes addiction. Joanna Ellison Rodgers discusses a new perspective on addictions and ponders the question of whether addiction is a disease or a behavior. She also elaborates on various productive and unproductive treatment methods for addiction.

"Stress, It's Worse Than You Think" offers another variation of a modern American plague. Stress seems to permeate many aspects of American life. As divulged here, stress affects our physical and psychological being. Fortunately, there are good techniques for managing stress, which are also detailed.

Finally, we examine happiness and optimism, ending the book on an upbeat note. In "The New Frontiers of Happiness," Peter Doskoch suggests that humor is important to good mental health. Although humor is not always effective, it can get us through many difficult moments. Closing this anthology, Michael Scheier and Charles Carver discuss optimism, a likely companion to happiness. Optimism as construed by these researchers enhances psychological and physical well-being. It is related also to an important concept, self-efficacy, which is the feeling that we can master our environments.

Looking Ahead: Challenge Questions

There are a myriad of definitions for maladjustment. List and discuss the pros and cons of each one. Discuss whether or not maladjustment is a fiction created by society to repress the few who are differently adjusted. In what way is mental health the absence of mental illness? How do idiosyncrasies and quirks differ from mental disorders? Explain whether or not there is a reason for psychic pain and for physical pain.

People often feel distressed at home or on the job, miss deadlines, feel moody, and gain weight. What are signs and symptoms of other everyday adjustments? How do most people cope with these situations? Explain whether or not these are the best ways to cope.

After reading "What You Can Change and What You Cannot Change," what does Martin Seligman suggest can be changed by self-determination? With professional assistance? Is one approach better than the other? Discuss what problems seem immune to change. Can most individuals successfully cope with everyday difficulties? When do you believe professional intervention is necessary? Can most of us effectively change on our own, so that professional help is not necessary? Explain.

What types of psychotherapy are available? Does one form seem better than another? Which type of therapy might suit you best, and why? How and why has the way therapy is delivered changed recently?

What is cybertherapy? Would you ever try cybertherapy? Why or why not? How is this form of therapy different from traditional psychotherapy? What are its advantages and disadvantages?

For depression and addiction, what are the major symptoms and forms of treatment? What seems to cause or exacerbate each problem? What are other causes of maladjustment?

What is stress? Is it always deleterious? Explain. Why is stress at epidemic proportions in modern American society? How can people better cope with stress?

What creates happiness? What role does humor play? When is humor not an effective coping mechanism, and why not?

What is optimism? What is self-efficacy? How are optimists and pessimists different? How does a positive attitude affect physical health?

What You Can Change & What You Cannot Change

There are things we can change about ourselves and things we cannot. Concentrate your energy on what is possible—too much time has been wasted.

Martin E. P. Seligman, Ph.D.

This is the age of psychotherapy and the age of self-improvement. Millions are struggling to change: We diet, we jog, we meditate. We adopt new modes of thought to counteract our depressions. We practice relaxation to curtail stress. We exercise to expand our memory and to quadruple our reading speed. We adopt draconian regimens to give up smoking. We raise our little boys and girls to androgyny. We come out of the closet or we try to become heterosexual. We seek to lose our taste for alcohol. We seek more meaning in life. We try to extend our life span.

Sometimes it works. But distressingly often, self-improvement and psychotherapy fail. The cost is enormous. We think we are worthless. We feel guilty and ashamed. We believe we have no willpower and that we are failures. We give up trying to change.

On the other hand, this is not only the age of self-improvement and therapy, but also the age of biological psychiatry. The human genome will be nearly mapped before the millennium is over. The brain systems underlying sex, hearing, memory, left-handedness, and sadness are now known. Psychoactive drugs quiet our fears, relieve our blues, bring us bliss, dampen our mania, and dissolve our delusions more effectively than we can on our own.

Our very personality—our intelligence and musical talent, even our religiousness, our conscience (or its absence), our politics, and our exuberance—turns out to be more the product of our genes than almost anyone would have believed a decade ago. The underlying message of the age of biological psychiatry is that our biology frequently makes changing, in spite of all our efforts, impossible.

But the view that all is genetic and biochemical and therefore unchangeable is also very often wrong. Many people surpass their IQs, fail to "respond" to drugs, make sweeping changes in their lives, live on when their cancer is "terminal," or defy the hormones and brain circuitry that "dictate" lust, femininity, or memory loss.

The ideologies of biological psychiatry and self-improvement are obviously colliding. Nevertheless, a resolution is apparent. There are some things about ourselves that can be changed, others that cannot, and some that can be changed only with extreme difficulty.

What can we succeed in changing about ourselves? What can we not? When can we overcome our biology? And when is our biology our destiny?

I want to provide an understanding of what you can and what you can't change about yourself so that you can concentrate your limited time and energy on what is possible. So much time has been wasted. So much needless frustration has been endured. So much of therapy, so much of child rearing, so much of self-improving, and even some of the great social movements in our century have come to nothing because they tried to change the unchangeable. Too often we have wrongly thought we were weak-willed failures, when the changes we wanted to make in ourselves were just not possible. But all this effort was necessary: Because there have been so many failures, we are now able to see the boundaries of the unchangeable; this in turn allows us to see clearly for the first time the boundaries of what *is* changeable.

With this knowledge, we can use our precious time to make the many rewarding changes that are possible. We can live with less self-reproach and less remorse. We can live with greater confidence. This knowledge is a new understanding of who we are and where we are going.

CATASTROPHIC THINKING: PANIC

S. J. Rachman, one of the world's leading clinical researchers and one of the founders of behavior therapy, was on the phone. He was proposing that I be the "discussant" at a conference about panic disorder sponsored by the National Institute of Mental Health (NIMH).

"Why even bother, Jack?" I responded. "Everyone knows that panic is biological and that the only thing that works is drugs."

"Don't refuse so quickly, Marty. There is a breakthrough you haven't yet heard about."

Breakthrough was a word I had never heard Jack use before.

"What's the breakthrough?" I asked.

"If you come, you can find out."

So I went.

I had known about and seen panic patients for many years, and had read the literature with mounting excitement during

> So much child rearing, therapy, and self-improvement have come to nothing.

the 1980s. I knew that panic disorder is a frightening condition that consists of recurrent attacks, each much worse than anything experienced before. Without prior warning, you feel as if you are going to die. Here is a typical case history:

The first time Celia had a panic attack, she was working at McDonald's. It was two days before her 20th birthday. As she was handing a customer a Big Mac, she had the worst experience of her life. The earth seemed to open up beneath her. Her heart began to pound, she felt she was smothering, and she was sure she was going to have a heart attack and die. After about 20 minutes of terror, the panic subsided. Trembling, she got in her car, raced home, and barely left the house for the next three months.

Since then, Celia has had about three attacks a month. She does not know when they are coming. She always thinks she is going to die.

Panic attacks are not subtle, and you need no quiz to find out if you or someone you love has them. As many as five percent of American adults probably do. The defining feature of the disorder is simple: recurrent awful attacks of panic that come out of the blue, last for a few minutes, and then subside. The attacks consist of chest pains, sweating, nausea, dizziness, choking, smothering, or trembling. They are accompanied by feelings of overwhelming dread and thoughts that you are having a heart attack, that you are losing control, or that you are going crazy.

THE BIOLOGY OF PANIC

There are four questions that bear on whether a mental problem is primarily "biological" as opposed to "psychological":
- Can it be induced biologically?
- Is it genetically heritable?
- Are specific brain functions involved?
- Does a drug relieve it?

Inducing panic. Panic attacks can be created by a biological agent. For example, patients who have a history of panic attacks are hooked up to an intravenous line. Sodium lactate, a chemical that normally produces rapid, shallow breathing and heart palpitations, is slowly infused into their bloodstream. Within a few minutes, about 60 to 90 percent of these patients have a panic attack. Normal controls—subjects with no history of panic—rarely have attacks when infused with lactate.

Genetics of panic. There may be some heritability of panic. If one of two identical twins has panic attacks, 31 percent of the cotwins also have them. But if one of two fraternal twins has panic attacks, none of the cotwins are so afflicted.

Panic and the brain. The brains of people with panic disorders look somewhat unusual upon close scrutiny. Their neurochemistry shows abnormalities in the system that turns on, then dampens, fear. In addition, the PET scan (positron-emission tomography), a technique that looks at how much blood and oxygen different parts of the brain use, shows that patients who panic from the infusion of lactate have higher blood flow and oxygen use in relevant parts of their brain than patients who don't panic.

Drugs. Two kinds of drugs relieve panic: tricyclic antidepressants and the antianxiety drug Xanax, and both work better than placebos. Panic attacks are dampened, and sometimes even eliminated. General anxiety and depression also decrease.

Since these four questions had already been answered "yes" when Jack Rachman called, I thought the issue had already been settled. Panic disorder was simply a biological illness, a disease of the body that could be relieved only by drugs.

A few months later I was in Bethesda, Maryland, listening once again to the same four lines of biological evidence. An inconspicuous figure in a brown suit sat hunched over the table. At the first break, Jack introduced me to him—David Clark, a young psychologist from Oxford. Soon after, Clark began his address.

"Consider, if you will, an alternative theory, a cognitive theory." He reminded all of us that almost all panickers believe that they are going to die during an attack. Most commonly, they believe that they are having heart attacks. Perhaps, Clark suggested, this is more than just a mere symptom. Perhaps it is the root cause. Panic may simply be the *catastrophic misinterpretation of bodily sensations.*

For example, when you panic, your heart starts to race. You notice this, and you see it as a possible heart attack. This makes you very anxious, which means

41. What You Can Change

What Can We Change?
When we survey all the problems, personality types, patterns of behavior, and the weak influence of childhood on adult life, we see a puzzling array of how much change occurs. From the things that are easiest to those that are the most difficult, this rough array emerges:

Panic	Curable
Specific Phobias	Almost Curable
Sexual Dysfunctions	Marked Relief
Social Phobia	Moderate Relief
Agoraphobia	Moderate Relief
Depression	Moderate Relief
Sex Role Change	Moderate
Obsessive–Compulsive Disorder	Moderate Mild Relief
Sexual Preferences	Moderate Mild Change
Anger	Mild, Moderate Relief
Everyday Anxiety	Mild Moderate Relief
Alcoholism	Mild Relief
Overweight	Temporary Change
Posttraumatic Stress Disorder (PTSD)	Marginal Relief
Sexual Orientation	Probably Unchangeable
Sexual Identity	Unchangeable

your heart pounds more. You now notice that your heart is *really* pounding. You are now *sure* it's a heart attack. This terrifies you, and you break into a sweat, feel nauseated, short of breath—all symptoms of terror, but for you, they're confirmation of a heart attack. A full-blown panic attack is under way, and at the root of it is your misinterpretation of the symptoms of anxiety as symptoms of impending death.

> We are now able to see the boundaries of the unchangeable.

6. ENHANCING HUMAN ADJUSTMENT: LEARNING TO COPE EFFECTIVELY

I was listening closely now as Clark argued that an obvious sign of a disorder, easily dismissed as a symptom, is the disorder itself. If he was right, this was a historic occasion. All Clark had done so far, however, was to show that the four lines of evidence for a biological view of panic could fit equally well with a misinterpretation view. But Clark soon told us about a series of experiments he and his colleague Paul Salkovskis had done at Oxford.

First, they compared panic patients with patients who had other anxiety disorders and with normals. All the subjects read the following sentences aloud, but the last word was presented blurred. For example:

dying
If I had palpitations, I could be
excited

choking
If I were breathless, I could be
unfit

When the sentences were about bodily sensations, the panic patients, but no one else, saw the catastrophic endings fastest. This showed that panic patients possess the habit of thinking Clark had postulated.

Next, Clark and his colleagues asked if activating this habit with words would induce panic. All the subjects read a series of word pairs aloud. When panic patients got to "breathlessness-suffocation: and "palpitations-dying," 75 percent suffered a full-blown panic attack right there in the laboratory. No normal people had panic attacks, no recovered panic patients (I'll tell you more in a moment about how they got better) had attacks, and only 17 percent of other anxious patients had attacks.

The final thing Clark told us was the "breakthrough" that Rachman had promised.

"We have developed and tested a rather novel therapy for panic," Clark continued in his understated, disarming way. He explained that if catastrophic misinterpretations of bodily sensation are the cause of a panic attack, then changing the tendency to misinterpret should cure the disorder. His new therapy was straightforward and brief:

Patients are told that panic results when they mistake normal symptoms of mounting anxiety for symptoms of heart attack, going crazy, or dying. Anxiety itself, they are informed, produces shortness of breath, chest pain, and sweating. Once

Issues of the soul can barely be changed by psychotherapy or drugs.

they misinterpret these normal bodily sensations as an imminent heart attack, their symptoms become even more pronounced because the misinterpretation changes their anxiety into terror. A vicious circle culminates in a full-blown panic attack.

Patients are taught to reinterpret the symptoms realistically as mere anxiety symptoms. Then they are given practice right in the office, breathing rapidly into a paper bag. This causes a buildup of carbon dioxide and shortness of breath, mimicking the sensations that provoke a panic attack. The therapist points out that the symptoms the patient is experiencing—shortness of breath and heart racing—are harmless, simply the result of overbreathing, not a sign of a heart attack. The patient learns to interpret the symptoms correctly.

"This simple therapy appears to be a cure," Clark told us. "Ninety to 100 percent of the patients are panic free at the end of therapy. One year later, only one person had had another panic attack."

This, indeed, was a breakthrough: a simple, brief psychotherapy with no side effects showing a 90-percent cure rate of a disorder that a decade ago was thought to be incurable. In a controlled study of 64 patients comparing cognitive therapy to drugs to relaxation to no treatment, Clark and his colleagues found that cognitive therapy is markedly better than drugs or relaxation, both of which are better than

Self-Analysis Questionnaire
Is your life dominated by anxiety? Read each statement and then mark the appropriate number to indicate *how you generally feel*. There are no right or wrong answers.

1. I am a steady person.

Almost never	Sometimes	Often	Almost always
4	3	2	1

2. I am satisfied with myself.

Almost never	Sometimes	Often	Almost always
4	3	2	1

3. I feel nervous and restless.

Almost never	Sometimes	Often	Almost always
1	2	3	4

4. I wish I could be as happy as others seem to be.

Almost never	Sometimes	Often	Almost always
1	2	3	4

5. I feel like a failure.

Almost never	Sometimes	Often	Almost always
1	2	3	4

6. I get in a state of tension and turmoil as I think over my recent concerns and interests.

Almost never	Sometimes	Often	Almost always
1	2	3	4

7. I feel secure.

Almost never	Sometimes	Often	Almost always
4	3	2	1

41. What You Can Change

nothing. Such a high cure rate is unprecedented.

How does cognitive therapy for panic compare with drugs? It is more effective and less dangerous. Both the antidepressants and Xanax produce marked reduction in panic in most patients, but drugs must be taken forever; once the drug is stopped, panic rebounds to where it was before therapy began for perhaps half the patients. The drugs also sometimes have severe side effects, including drowsiness, lethargy, pregnancy complications, and addictions.

After this bombshell, my own "discussion" was an anticlimax. I did make one point that Clark took to heart. "Creating a cognitive therapy that works, even one that works as well as this apparently does, is not enough to show that the *cause* of panic is cognitive." I was niggling. "The biological theory doesn't deny that some other therapy might work well on panic. It merely claims that panic is caused at the bottom by some biochemical problem."

Two years later, Clark carried out a crucial experiment that tested the biological theory against the cognitive theory. He gave the usual lactate infusion to 10 panic patients, and nine of them panicked. He did the same thing with another 10 patients, but added special instructions to allay the misinterpretation of the sensations. He simply told them: "Lactate is a natural bodily substance that produces sensations similar to exercise or alcohol. It is normal to experience intense sensations during infusion, but these do not indicate an adverse reaction." Only three out of the 10 panicked. This confirmed the theory crucially.

The therapy works every well, as it did for Celia, whose story has a happy ending. She first tried Xanax, which reduced the intensity and the frequency of her panic attacks. But she was too drowsy to work, and she was still having about one attack every six weeks. She was then referred to Audrey, a cognitive therapist who explained that Celia was misinterpreting her heart racing and shortness of breath as symptoms of a heart attack, that they were actually just symptoms of mounting anxiety, nothing more harmful. Audrey taught Celia progressive relaxation, and then she demonstrated the harmlessness of Celia's symptoms of overbreathing. Celia then relaxed in the presence of the symptoms and found that they gradually subsided. After several more practice sessions, therapy terminated. Celia has gone two years without another panic attack.

Everyday Anxiety

Attend to your tongue—right now. What is it doing? Mine is swishing around near my lower right molars. It has just found a minute fragment of last night's popcorn (debris from *Terminator 2*). Like a dog at a bone, it is worrying the firmly wedged flake.

Attend to your hand—right now. What's it up to? My left hand is boring in on an itch it discovered under my earlobe.

Your tongue and your hands have, for the most part, a life of their own. You can bring them under voluntary control by consciously calling them out of their "default" mode to carry out your commands:

8. I have self-confidence.			
Almost never	Sometimes	Often	Almost always
4	3	2	1
9. I feel inadequate.			
Almost never	Sometimes	Often	Almost always
1	2	3	4
10. I worry too much over something that does not matter.			
Almost never	Sometimes	Often	Almost always
1	2	3	4

To score, simply add up the numbers under your answers. Notice that some of the rows of numbers go up and others go down. The higher your total, the more the trait of anxiety dominates your life. If your score was:

10–11, you are in the lowest 10 percent of anxiety.

13–14, you are in the lowest quarter.

16–17, your anxiety level is about average.

19–20, your anxiety level is around the 75th percentile.

22–24 (and you are male) your anxiety level is around the 90th percentile.

24–26 (and you are female) your anxiety level is around the 90th percentile.

25 (and you are male) your anxiety level is at the 95th percentile.

27 (and you are female) your anxiety level is at the 95th percentile.

Should you try to change your anxiety level? Here are my rules of thumb:

• If your score is at the 90th percentile or above, you can probably improve the quality of your life by lowering your general anxiety level—regardless of paralysis and irrationality.

• If your score is at the 75th percentile or above, and you feel that anxiety is either paralyzing you or that it is unfounded, you should probably try to lower your general anxiety level.

• If your score is 18 or above, and you feel that anxiety is unfounded and paralyzing, you should probably try to lower your general anxiety level.

Anxiety scans your life for imperfections. When it finds one, it won't let go.

6. ENHANCING HUMAN ADJUSTMENT: LEARNING TO COPE EFFECTIVELY

"Pick up the phone" or "Stop picking that pimple." But most of the time they are on their own. They are seeking out small imperfections. They scan your entire mouth and skin surface, probing for anything going wrong. They are marvelous, nonstop grooming devices. They, not the more fashionable immune system, are your first line of defense against invaders.

Anxiety is your mental tongue. Its default mode is to search for what may be about to go wrong. It continually, and without your conscious consent, scans your life—yes, even when you are asleep, in dreams and nightmares. It reviews your work, your love, your play—until it finds an imperfection. When it finds one, it worries it. It tries to pull it out from its hiding place, where it is wedged inconspicuously under some rock. It will not let go. If the imperfection is threatening enough, anxiety calls your attention to it by making you uncomfortable. If you do not act, it yells more insistently—disturbing your sleep and your appetite.

You can reduce daily, mild anxiety. You can numb it with alcohol, Valium, or marijuana. You can take the edge off with meditation or progressive relaxation. You can beat it down by becoming more conscious of the automatic thoughts of danger that trigger anxiety and then disputing them effectively.

But do not overlook what your anxiety is trying to do for you. In return for the pain it brings, it prevents larger ordeals by making you aware of their possibility and goading you into planning for and forestalling them. It may even help you avoid them altogether. Think of your anxiety as the "low oil" light flashing on the dashboard of your car. Disconnect it and you will be less distracted and more comfortable for a while. But this may cost you a burned-up engine. Our *dysphoria,* or bad feeling, should, some of the time, be tolerated, attended to, even cherished.

Guidelines for When to Try to Change Anxiety

Some of our everyday anxiety, depression, and anger go beyond their useful function. Most adaptive traits fall along a normal spectrum of distribution, and the capacity for internal bad weather for everyone some of the time means that some of us may have terrible weather all of the time. In general, when the hurt is pointless and recurrent—when, for example, anxiety insists we formulate a plan but no plan will work—it is time to take action to relieve the hurt. There are three hallmarks indicating that anxiety has become a burden that wants relieving:

First, is it *irrational?*

We must calibrate our bad weather inside against the real weather outside. Is what you are anxious about out of proportion to the reality of the danger? Here are some examples that may help you answer this question. All of the following are not irrational:

• A fire fighter trying to smother a raging oil well burning in Kuwait repeatedly wakes up at four in the morning because of flaming terror dreams.

• A mother of three smells perfume on her husband's shirts and, consumed by jealousy, broods about his infidelity, reviewing the list of possible women over and over.

• A student who had failed two of his midterm exams finds, as finals approach, that he can't get to sleep for worrying. He has diarrhea most of the time.

The only good thing that can be said about such fears is that they are well-founded.

In contrast, all of the following are irrational, out of proportion to the danger:

• An elderly man, having been in a fender bender, broods about travel and will no longer take cars, trains, or airplanes.

• An eight-year-old child, his parents having been through an ugly divorce, wets his bed at night. He is haunted with visions of his bedroom ceiling collapsing on him.

• A housewife who has an MBA and who accumulated a decade of experience as a financial vice president before her twins were born is sure her job search will be fruitless. She delays preparing her résumés for a month.

The second hallmark of anxiety out of control is *paralysis.* Anxiety intends action: Plan, rehearse, look into shadows for lurking dangers, change your life. When anxiety becomes strong, it is unproductive; no problem-solving occurs. And when anxiety is extreme, it paralyzes you. Has your anxiety crossed this line? Some examples:

• A woman finds herself housebound because she fears that if she goes out, she will be bitten by a cat.

• A salesman broods about the next customer hanging up on him and makes no more cold calls.

• A writer, afraid of the next rejection slip, stops writing.

The final hallmark is *intensity.* Is your life dominated by anxiety? Dr. Charles Spielberger, one of the world's foremost

> 'Dieting below your natural weight is a necessary condition for bulimia. Returning to your natural weight will cure it.'

testers of emotion, has developed well-validated scales for calibrating how severe anxiety is. To find out how anxious *you* are, use the self-analysis questionnaire.

Lowering Your Everyday Anxiety

Everyday anxiety level is not a category to which psychologists have devoted a great deal of attention. Enough research has been done, however, for me to recommend two techniques that quite reliably lower everyday anxiety levels. Both techniques are cumulative, rather than one-shot fixes. They require 20 to 40 minutes a day of your valuable time.

The first is *progressive relaxation,* done once or, better, twice a day for at least 10 minutes. In this technique, you tighten and then turn off each of the major muscle groups of your body until you are wholly flaccid. It is not easy to be highly anxious when your body feels like Jell-O. More formally, relaxation engages a response system that competes with anxious arousal.

The second technique is regular *meditation.* Transcendental meditation ™ is one useful, widely available version of this. You can ignore the cosmology in which it is packaged if you wish, and treat it simply as the beneficial technique it is. Twice a day for 20 minutes, in a quiet setting, you close your eyes and repeat a *mantra* (a syllable whose "sonic properties are known") to yourself. Meditation works by blocking thoughts that produce anxiety. It complements relaxation, which blocks the motor components of anxiety but leaves the anxious thoughts untouched.

Done regularly, meditation usually induces a peaceful state of mind. Anxiety at other times of the day wanes, and hyperarousal from bad events is dampened. Done religiously, TM probably works better than relaxation alone.

There's also a quick fix. The minor tranquilizers—Valium, Dalmane, Librium, and their cousins—relieve everyday anxiety. So does alcohol. The advantage of all these is that they work within minutes and require no discipline to use. Their disadvantages outweigh their advantages, however. The minor tranquilizers make you fuzzy and somewhat uncoordinated as they work (a not uncommon side effect is an automobile accident). Tranquilizers soon lose their effect when taken regularly, and they are habit-forming—probably addictive. Alcohol, in addition, produces gross cognitive and motor disability in lockstep with its anxiety relief. Taken regularly over long periods, deadly damage to liver and brain ensue.

If you crave quick and temporary relief from acute anxiety, either alcohol or minor tranquilizers, taken in small amounts and only occasionally, will do the job. They are, however, a distant second-best to progressive relaxation and meditation, which are each worth trying before you seek out psychotherapy or in conjunction with therapy. Unlike tranquilizers and alcohol, neither of these techniques is likely to do you any harm.

Weigh your everyday anxiety. If it is not intense, or if it is moderate and not irrational or paralyzing, act now to reduce it. In spite of its deep evolutionary roots, intense everyday anxiety is often changeable. Meditation and progressive relaxation practiced regularly can change it forever.

DIETING: A WAIST IS A TERRIBLE THING TO MIND

I have been watching my weight and restricting my intake—except for an occasional binge like this—since I was 20. I weighed about 175 pounds then, maybe 15 pounds over my official "ideal" weight. I weigh 199 pounds now, 30 years later, about 25 pounds over the ideal. I have tried about a dozen regimes—fasting, the Beverly Hills Diet, no carbohydrates, Metrecal for lunch, 1,200 calories a day, low fat, no lunch, no starches, skipping every other dinner. I lost 10 or 15 pounds on each in about a month. The pounds always came back, though, and I have gained a net of about a pound a year—inexorably.

This is the most consistent failure in my life. It's also a failure I can't just put out of mind. I have spent the last few years reading the scientific literature, not the parade of best-selling diet books or the flood of women's magazine articles on the latest way to slim down. The scientific findings look clear to me, but there is not yet a consensus. I am going to go out on a limb, because I see so many signs all pointing in one direction. What I have concluded will, I believe, soon be the consensus of the scientists. The conclusions surprise me. They will probably surprise you, too, and they may change your life.

Her[e] is what the picture looks like to me:
- Dieting doesn't work.
- Dieting may make overweight worse, not better.
- Dieting may be bad for health.
- Dieting may cause eating disorders—including bulimia and anorexia.

ARE YOU OVERWEIGHT?

Are you above the ideal weight for your sex, height, and age? If so, you are "overweight." What does this really mean? Ideal weight is arrived at simply. Four million people, now dead, who were insured by the major American life-insurance companies, were once weighed and had their height measured. At what weight on average do people of a given height turn out to live longest? That weight is called ideal. Anything wrong with that?

You bet. The real use of a weight table, and the reason your doctor takes it seriously, is that an ideal weight implies that, on average, if you slim down to yours, you will live longer. This is the crucial claim. Lighter people indeed live longer, on average, than heavier people, but how much longer is hotly debated.

But the crucial claim is unsound because weight (at any given height) has a normal distribution, *normal* both in a statistical sense and in the biological sense. In the biological sense, couch potatoes who overeat and never exercise can legitimately be called overweight, but the buxom, "heavy-boned" slow people deemed overweight by the ideal table are at their natural and healthiest weight. If you are a 155-pound woman and 64 inches in height, for example, you are "overweight" by around 15 pounds. This means nothing more than that the average 140-pound, 64-inch-tall woman lives somewhat longer than the average 155-pound woman of your height. It does not follow that if you slim down to 125 pounds, *you* will stand any better chance of living longer.

In spite of the insouciance with which dieting advice is dispensed, no one has properly investigated the question of whether slimming down to "ideal" weight produces longer life. The proper study would compare the longevity of people who are at their ideal weight without dieting to people who achieve their ideal weight by dieting. Without this study the common medical advice to diet down to your ideal weight is simply unfounded.

This is not a quibble; there is evidence that dieting damages your health and that this damage may shorten your life.

MYTHS OF OVERWEIGHT

The advice to diet down to your ideal weight to live longer is one myth of overweight. Here are some others:

- *Overweight people overeat.* Wrong. Nineteen out of 20 studies show that obese people consume no more calories each day than nonobese people. Telling a fat person that if she would change her eating habits and eat "normally" she would lose weight is a lie. To lose weight and stay there, she will need to eat excruciatingly less than a normal person, probably for the rest of her life.

- *Overweight people have an overweight personality.* Wrong. Extensive research on personality and fatness has proved little. Obese people do not differ in any major personality style from nonobese people.

- *Physical inactivity is a major cause of obesity.* Probably not. Fat people are indeed less active than thin people, but the inactivity is probably caused more by the fatness than the other way around.

- *Overweight shows a lack of willpower.* This is the granddaddy of all the myths. Fatness is seen as shameful because we hold people responsible for their weight. Being overweight equates with being a weak-willed slob. We believe this primarily because we have seen people decide to lose weight and do so in a matter of weeks.

But almost everyone returns to the old weight after shedding pounds. Your body has a natural weight that it defends vigorously against dieting. The more diets tried, the harder the body works to defeat the next diet. Weight is in large part genetic. All this gives the lie to the "weak-willed" interpretations of overweight. More accurately, dieting is the conscious will of the individual against a more vigilant opponent: the species' biological defense against starvation. The body can't tell the difference between self-imposed starvation and actual famine, so it defends its weight by refusing to release fat, by lowering its metabolism, and by demanding food. The harder the creature tries not to eat, the more vigorous the defenses become.

BULIMIA AND NATURAL WEIGHT

A concept that makes sense of your body's vigorous defense against weight loss is *natural weight*. When your body screams "I'm hungry," makes you lethargic, stores fat, craves sweets and renders them more delicious than ever, and makes you obsessed with food, what it is defending is your natural weight. It is signaling that you have dropped into a range it will not accept. Natural weight prevents you from gaining too much weight or losing too much. When you eat too much for too long, the opposite defenses are activated and make long-term weight gain difficult.

There is also a strong genetic contribution to your natural weight. Identical twins reared apart weigh almost the same throughout their lives. When identical twins are overfed, they gain weight and add fat in lockstep and in the same places. The fatness or thinness of adopted children resembles their biological parents—particularly their mother—very closely but does not at all resemble their adoptive parents. This suggests that you have a genetically given natural weight that your body wants to maintain.

The idea of natural weight may help cure the new disorder that is sweeping young America. Hundreds of thousands of young women have contracted it. It consists of bouts of binge eating and purging alternating with days of undereating. These young women are usually normal in weight or a bit on the thin side, but they are terrified of becoming fat. So they diet. They exercise. They take laxatives by the cup. They gorge. Then they vomit and take more laxatives. This malady is called *bulimia nervosa* (bulimia, for short).

Therapists are puzzled by bulimia, its causes, and treatment. Debate rages about whether it is an equivalent of depression, or an expression of a thwarted desire for control, or a symbolic rejection of the feminine role. Almost every psychotherapy has been tried. Antidepressants and other drugs have been administered with some effect but little success has been reported.

I don't think that bulimia is mysterious, and I think that it will be curable. I believe that bulimia is caused by dieting. The bulimic goes on a diet, and her body attempts to defend its natural weight. With repeated dieting, this defense becomes more vigorous. Her body is in massive revolt—insistently demanding food, storing fat, craving sweets, and lowering metabolism. Periodically, these biological defenses will overcome her extraordinary willpower (and extraordinary it must be to even approach an ideal weight, say, 20 pounds lighter than her natural weight). She will then binge. Horrified by what this will do to her figure, she vomits and takes laxatives to purge calories. Thus, bulimia is a natural consequence of self-starvation to lose weight in the midst of abundant food.

The therapist's task is to get the patient to stop dieting and become comfortable with her natural weight. He should first convince the patient that her binge eating is caused by her body's reaction to her diet. Then he must confront her with a question: Which is more important, staying thin or getting rid of bulimia? By stopping the diet, he will tell her, she can get rid of the uncontrollable binge–purge cycle. Her body will now settle at her natural weight, and she need not worry that she will balloon beyond that point. For some patients, therapy will end there because they would rather be bulimic than "loathsomely fat." For these patients, the central issue—ideal weight versus natural weight—can now at least become the focus of therapy. For others, defying the social and sexual pressure to be thin will be possible, dieting will be abandoned, weight will be gained, and bulimia should end quickly.

These are the central moves of the cognitive-behavioral treatment of bulimia. There are more than a dozen outcome studies of this approach, and the results are good. There is about 60 percent reduction in binging and purging (about the same as with antidepressant drugs). But unlike drugs, there is little relapse after treatment. Attitudes toward weight and shape relax, and dieting withers.

Of course, the dieting theory cannot fully explain bulimia. Many people who diet don't become bulimic; some can avoid it because their natural weight is close to their ideal weight, and therefore the diet they adopt does not starve them. In addition, bulimics are often depressed, since binging-purging leads to self-loathing. Depression may worsen bulimia by making it easier to give in to temptation. Further, dieting may just be another symptom of bulimia, not a cause. Other factors aside, I can speculate that dieting below your natural weight is a necessary condition for bulimia, and that returning to your natural weight and accepting that weight will cure bulimia.

OVERWEIGHT VS. DIETING: THE HEALTH DAMAGE

Being heavy carries some health risk. There is no definite answer to how much, because there is a swamp of inconsistent findings. But even if you could just wish pounds away, never to return, it is not certain you should. Being somewhat above your "ideal" weight may actually be your healthiest natural condition, best for your particular constitution and your particular metabolism. Of course you can diet, but the odds are overwhelming that most of the weight will return, and that you will have to diet again and again. From a health and mortality perspective, should you? *There is, probably, a serious health risk from losing weight and regaining it.*

In one study, more than five thousand men and women from Framingham, Massachusetts, were observed for 32 years. People whose weight fluctuated over the years had 30 to 100 percent greater risk of death from heart disease than people whose weight was stable. When corrected for smoking, exercise, cholesterol level, and blood pressure, the findings became more convincing, suggesting that weight fluctuation (the primary cause of which is presumably dieting) may itself increase the risk of heart disease.

If this result is replicated, and if dieting is shown to be the primary cause of weight cycling, it will convince me that you should not diet to reduce your risk of heart disease.

DEPRESSION AND DIETING

Depression is yet another cost of dieting, because two root causes of depression are failure and helplessness. Dieting sets you up for failure. Because the goal of slimming down to your ideal weight pits your fallible willpower against untiring biological defenses, you will often fail. At first you will lose weight and feel pretty good about it. Any depression you had about your figure will disappear. Ultimately, however, you will probably not reach your goal; and then you will be dismayed as the pounds return. Every time you look in the mirror or vacillate over a white chocolate mousse, you will be reminded of your failure, which in turn brings depression.

On the other hand, if you are one of the fortunate few who can keep the weight from coming back, you will probably have to stay on an unsatisfying low-calorie diet for the rest of your life. A side effect of prolonged malnutrition is depression. Either way, you are more vulnerable to it.

If you scan the list of cultures that have a thin ideal for women, you will be struck by something fascinating. All thin-ideal cultures also have eating disorders. They also have roughly twice as much depression in women as in men. (Women diet twice as much as men. The best estimate is that 13 percent of adult men and 25 percent of adult women are now on a diet.) The cultures without the thin ideal have no eating disorders, and the amount of depression in women and men in these cultures is the same. This suggests that around the world, the thin ideal and dieting not only cause eating disorders, but they may also cause women to be more depressed than men.

THE BOTTOM LINE

I have been dieting off and on for 30 years because I want to be more attractive, healthier, and more in control. How do these goals stack up against the facts?

Attractiveness. If your attractiveness is a high-enough priority to convince you to diet, keep three drawbacks in mind. First, the attractiveness you gain will be temporary. All the weight you lose and maybe more will likely come back in a few years. This will depress you. Then you will have to lose it again and it will be harder the second time. Or you will have to resign yourself to being less attractive. Second, when women choose the silhouette figure they want to achieve, it turns out to be thinner than the silhouette that men label most attractive. Third, you may well become bulimic particularly if your natural weight is substantially more than your ideal weight. On balance, if short-term attractiveness is your overriding goal, diet. But be prepared for the costs.

Health. No one has ever shown that losing weight will increase my longevity. On balance, the health goal does not warrant dieting.

Control. For many people, getting to an ideal weight and staying there is just as biologically impossible as going with much less sleep. This fact tells me not to diet, and defuses my feeling of shame. My bottom line is clear: I am not going to diet anymore.

DEPTH AND CHANGE: THE THEORY

Clearly, we have not yet developed drugs or psychotherapies that can change all the problems, personality types, and patterns of behavior in adult life. But I believe that success and failure stems from something other than inadequate treatment. Rather, it stems from the depth of the problem.

We all have experience of psychological states of different depths. For example, if you ask someone, out of the blue, to answer quickly, "Who are you?" they will usually tell you—roughly in this order—their name, their sex, their profession, whether they have children, and their religion or race. Underlying this is a continuum of depth from surface to soul—with all manner of psychic material in between.

I believe that issues of the soul can barely be changed by psychotherapy or by drugs. Problems and behavior patterns somewhere between soul and surface can be changed somewhat. Surface problems can be changed easily, even cured. What is changeable, by therapy or drugs, I speculate, varies with the depth of the problem.

My theory says that it does not matter *when* problems, habits, and personality are acquired; their depth derives only from their biology, their evidence, and their power. Some childhood traits, for example, are deep and unchangeable but not because they were learned early and therefore have a privileged place.

Rather, those traits that resist change do so either because they are evolutionarily prepared or because they acquire great power by virtue of becoming the framework around which later learning crystallizes. In this way, the theory of depth carries the optimistic message that we are not prisoners of our past.

41. What You Can Change

When you have understood this message, you will never look at your life in the same way again. Right now there are a number of things that you do not like about yourself and that you want to change: your short fuse, your waistline, your shyness, your drinking, your glumness. You have decided to change, but you do not know what you should work on first. Formerly you would have probably selected the one that hurts the most. Now you will also ask yourself which attempt is most likely to repay your efforts and which is most likely to lead to further frustration. Now you know your shyness and your anger are much more likely to change than your drinking, which you now know is more likely to change than your waistline.

Some of what does change is under your control, and some is not. You can best prepare yourself to change by learning as much as you can about what you can change and how to make those changes. Like all true education, learning about change is not easy; harder yet is surrendering some of our hopes. It is certainly not my purpose to destroy your optimism about change. But it is also not my purpose to assure everybody they can change in every way. My purpose is to instill a new, warranted optimism about the parts of your life you can change and so help you focus your limited time, money, and effort on making actual what is truly within your reach.

Life is a long period of change. What you have been able to change and what has resisted your highest resolve might seem chaotic to you: for some of what you are never changes no matter how hard you try, and other aspects change readily. My hope is that this essay has been the beginning of wisdom about the difference.

Frontiers of psychotherapy

Psychotherapy has invented new forms of dialogue

Saúl Fuks

SAÚL FUKS, an Argentine psychologist, is director of the research institute of the faculty of psychology at the University of Rosario, where he teaches a specialist course in clinical psychology for postgraduate students.

Psychotherapy that takes account of complexity must be based on a form of dialogue that enables those involved to question their convictions and dare to explore new approaches to reality.

This means that the psychotherapist must agree to come down from his or her pedestal. If psychotherapists really want their patients to rediscover the capacity to assume responsibility for their lives, they must reject the position of power their patients attribute to them at the outset.

The therapeutic relationship tends to function according to a socio-cultural pattern in which the psychotherapist is regarded as the heir of the shaman, the healer or the sage—as a person with special powers associated with a vast and diffuse corpus of knowledge.

'Psychotherapists have had to become explorers of the unknown territories of existence.'

The state of desperation and extreme vulnerability that induces people to consult a psychotherapist makes them extremely receptive to the image of the therapist as an omniscient person with unlimited powers to cure mental suffering.

Because people who suffer in this way feel weak, they tend to entrust themselves fully to the psychotherapist, who is regarded as someone who can answer all their questions (and thus, they hope, solve all their problems).

The only way to modify the balance of power between the person who has all the knowledge and the person who has none is to redefine psychotherapy and first of all what society expects from the psychotherapist.

A co-operative relationship

Long before psychotherapy became a profession, a variety of practices existed to put right those who "deviated" from the social norm, either by going too far (agitation, manic states, madness) or not far enough (loss of contact, unsociability, inertia).

"Madness" and "delinquency" are the terms society uses to describe these deviations from the line it considers to be "normal" at a given moment in its history. A penal system and a security apparatus exist to take steps against delinquency; machinery for control and isolation exists to deal with madness. On the other hand, society makes allowances for those it regards as "visionary" or "inspired" people whose ways of life are accompanied by certain deviant forms of behaviour.

In the 1960s questions began to be asked about the power relationships that exist in psychotherapy, paving the way for exploration of other aspects of the therapeutic relationship.

This relationship gradually ceased to be considered as a contract between a professional possessing a specific body of knowledge and a patient ready to accept and absorb that knowledge, but rather as the confrontation of two different, but equally valid, types of knowledge. These forms of knowledge may or may not coincide, but their degree of convergence or divergence does not affect the idea that the therapeutic relationship is by nature co-operative.

This approach has led to a transformation of the roles, identities, practices, context and forms that exist in this type of relationship. Today, those involved in psychotherapy are no longer simply people telling a story, true or false as the case may be, but have become architects of their own lives.

The complexities of psychotherapy

This new approach to the alleviation of psychological distress has naturally transformed the possibilities and the operational capacity of psychotherapy.

Crises, troubles and disorders are no longer considered as "risk situations" but as "fields of possibility". This being so, a rich array of intensely felt choices, decisions, and hesitations between "future and possible" worlds comes into play and obliges psychotherapists to invent new forms of dialogue.

When their inherent complexities are taken into account, deviant symptoms and forms of behaviour become part of a contextual dynamic based on language. Verbal exchanges bring into play factors large and small, subjectivity and intersubjectivity, and all the building blocks of reality available to the protagonist and to the person who is seemingly a mere observer.

Before it began to explore these different ways of being and their contexts, psychotherapy first had to re-examine the function of "social control". This meant that therapists had to abandon the role whereby they made a diagnosis based on a system of theoretical knowledge and become explorers of the unknown territories of existence. They had to use their ignorance and their capacity for surprise, in order to explore the mysteries of what seems "obvious", "natural", and "common knowledge".

This joint construction of a shared reality involved the creation of new mechanisms: a form of dialogue in which the questions are more important than the answers; an atmosphere of co-operation conducive to the exploration of possible futures and ways leading to them.

The "essentialist" approach whereby persons are considered as possessors of *an* identity was based on the coherence and permanence of a uniform "mode of existing". The idea that each of us is the sum of *multiple* identities, on the other hand, makes it possible for both therapists and their patients to use all these complex and multidimensional aspects of their personality.

This is not a purely theoretical question: multiple identities also define our possibilities and limits in the worlds of the emotions, the intellect and action. What people allow or refuse to allow themselves to think, feel and do is closely linked to the structure of their identities and to the degree of flexibility, creativity and reflection that it allows, and to their possibilities of further development.

Psychotherapy has become a field in which all those involved can explore and discover their resources in order to redefine their lives.

> *'The idea that each of us is the sum of multiple identities makes it possible for both therapists and their patients to use all the multidimensional aspects of their personalities.'*

PROZAC. ZOLOFT. PAXIL. WELLBUTRIN.

Prescriptions for Happiness?

The biological approach to treating unhappiness is booming. But is it all it's cracked up to be? Two noted researchers demonstrate that the "scientific" studies that underpin claims of drug effectiveness are seriously flawed—undone by signals from our bodies. Perhaps the studies really prove the power of placebo—and the absurdity of drawing any line between what is biological and what is psychological.

Seymour Fisher, Ph.D., and Roger P. Greenberg, Ph.D.

The air is filled with declarations and advertisements of the power of biological psychiatry to relieve people of their psychological distress. Some biological psychiatrists are so convinced of the superiority of their position that they are recommending young psychiatrists no longer be taught the essentials of doing psychotherapy. Feature stories in such magazines as *Newsweek* and *Time* have portrayed drugs like Prozac as possessing almost a mystical potency. The best-selling book *Listening to Prozac* by psychiatrist Peter Kramer, M.D., projects the idyllic possibility that psychotropic drugs may eventually be capable of correcting a spectrum of personality quirks and lacks.

As longtime faculty members of a number of psychiatry departments, we have personally witnessed the gradual but steadily accelerated dedication to the idea that "mental illness" can be mastered with biologically based substances. Yet a careful sifting of the pertinent literature indicates that modesty and skepticism would be more appropriate responses to the research accumulated thus far. In 1989, we first raised radical questions about such biological claims in a book, *The Limits of Biological Treatments for Psychological Distress: Comparisons with Psychotherapy and Placebo* (Lawrence Erlbaum). Our approach has been to filter the studies that presumably anchor them through a series of logical and quantitative (meta-analytic) appraisals.

HOW EFFECTIVE ARE ANTIDEPRESSANT DRUGS?

Antidepressants, one of the major weapons in the biological therapeutic arsenal, illustrate well the largely unacknowledged uncertainty that exists in the biological approach to psychopathology. We suggest that, at present, no one actually knows how effective antidepressants are. Confident declarations about their potency go well beyond the existing evidence.

To get an understanding of the scientific status of antidepressants, we analyzed how much more effective the antidepressants are than inert pills called "placebos." That is, if antidepressants are given to one depressed group and a placebo to another group, how much greater is the recovery of those taking the active drug as compared to those taking the inactive placebo? Generous claims that antidepressants usually produce improvement in about 60 to 70 percent of patients are not infrequent, whereas placebos are said to benefit 25 to 30 percent. If antidepressants were, indeed, so superior to placebos, this would be a persuasive advertisement for the biological approach.

We found 15 major reviews of the antidepressant literature. Surprisingly, even the most positive reviews indicate that 30 to 40 percent of studies show no significant difference in response to drug versus placebo! The reviews indicate overall that one-third of patients do not improve with antidepressant treatment, one-third improve with placebos, and an additional third show a response to medication they would not have attained with placebos. In the most optimistic view of such findings, two-thirds of the cases (placebo responders and those who do not respond to anything) do as well with placebo as with active medication.

We also found two large-scale quantitative evaluations (meta-analyses) integrating the outcomes of multiple studies of antidepressants. They clearly indicated, on the average, quite modest therapeutic power.

We were particularly impressed by the large variation in outcomes of studies conducted at multiple clinical sites or centers. Consider a study that compared the effectiveness of an antidepressant among patients at five different research centers. Although the pooled results demonstrate that the drug was generally more effective than placebo, the results from individual centers reveal much variation. After six weeks of treatment, every one of the six measures of effectiveness showed the antidepressant (imipramine) to be merely equivalent to placebo in two or more of the centers. In two of the settings, a difference favoring the medication was detected on only one of 12 outcome comparisons.

In other words, the pooled, apparently favorable, outcome data conceal that dramatically different results could be obtained as a function of who conducted the study and the specific conditions at each locale. We can only conclude that a good deal of fragility characterized the apparent superiority of drug over placebo. The scientific literature is replete with analogous examples.

Incidentally, we also looked at whether modern studies, which are presumably better protected against bias, use higher doses, and often involve longer treatment periods, show a greater superiority of the antidepressant than did earlier studies. The literature frequently asserts that failures to demonstrate antidepressant superiority are due to such methodological failures as not using high enough doses, and so forth.

We examined this issue in a pool of 16 studies assembled by psychiatrists John Kane and Jeffrey Lieberman in 1984. These studies all compare a standard drug, such as imipramine or amitriptyline, to a newer drug and a placebo. They use clearer diagnostic definitions of depression than did the older studies and also adopt currently accepted standards for dosage levels and treatment duration. When we examined the data, we discovered that the advantage of drug over placebo was modest. Twenty-one percent more of the patients receiving a drug improved as compared to those on placebo. Actually, most of the studies showed no difference in the percentage of patients significantly improved by drugs. There was no indication that these studies, using more careful methodology, achieved better outcomes than older studies.

Finally, it is crucial to recognize that several studies have established that there is a high rate of relapse among those who have responded positively to an antidepressant but then are taken off treatment. The relapse rate may be 60 percent or more during the first year after treatment cessation. Many studies also show that any benefits of antidepressants wane in a few months, even while the drugs are still being taken. This highlights the complexity of evaluating antidepressants. They may be effective initially, but lose all value over a longer period.

Are Drug Trials Biased?

As we burrowed deeper into the antidepressant literature, we learned that there are also crucial problems in the methodology used to evaluate psychotropic drugs. Most central is the question of whether this methodology properly shields drug trials from bias. Studies have shown that the more open to bias a drug trial is, the greater the apparent superiority of the drug over placebo. So questions about the trustworthiness of a given drug-testing procedure invite skepticism about the results.

The question of potential bias first came to our attention in studies comparing inactive placebos to active drugs. In the classic double-blind design, neither patient nor researcher knows who is receiving drug or placebo. We were struck by the fact that the presumed protection provided by the double-blind design was undermined by the use of placebos that simply do not arouse as many body sensations as do active drugs. Research shows that patients learn to discriminate between drug and placebo largely from body sensations and symptoms.

A substance like imipramine, one of the most frequently studied antidepressants, usually causes clearly defined sensations, such as dry mouth, tremor, sweating, constipation. Inactive placebos used in studies of antidepressants also apparently initiate some body sensations, but they are fewer, more inconsistent, and less intense as indicated by the fact that they are less often cited by patients as a source of discomfort causing them to drop out of treatment.

Vivid differences between the body sensations of drug and placebo groups could signal to patients as to whether they are receiving an active or inactive agent. Further, they could supply discriminating cues to those responsible for the patients's day-to-day treatment. Nurses, for example, might adopt different attitudes toward patients they identify as being "on" versus "off" active treatment—and consequently communicate contrasting expectations.

The Body of Evidence

This is more than theoretical. Researchers have reported that in a double-blind study of imipramine, it was possible by means of side effects to identify a significant number of the patients taking the active drug. Those patients receiving a placebo have fewer signals (from self and others) indicating they are being actively treated and should be improving. By the same token, patients taking an active drug receive multiple signals that may well amplify potential placebo effects linked to the therapeutic context. Indeed, a doctor's strong belief in the power of the active drug enhances the apparent therapeutic power of the drug or placebo.

Is it possible that a large proportion of the difference in effectiveness often reported between antidepressants and placebos can be explained as a function of body sensation discrepancies? It is conceivable, and fortunately there are research findings that shed light on the matter.

Consider an analysis by New Zealand psychologist Richard Thomson. He reviewed double-blind, placebo-controlled studies of antidepressants completed between 1958 and 1972. Sixty-eight had employed an inert placebo and seven an active one (atropine) that produced a variety of

Vivid differences between the body sensations of drug and placebo could signal to patients whether they are receiving an active or inactive agent.

6. ENHANCING HUMAN ADJUSTMENT: LEARNING TO COPE EFFECTIVELY

A patient's attitude toward the therapist is just as biological in nature as a patient's response to an antidepressant drug.

body sensations. The antidepressant had a superior therapeutic effect in 59 percent of the studies using inert placebo—but in only one study (14 percent) using the active placebo. The active placebo eliminated any therapeutic advantage for the antidepressants, apparently because it convinced patients they were getting real medication.

How Blind Is Double-Blind?

Our concerns about the effects of inactive placebos on the double-blind design led us to ask just how blind the double-blind really is. By the 1950s reports were already surfacing that for psychoactive drugs, the double-blind design is not as scientifically objective as originally assumed. In 1993 we searched the world literature and found 31 reports in which patients and researchers involved in studies were asked to guess who was receiving the active psychotropic drug and who the placebo. In 28 instances the guesses were significantly better than chance—and at times they were surprisingly accurate. In one double-blind study that called for administering either imipramine, phenelzine, or placebo to depressed patients, 78 percent of patients and 87 percent of psychiatrists correctly distinguished drug from placebo.

One particularly systematic report in the literature involved the administration of alprazolam, imipramine, and placebo over an eight-week period to groups of patients who experienced panic attacks. Halfway through the treatment and also at the end, the physicians and the patients were asked to judge independently whether each patient was receiving an active drug or a placebo. If they thought an active drug was being administered, they had to decide whether it was alprazolam or imipramine. Both physicians (with an 88 percent success rate) and patients (83 percent) substantially exceeded chance in the correctness of their judgments. Furthermore, the physicians could distinguish alprazolam from imipramine significantly better than chance. The researchers concluded that "double-blind studies of these pharmacological treatments for panic disorder are not really 'blind.'"

Yet the vast majority of psychiatric drug efficacy studies have simply *assumed* that the double-blind design is effective; they did not test the blindness by determining whether patients and researchers were able to differentiate drug from placebo.

We take the somewhat radical view that this means most past studies of the efficacy of psychotropic drugs are, to unknown degrees, scientifically untrustworthy. At the least, we can no longer speak with confidence about the true differences in therapeutic power between active psychotropic drugs and placebos. We must suspend judgment until future studies are completed with more adequate controls for the defects of the double-blind paradigm.

Other bothersome questions arose as we scanned the cascade of studies focused on antidepressants. Of particular concern is how unrepresentative the patients are who end up in the clinical trials. There are the usual sampling problems having to do with which persons seek treatment for their discomfort, and, in addition, volunteer as subjects for a study. But there are others. Most prominent is the relatively high proportion of patients who "drop out" before the completion of their treatment programs.

Numerous dropouts occur in response to unpleasant side effects. In many published studies, 35 percent or more of patients fail to complete the research protocol. Various procedures have been developed to deal fairly with the question of how to classify the therapeutic outcomes of dropouts, but none can vitiate the simple fact that the final sample of fully treated patients has often been drastically reduced.

There are still other filters that increase sample selectivity. For example, studies often lose sizable segments of their samples by not including patients who are too depressed to speak, much less participate in a research protocol, or who are too disorganized to participate in formal psychological testing. We also found decisions not to permit particular racial or age groups to be represented in samples or to avoid using persons below a certain educational level. Additionally, researchers typically recruit patients whose depression is not accompanied by any other type of physical or mental disorder, a situation that does not hold for the depressed in the general population.

So we end up wondering about the final survivors in the average drug trial. To what degree do they typify the average individual in real life who seeks treatment? How much can be generalized from a sample made up of the "leftovers" from multiple depleting processes? Are we left with a relatively narrow band of those most willing to conform to the rather rigid demands of the research establishment? Are the survivors those most accepting of a dependent role?

The truth is that there are probably multiple kinds of survivors, depending upon the specific local conditions prevailing where the study was carried out. We would guess that some of the striking differences in results that appear in multicenter drug studies could be traced to specific forms of sampling bias. We do not know how psychologically unique the persons are who get recruited into, and stick with, drug research enterprises. We are not the first to raise this question, but we are relatively more alarmed about the potential implications.

Researcher Motivation and Outcome

We recently conducted an analysis that further demonstrates how drug effectiveness diminishes as the opportunity for bias in research design wanes. This analysis seized on studies in which a newer antidepressant is compared (under double-blind conditions) with an older, standard antidepressant and a placebo. In such a context the efficacy of the newer drug (which the drug company hopes to introduce) is of central interest to the researcher, and the effectiveness of the older drug of peripheral import. Therefore, if the double-blind is breached (as is likely), there would presumably be less bias to enhance the efficacy of the older drug than occurred in the original trials of that drug.

We predicted that the old drug would appear significantly less powerful in the newer studies than it had in earlier designs, where it was of central interest of the researcher. To test this hypothesis, we located 22 double-blind studies in which newer antidepressants were compared with an older antidepressant drug (usually imipramine) and a placebo. Our meta-analysis revealed, as predicted, that the efficacy rates, based on clinicians's judgments of outcome, were quite modest for the older antidepressants. In fact, they were approximately one-half to one-quarter the average size of the effects reported in earlier studies when the older drug was the only agent appraised.

Let us be very clear as to what this signifies: When researchers were evaluating the

43. Prescriptions for Happiness?

antidepressant in a context where they were no longer interested in proving its therapeutic power, there was a dramatic decrease in that apparent power, as compared to an earlier context when they were enthusiastically interested in demonstrating the drug's potency. A change in researcher motivation was enough to change outcome. Obviously this means too that the present double-blind design for testing drug efficacy is exquisitely vulnerable to bias.

Another matter of pertinence to the presumed biological rationale for the efficacy of antidepressants is that no consistent links have been demonstrated between the concentration of drug in blood and its efficacy. Studies have found significant correlations for some drugs, but of low magnitude. Efforts to link plasma levels to therapeutic outcome have been disappointing.

Similarly, few data show a relationship between antidepressant dosage levels and their therapeutic efficacy. That is, large doses of the drug do not necessarily have greater effects than low doses. These inconsistencies are a bit jarring against the context of a biological explanatory framework.

We have led you through a detailed critique of the difficulties and problems that prevail in the body of research testing the power of the antidepressants. We conclude that it would be wise to be relatively modest in claims about their efficacy. Uncertainty and doubt are inescapable.

While we have chosen the research on the antidepressants to illustrate the uncertainties attached to biological treatments of psychological distress, reviews of other classes of psychotropic drugs yield similar findings. After a survey of anti-anxiety drugs, psychologist Ronald Lipman concluded there is little consistent evidence that they help patients with anxiety disorders: "Although it seems natural to assume that the anxiolytic medications would be the most effective psychotropic medications for the treatment of anxiety disorders, the evidence does not support this assumption."

Biological Versus Psychological?

The faith in the biological approach has been fueled by a great burst of research. Thousands of papers have appeared probing the efficacy of psychotropic drugs. A good deal of basic research has attacked fundamental issues related to the nature of brain functioning in those who display psychopathology. Researchers in these areas are dedicated and often do excellent work. However, in their zeal, in their commitment to the so-called biological, they are at times overcome by their expectations. Their hopes become rigidifying boundaries. Their vocabulary too easily becomes a jargon that camouflages over-simplified assumptions.

A good example of such oversimplification is the way in which the term "biological" is conceptualized. It is too often viewed as a realm distinctly different from the psychological. Those invested in the biological approach all too often practice the ancient Cartesian distinction between somatic-stuff and soul-stuff. In so doing they depreciate the scientific significance of the phenomena they exile to the soul-stuff category.

But paradoxically, they put a lot of interesting phenomena out of bounds to their prime methodology and restrict themselves to a narrowed domain. For example, if talk therapy is labeled as a "psychological" thing—not biological—this implies that biological research can only hover at the periphery of what psychotherapists do. A sizable block of behavior becomes off limits to the biologically dedicated.

In fact, if we adopt the view that the biological and psychological are equivalent (biological monism), there is no convincing real-versus-unreal differentiation between the so-called psychological and biological. It *all* occurs in tissue and one is not more "real" than the other. A patient's attitude toward the therapist is just as biological in nature as a patient's response to an antidepressant. A response to a placebo is just as biological as a response to an antipsychotic drug. This may be an obvious point, but it has not yet been incorporated into the world views of either the biologically or psychologically oriented.

Take a look at a few examples in the research literature that highlight the overlap or identity of what is so often split apart. In 1992, psychiatrist Lewis Baxter and colleagues showed that successful psychotherapy of obsessive-compulsive patients results in brain imagery changes equivalent to those produced by successful drug treatment. The brain apparently responds in equivalent ways to both the talk and drug approaches. Even more dramatic is a finding that instilling in the elderly the illusion of being in control of one's surroundings (by putting them in charge of some plants) significantly increased their life span compared to a control group. What could be a clearer demonstration of the biological nature of what is labeled as a psychological expectation than the postponement of death?

Why are we focusing on this historic Cartesian confusion? Because so many who pursue the so-called biological approach are by virtue of their tunnel vision motivated to overlook the psychosocial variables that mediate the administration of such agents as psychotropic drugs and electroconvulsive therapy. They do not permit themselves to seriously grasp that psychosocial variables are just as biological as a capsule containing an antidepressant. It is the failure to understand this that results in treating placebo effects as if they were extraneous or less of a biological reality than a chemical agent.

Placebo Effects

Indeed, placebos have been shown to initiate certain effects usually thought to be reserved for active drugs. For example, placebos clearly show dose-level effects. A larger dose of a placebo will have a greater impact than a lower dose. Placebos can also create addictions. Patients will poignantly declare that they cannot stop taking a particular placebo substance (which they assume is an active drug) because to do so causes them too much distress and discomfort.

Placebos can produce toxic effects such as rashes, apparent memory loss, fever, headaches, and more. These "toxic" effects may be painful and even overwhelming in their intensity. The placebo literature is clear: Placebos are powerful body-altering substances, especially considering the wide range of body systems they can influence.

Actually, the power of the placebo complicates all efforts to test the therapeutic efficacy of psychotropic drugs. When placebos alone can produce positive curative effects in the 40 to 50 percent range (occasionally even up to 70–80 percent), the active drug being tested is hard-pressed to demonstrate its superiority. Even if the active drug exceeds the placebo in potency, the question remains whether the advantage is at least partially due to the superior potential of the active drug itself to mobilize placebo effects be-

---

Administering a therapeutic drug is not simply a medical, biological act. It is also a complex social act, its effectiveness mediated by the patient's expectations.

> **If a stimulant drug is administered with the deceptive instruction that it is a sedative, it can initiate a physiological response characteristic of a sedative, such as decreased heart rate.**

cause it is an active substance that stirs vivid body sensations. Because it is almost always an inactive substance (sugar pill) that arouses fewer genuine body sensations, the placebo is less convincingly perceived as having therapeutic prowess.

Drug researchers have tried, in vain, to rid themselves of placebo effects, but these effects are forever present and frustrate efforts to demonstrate that psychoactive drugs have an independent "pure" biological impact. This state of affairs dramatically testifies that the labels "psychological" and "biological" refer largely to different perspectives on events that all occur in tissue. At present, it is somewhat illusory to separate the so-called biological and psychological effects of drugs used to treat emotional distress.

The literature is surprisingly full of instances of how social and attitudinal factors modify the effects of active drugs. Antipsychotic medications are more effective if the patient likes rather than dislikes the physician administering them. An antipsychotic drug is less effective if patients are led to believe they are only taking an inactive placebo. Perhaps even more impressive, if a stimulant drug is administered with the deceptive instruction that it is a sedative, it can initiate a pattern of physiological response, such as decreased heart rate, that is sedative rather than arousing in nature. Such findings reaffirm how fine the line is between social and somatic domains.

What are the practical implications for distressed individuals and their physicians? Administering a drug is not simply a medical (biological) act. It is, in addition, a complex social act whose effectiveness will be mediated by such factors as the patient's expectations of the drug and reactions to the body sensations created by that drug, and the physician's friendliness and degree of personal confidence in the drug's power. Practitioners who dispense psychotropic medications should become thoroughly acquainted with the psychological variables modifying the therapeutic impact of such drugs and tailor their own behavior accordingly. By the same token, distressed people seeking drug treatment should keep in mind that their probability of benefiting may depend in part on whether they choose a practitioner they truly like and respect. And remember this: You are the ultimate arbiter of a drug's efficacy.

How to go about mastering unhappiness, which ranges from "feeling blue" to despairing depression, puzzles everyone. Such popular quick fixes as alcohol, conversion to a new faith, and other splendid distractions have proven only partially helpful. When antidepressant drugs hit the shelves with their seeming scientific aura, they were easily seized upon. Apparently serious unhappiness (depression) could now be chemically neutralized in the way one banishes a toothache.

But the more we learn about the various states of unhappiness, the more we recognize that they are not simply "symptoms" awaiting removal. Depressed feelings have complex origins and functions. In numerous contexts—for example, chronic conflict with a spouse—depression may indicate a realistic appraisal of a troubling problem and motivate a serious effort to devise a solution.

While it is true that deep despair may interfere with sensible problem-solving, the fact is that, more and more, individuals are being instructed to take antidepressants at the earliest signs of depressive distress and this could interfere with the potentially constructive signaling value of such distress. Emotions are feelings full of information. Unhappiness is an emotion, and despite its negativity, should not be classified single-mindedly as a thing to tune out. This in no way implies that one should submit passively to the discomfort of feeling unhappy. Actually, we all learn to experiment with a variety of strategies for making ourselves feel better, but the ultimate aim is long-term effective action rather than a depersonalized "I feel fine."

Seymour Fisher, Ph.D., is professor of psychology and coordinator of research training in the Department of Psychiatry and Behavioral Sciences at the University of New York Health Science Center, Syracuse.

Roger P. Greenberg, Ph.D., is professor and head of the Division of Clinical Psychology, as well as director of psychology internship training, at the State University of New York Health Science Center, Syracuse.

UPSET? TRY CYBERTHERAPY

An online visit to the psychologist may provide an answer, cheap

KERRY HANNON

Got the blues? Can't stop scarfing down bags of potato chips? Your spouse is always hostile, and you and the kids are, too? Therapy might help—at $125 a session. Or you could test a '90s solution: E-mail your way to mental health for a fraction of the cost.

In the past year, angst has become a thriving niche on the World Wide Web. Many psychologists who are setting up home pages see electronic consultation as a way to plump up incomes hit by managed care and to attract new patients to the office. For the most part, these cyberpractitioners are careful to warn potential patients that the medium doesn't allow for detailed probing. "I give advice like Ann Landers and Dear Abby do," explains Dorothy Litwin, a New York psychologist who specializes in substance abuse, women's issues and couples therapy.

Litwin is one of five women who joined forces about a year ago to form an electronic practice, Shrink-Link (see box, "A few routes to mental health"). Four are New York State-licensed psychologists; one is a psychiatrist. Each has her own regular practice and specializes in a particular area of psychotherapy. For $20—you pay upfront by typing in your credit card number—you can send off your 200-word (or less) question; it is then routed to the appropriate therapist. Within 72 hours (often within 24 hours), you get back two or three paragraphs of privately E-mailed advice.

The cybercouch is best at giving people who can clearly identify the dilemma a start toward a solution.

The short answer. The cybercouch is most effective at giving people who can clearly identify the dilemma (my daughter is anorexic; I'm deep in debt and can't stop spending) a start toward a solution. A typical Shrink-Link question: "My 5-year-old was diagnosed with attention deficit disorder (ADD) in 1993 and has been on Ritalin ever since. She has been having trouble falling asleep for the past several months and has been moodier than usual of late. What do you think?"

The gist of the response: "Some trial and error is often required before the correct dosage and timing are found, and symptoms such as sleep disturbance and moodiness often occur in the interim. Moreover, since children's rates of metabolism change, dosages often need to be adjusted. Even if the dosage is correct, the behavior irregularities you describe could be caused by administering the drug too late in the afternoon or by a host of other factors, such as nighttime fears. These possibilities need to be ruled out one by one until the culprit is found."

The advice could well be to seek face-to-face counseling. E-mail exchanges are no basis for a diagnosis, for example, warns Marlene Maheu, a San Diego clinical psychologist who headed the American Psychological Association's subcommittee that recently looked into the ethics of cybertherapy. "It's impossible to get an anonymous patient's complete family history in a 200-word question," she says. And without such cues as voice tone, facial expressions and body language, how can a therapist be sure what the problems really are? "Smiley screen faces are a poor substitute for real communication," agrees Leonard Holmes, a therapist based in Newport News, Va., who says his online services are not therapy but "E-mail discussions." ("It's a bit more private than a call-in radio show," he notes.) Holmes charges $1.50 per minute and will spend as much time "with" a patient as the patient desires.

Maheu's subcommittee and other psychology professionals worry that a lack of standards makes people seeking online help vulnerable. "When you are answering questions by E-mail, it's tempting to stray beyond your area of expertise," says Maheu. "The APA's ethical principles prohibit that." Critics also worry that confidentiality is at risk. While patients remain anonymous, a hacker could conceivably identify them. And these Internet sessions aren't encrypted. "You have no way of knowing who is printing the E-mail message out or where it is stored," says Thomas Nagy, a psychologist and Stanford University School of Medicine psychiatry professor. Nagy also worries that people with really significant problems will stop with an online Band-Aid.

Troubling, too, is the fact that patients may know little about the therapist and his or her qualifications. Many sites don't disclose details about the counselors' experience and where they earned their credentials. Leonard Holmes, by contrast, provides a complete biography on his Web page that includes his educational background, what state he is licensed in, as well as areas of expertise. That way, interested patients can check out his professional background before a session.

Beyond the couch. Aside from the various psychologists' couches, other Net offerings can be a great resource for someone trying to research a particular mental illness. One of the richest sites is the American Psychological Association's PsychNET, where you can find a wealth of downloadable material on topics from eating disorders to panic disorders to childhood abuse to how to choose a psychologist. A list of state psychological and mental health organizations is provided, and you can link to related home pages of interest. Other sites that provide entree to a comprehensive list of psychology-related pages: the online *Self-Help & Psychology Magazine*, Psychology.Com's Cyber-Psych link and the Psych Central page. You might look up an article in the *American Journal of Psychology*, for example—or check out the services of the National Alliance for the Mentally Ill or take the Myers Briggs Personality Profile.

Much of the Internet action takes place on a portion of the Web dedicated to a collection of electronic bulletin boards, or newsgroups, where people can look to their peers for support and advice. Each such mental health forum is dedicated to a specific topic: depression (*news:alt.support.depression*), shyness (*news:alt.support.shyness*), loneliness (*news:alt.support.loneliness*), for example. "For consumers who want to compare notes, exchange information and have a virtual shoulder to cry on, these can offer some real solace," says Maheu. All three major online services—America Online, CompuServe and Prodigy—offer similar mental health forums, with lengthy lists of links to other sites. For many people, the knowledge and companionship to be tapped online will be worth much more than byte-size advice.

A few routes to mental health

- **Shrink-Link** (*http://www.westnet.com/shrink*). These New York women—four psychologists and one psychiatrist—offer E-mail advice for $20 a pop.
- **Leonard Holmes** (*http://www.psychology.com/holmes.htm*). Holmes is a therapist in Newport News, Va., who answers E-mail questions for $1.50 per minute and provides links to other sites.
- **PsychNET** (*http://www.apa.org*). The American Psychological Association offers downloadable mental health information and other Web links.
- **Self-Help & Psychology Magazine** (*http://www.well.com/user/selfhelp*). It carries articles on a range of mental health topics, and links to hundreds of pages.
- **Psychology.Com's Cyber-Psych link** (*http://www.psychology.com*). You get access to psychology journals, newsgroups and more.
- **Psych Central** (*http://www.coil.com/~grohol/*). Dr. John Grohol, a Columbus, Ohio-based therapist offers no counseling but features articles on mental health and hundreds of links.

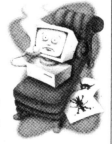

ILLUSTRATION BY DOUG STERN FOR *USN&WR*

Article 45

DEFEATING Depression

An array of new treatments combats the "common cold of mental illness"

Nancy Wartik

Nancy Wartik is a Contributing Editor at AMERICAN HEALTH.

For Charles Kennedy* of Princeton, N.J., the overwhelming sensation was a leaden slowness, as if a heavy weight were bearing down on him. Just beginning a competitive retraining program, the 51-year-old banker needed all his wits about him. Instead Kennedy found it harder and harder to function.

"Usually a challenge triggers my adrenaline," he says. "This time I found it difficult to respond. I couldn't understand the course assignments, much less complete them, which made me feel helpless and hopeless. Everything became very slow." At night Kennedy tossed and turned. He plodded through days in a pall of indifference. "The feeling was, 'Oh yeah, a bus is coming right at me. Should I move or not?' " he says. It was not until a therapist suggested he try an antidepressant drug that Kennedy found relief. "I could sleep better, proceed with initiative," he says. "My indifference disappeared. I became much more of a player again."

Everyone falls into the doldrums at times, or luxuriates in a bit of self-pity or melancholy. But depression is different. A mind-warping, energy-sapping malady, it unbalances the normal rhythms of the body and turns the psychic landscape bleak, robbing a person of vigor and hope. For someone afflicted with clinical (also called unipolar) depression, the sensations of sadness and loss, familiar to everyone on occasion, stretch into weeks or months. Nor does there seem to be an end in sight: Perhaps depression's worst torment is the conviction that things will never change. The depressed feel they will be mired in numbing despair forever.

The trappings of good fortune—wealth, talent or power—confer no immunity. "I am now the most miserable man living," wrote Abraham Lincoln. "If what I feel were equally distributed to the whole human family, there would not be one cheerful face on earth." Sir Winston Churchill, writer Sylvia Plath and actress Jean Seberg were similarly visited with bouts of despair. More recently, TV journalist Mike Wallace, author William Styron and talk show host Dick Cavett went public about their struggles with depression. Last summer, White House aide Vincent Foster committed suicide in the throes of depression apparently triggered by the Capitol Hill pressure cooker. Like Foster, 15% of those suffering from the more severe form of the disorder, which doctors call major depression, will ultimately take their own lives.

Not so long ago, the prevailing belief was that depressed people simply needed to pull themselves together and snap out of it. But an explosion of new research in recent decades has shown depression to be a real disorder that can be diagnosed and successfully treated. "Depression used to be viewed as some sort of moral weakness or personal failure," says Dr. Ewald Horwath, director of the intensive care unit at the New York State Psychiatric Institute in New York City. "Now there's more of a tendency to think of it as a disease, and that's a big improvement."

Most scientists think depression results from an interaction of biochemical, genetic and psychological factors, often, although not always, combined with a change in life circumstances—from the failure of a relationship to the loss of a job. In other words, depression is like many other diseases. "The factors that cause a physical illness such as coronary artery disease include diet, genetics and the way people who have a Type A personality put pressure on themselves," says Horwath. "Cultural factors influence who gets it, how frequent it is in each sex, and how prevalent it is in different epochs. It's the same kind of thing with depression."

Treatments for depression have expanded along with knowledge of its origins. There are now more than 20 antidepressants on the market, many of them "cleaner" drugs with fewer side effects than their predecessors. The most popular is the much-ballyhooed Prozac, already prescribed to more than 5 million Americans. Not that pills are the only antidote to depression: Cognitive psychotherapy, developed specifically to attack the disorder, teaches people how to correct the thought patterns that generate black moods. There's now evidence that regular exercise can alleviate more moderate cases of depression, perhaps because it increases levels of certain brain chemicals that mediate mood,

[*Real names are not used in this article.]

6. ENHANCING HUMAN ADJUSTMENT: LEARNING TO COPE EFFECTIVELY

and has arousing effects on body metabolism and energy. Victims of seasonal affective disorder, whose despondency comes and goes as the seasons change, often benefit from light therapy. And in some extreme cases of depression, electroconvulsive therapy, a much refined and milder form of the "shock therapy" first used here in the 1940s, can help when other treatments fail or would take too long—as when there is a likelihood of suicide. Through one or more of these treatments, the National Institute of Mental Health estimates that 80% to 90% of the depressed can find relief. As researchers sometimes say jokingly, today is the best time in history to feel miserable.

That's fortunate, because huge numbers of Americans do. More than 9 million people endure major depression yearly in this country, and about one in 20 will face the struggle at some point in his or her life. So ubiquitous is depression that researchers now refer to it as the "common cold of mental illness." And millions more are affected by other mood-related disorders. Victims of dysthymia, a recently identified form of chronic, milder depression, may battle gloom for years at a time (see "Long-Term Blues"). People with manic depression (also called bipolar disorder) veer dizzyingly between protracted emotional heights and depths, and cyclothymics go through less intense but more frequent ups and downs.

Many more women than men experience depression. Puberty is the dividing line: Before it, young boys and girls feel gloomy in almost equal numbers, but at adolescence, girls' depression rates begin to soar. At least twice as many women as men will fall prey to the disorder over the course of a lifetime, most studies have shown. Recent research by Johns Hopkins University psychiatrist Alan Romanoski paints an even more alarming picture: Although women and men have a similar risk of major depression, women suffer from more moderate depressions at *10 times* the rate men do. Researchers hotly debating the reason for this disparity have focused on three areas: physiological causes, such as genetic factors or hormonal imbalances; psychological factors, including differences in how men and women learn to deal with emotions; and social issues, from women's greater susceptibility to sexual abuse and battering to their lower economic status.

Sadly, the greatest obstacles to eliminating depression are ignorance and lack of understanding. For all its prevalence, and despite the many therapies available, two-thirds of those who have it don't get the help they need, often because they don't want to admit the problem or don't recognize its signs. "Many people who have major depression wouldn't even call themselves depressed," says psychiatrist A. John Rush of the University of Texas Southwestern Medical Center in Dallas. "If you ask them, 'Do you know you have clinical depression?'—depression serious enough to need treatment—they say, 'I don't know what that is.' " Trying to intervene in more cases, the Department of Health and Human Services (HHS) this year issued guidelines to alert general practitioners and other primary-care physicians to depression's warning signs.

As yet, there's no physical test to pinpoint the disease. Instead doctors look for a constellation of symptoms that persist for longer than two weeks. These include deep sadness or numbing apathy, a lack of interest in things that

---

DESPAIR BEYOND DESPAIR

William Styron

The pain is unrelenting, and what makes the condition intolerable is the foreknowledge that no remedy will come—not in a day, an hour, a month or a minute. If there is mild relief, one knows that it is only temporary; more pain will follow. It is hopelessness even more than pain that crushes the soul. So the decision-making of daily life involves not, as in normal affairs, shifting from one annoying situation to another less annoying—or from discomfort to relative comfort, or from boredom to activity—but moving from pain to pain. One does not abandon, even briefly, one's bed of nails, but is attached to it wherever one goes. And this results in a striking experience—one which I have called, borrowing military terminology, the situation of the walking wounded. For in virtually any other serious sickness, a patient who felt similar devastation would be lying flat in bed, possibly sedated and hooked up to the tubes and wires of life-support systems, but at the very least in a posture of repose and in an isolated setting. His invalidism would be necessary, unquestioned and honorably attained. The sufferer from depression has no option and therefore finds himself, like a walking casualty of war, thrust into the most intolerable social situations. There he must, despite the anguish devouring his brain, present a face approximating the one that is associated with ordinary events and companionship. He must try to utter small talk, and be responsive to questions, and knowingly nod and frown and, God help him, even smile. But it is a fierce trial attempting to speak a few simple words.

That December evening, for example, I could have remained in bed as usual during those worst hours, or agreed to the dinner party my wife had arranged downstairs. But the very idea of a decision was academic. Either course was torture, and I chose the dinner not out of any particular merit but through indifference to what I knew would be indistinguishable ordeals of fogbound horror. At dinner I was barely able to speak, but the quartet of guests, who were all good friends, were aware of my condition and politely ignored my catatonic muteness. Then, after dinner, sitting in the living room, I experienced a curious inner convulsion that I can describe only as despair beyond despair. It came out of the cold night; I did not think such anguish possible.

Excerpted from Darkness Visible: A Memoir of Madness, © *1990 by William Styron. Reprinted by permission of Random House.*

once brought pleasure—from sex to socializing—and at least four of seven other markers: appetite disturbances, sleep problems, fatigue, difficulty concentrating, undue restlessness or lethargy, feelings of worthlessness, or suicidal thoughts. (Someone mourning a death may have one or more of these symptoms for several months without necessarily being clinically depressed.) Many depressed people are also afflicted with vague physical symptoms or complaints.

Exercise can alleviate moderate cases.

"They come into the doctor's office with stomachaches or joint pain, or they feel blah," says Dr. Rush. "Many of these patients turn out to have major depression." Untreated, the disorder typically lasts for six months or longer.

Researchers now know several risk factors that raise a person's vulnerability to depression, including a family history of the disorder. Research with twins has provided evidence that depression's roots are at least partially inherited. A 1992 study of more than 1,000 pairs of female twins showed that if one identical twin (who shares all of her sister's genes) suffered major depression, the other's risk was 66% higher than that of someone from the general population. If a fraternal twin was depressed, however, her twin (who is no more genetically similar to her than any other sibling) had a risk only 27% higher. While such statistics suggest genetics play a significant role in depression, Medical College of Virginia psychiatrist Kenneth Kendler, who conducted the study, notes that "depression isn't something you inherit 100%, as you do eye color or height. It's probably about 40% influenced by your genes."

Inheritance may also influence certain personality traits that can make a person depression-prone. Some researchers now argue for the existence of a syndrome—at least partially innate—known as depressive personality disorder, which predisposes those who have it to depression problems. People with this disorder, explains psychiatrist Robert Hirschfeld of the University of Texas Medical Branch in Galveston, tend to be pessimistic and brooding, critical of themselves and others. The probability that such individuals will develop clinical depression is correspondingly higher than the average person's.

Genetics or personality structure may prime a person for depression, but life's travails often play a marked role in pushing someone over the brink. Although some people fall into depressions with no apparent cause, the experience of Angela Wolf* is more typical. A vice president at a Manhattan marketing firm, she plunged into paralyzing despair after she discovered that her husband of 16 years was cheating on her. She was unable to work efficiently or sleep soundly; she cried often and paced restlessly. Not until a friend referred her to a cognitive therapist did Wolf realize what was happening to her. "It was a relief when he told me I was depressed," she says. "I could say, 'No wonder! So there's a reason I feel this way.'"

A growing body of research supports the idea that major depressions are often triggered by stressful events of the kind Wolf experienced. A study of 680 pairs of female twins, published this year in *The American Journal of Psychiatry*, ranked the importance of nine risk factors for serious depression, including recent upsetting events, genetics, lack of social support, traumas suffered over a lifetime (for example, rape or sexual abuse), and childhood loss of a parent. Of all the variables, recent stress—divorce, illness, legal troubles, bereavement—was the best predictor of a depressive episode. A family history of the disorder ranked second. Similarly, Dr. Romanoski's study, based on data gathered from 800 Baltimore residents, found that 86% of major depressions were precipitated by a real-life event or situation. This research contradicts a prevailing belief that depressions triggered by an identifiable event aren't really illnesses and don't need professional treatment. "Just because we can understand why a person is depressed doesn't mean we shouldn't treat the problem seriously," says psychiatrist Sidney Zisook of the University of California at San Diego. "Depression can develop a life of its own, and once it does, it needs to be addressed, because it's still associated with decreased functioning and suicide."

Painful experiences in early life can also sow the seeds of future gloom. A 1991 Stanford University study attributed up to 35% of the discrepancy between male and female depression rates to sexual abuse of women in childhood. Other research suggests that growing up in the wake of a divorce may also predispose a person to depression. Such trauma may literally be etched into a young brain, some scientists speculate. "Life experiences might create enduring changes in the central nervous system," says Horwath, "and that might alter neurochemistry and place the person at higher risk for depression. The environmental factor ultimately has a biological effect."

Studies have long linked alcoholism and depression, but it's not always clear which is cause and which is effect. Logic would suggest that people in pain drink to ease their sorrow. Yet many studies show that people who are already alcoholic—men in particular—go on to develop major depression, perhaps because high levels of prolonged intoxication eventually unbalance brain chemistry. For women, the cause-and-effect pattern tends to go the other way, although researchers aren't sure why as yet.

No matter what its origins are, the neurochemistry of despair is the same. Imbalances of certain mood-regulating neurotransmitters—chemical messengers that transmit electrochemical signals between brain cells—are thought to underlie depression at its most fundamental level. Among possible scenarios of what goes awry in the brain: Levels of the neurotransmitters that control mood may be abnormally low, or the neural receptors that normally intercept neurotransmitters as they pass from cell to cell may malfunction.

Scientists have so far identified about 100 of the brain's many neurotransmitters. Two of these, norepinephrine and serotonin, appear to be most closely tied to depression. Says psychiatrist Elliott Richelson, director of research at a branch of the Mayo Clinic in Jacksonville, Fla., "It could be that changes in norepinephrine or serotonin levels affect some other neurotransmitter more directly involved in depression. There are probably at least 100 neurotransmitters we haven't even identified yet, so it's highly possible we still have to find the one that's absolutely key in regulating depression."

Antidepressants, which correct brain chemistry imbalances, have been on the market for over 30 years. Some early ones—specifically the tricyclic drugs, such as imipramine—affect neurochemicals other than serotonin and norepinephrine, causing a wide range of potential side effects, including dry mouth, weight gain and drowsiness. Other early antidepressants, the so-called monoamine oxidase (MAO) inhibitors, are inconvenient to take: Patients must avoid cheese, wine and a long list of other foods containing a chemical that reacts with the drug and can send blood pressure soaring. More targeted medications that act solely on mood-regulating neurotransmitters are generally easier on patients' systems. For example, Prozac and another relatively new drug, Zoloft, act only on serotonin. Fewer side effects combined with tales of miracle cures have made these new drugs more popular than the previous generations of antidepressants, which may nonetheless work as well or better in some people.

Researchers estimate that about 75% of those suffering from major depression can benefit from one of these medications. "In the last decade, there's been a shift toward using antidepressants, and I think that's good," says Brown University psychologist Tracie Shea. "They can be extremely helpful when depression has started to affect functioning. Pills don't solve life's problems, but they can put people in a better position to solve the problems themselves. They give people the energy to look at issues going on in their lives, and that gives them more choice and control."

This sort of talk alarms some mental health professionals, who worry that antidepressants are turning into the latest pharmaceutical fad, used in ever milder cases of the blues, rather than for the severe disorders they were developed to treat. "I'm not saying they should never be used," says Dr. Roger Greenberg, a psychologist at the State University of New York Health Science Center in Syracuse, "but I'm concerned at the promise being held out for drugs. I think people should be more cautious about taking them than they have

About 75% can benefit from medication.

been up to now. We want quick and easy solutions for complex and difficult problems—it's a fast-food kind of mentality. Drugs have a natural appeal, they help people say, 'I'm not responsible for my actions, it's my body chemistry.' "

Psychiatrist Peter Kramer, author of the best-selling book *Listening to Prozac*, views drug treatment differently. "There's an idea that there's a moral price to be paid if you're on medication, and that it's better to do things by other means. Is it more comfortable and easier to believe that disorders can be treated through honesty and hard work? Yes. But if you have someone in front of you who's suffering, you have to be realistic about choosing the best way to alleviate their pain."

Patients who've benefited from antidepressants tend to agree with Dr. Kramer. Charlotte Goldberg*, 30, of New York City was plagued by depression after she separated

---

Long-Term Blues

a milder form of depression known as dysthymia can dog a sufferer for years on end. "It's like a low-grade infection people just can't get rid of," says psychologist James McCullough, director of the Unipolar Mood Disorders Institute at Virginia Commonwealth University in Richmond. "They're not taken out of the work force or the home—they just feel bad most of the time. They don't know why, but they've felt that way for as long as they can remember."

An estimated 3% to 4% of Americans—two out of three of them women—experience dysthymia during their lifetime. Like victims of major depression, they may have sleep, appetite, energy and concentration problems. The disorder often strikes early in life: Dr. James Kocsis, a dysthymia expert at Cornell Medical Center in New York City, says his average patient has been despondent for 20 years, usually beginning in childhood or adolescence. Only about 10% to 15% of cases clear up on their own. Not surprisingly, dysthymics tend to have interpersonal problems, poor self-esteem and difficulty asserting themselves. They're also at significantly increased risk of major depression: Those who experience a severe slump are said to have "double depression."

Prior to 1980, when the disorder was first identified, dysthymics were typically dismissed as dark, gloomy people. Now mental health practitioners increasingly treat dysthymia like depression, with promising results. A 1988 study by Kocsis published in the *Archives of General Psychiatry* showed that six out of 10 dysthymics respond to antidepressants. "Patients say, 'This is the first time in my life I've ever felt normal,' " says Kocsis. "Their occupational underachievement and social problems tend to improve rapidly. One of the outcomes of treating dysthymia is that you start receiving wedding invitations. Patients get married and invite their psychiatrists to their weddings."

Unfortunately, even after a year of drug treatment, 60% to 70% of patients who discontinue medication will relapse. So far, there have been no controlled clinical trials of psychotherapy's effectiveness against the disorder. But Dr. McCullough, who has treated some 150 dysthymics with a combination of cognitive and behavioral therapy, says he's encouraged by the outcome. Of 20 therapy patients on whom he's kept systematic records, 70% were still depression-free after two years. "If their basic thought and behavior patterns don't change, dysthymics will stay depressed no matter what good things happen to them," notes McCullough. "These are issues that therapy can address."

from her husband and switched careers. Yet she had reservations about trying an antidepressant. "I was very hesitant," she recalls. "I was afraid I'd become falsely happy, that it wouldn't really be me. It bothered me to think of being chemically altered." But after she began taking Zoloft, Goldberg changed her mind: "I feel good but not in a stupid, high way," she says. "I can think more clearly, I'm calmer, not as anxious. Being less moody and having more energy has helped me to work through my problems better."

In sum, antidepressants can often restore emotional and physical equilibrium, but they don't make people euphoric or eliminate life stresses. After reviewing more than 400 clinical trials of antidepressants, a panel of distinguished researchers who developed the HHS depression treatment guidelines concluded that "no one antidepressant is clearly more effective than another. No single medication results in remission for all patients." Only 50% to 60% of patients respond to the first drug they try; the rest need to experiment until they find a drug that works for them. Moreover, for reasons researchers still don't understand, it usually takes four to six weeks before patients begin to feel the medication's full effects.

When the HHS guidelines were issued, the American Psychological Association, whose members specialize in talk therapy, issued a press release disassociating the organization from the guidelines on the grounds that they "do not encourage sufficient collaboration with mental health specialists and appear to be biased toward medication." In fact, says Rush of Texas Southwestern Medical Center, who chaired the government panel, 60% of antidepressants are now distributed by primary-care doctors, meaning that many people already take the drugs without accompanying psychotherapy. Some experts see no problem with that. "For the severely depressed patient, I don't think talk therapy is helpful," says the Mayo Clinic's Richelson. "The folks I see are really ill, and they're not going to be helped by the addition of a 50-minute hour."

Still, when the HHS panel compared the efficacy of talk therapy *and* medication with drug treatment alone, they found the combination treatment to be somewhat more effective. And a number of studies show that in less severe depressions psychotherapy by itself may work just as well as antidepressants. "My hunch is that whatever drugs are doing to brain chemistry, effective therapy can do also," notes Vanderbilt University clinical psychologist Steven Hollon, a specialist in cognitive therapy. "You're changing an attitude and that changes biology—just as biology changes attitude. I think the two are interactive processes."

A 1989 National Institute of Mental Health study of people with mild to moderate depressions found therapy to be as successful as medication in helping patients recover over a 16-week period. Overall, research suggests that some 50% of the depressed can alleviate the symptoms of depression with either cognitive therapy or other types.

Cognitive therapy was developed in the '60s by psychiatrist Aaron Beck, now at the University of Pennsylvania. Its premise is that thoughts create feelings: Change destructive ideas, Beck said, and unhappy emotions will change too. One such destructive pattern is a tendency to blame oneself exclusively when something goes wrong. Explains Dr. Hollon, "Someone who loses his job and says, 'I'm not good enough,' is more likely to get depressed than someone who says, 'It's a lousy economy and Bill Clinton is to blame.'"

The inclination to brood rather than act on difficulties is another pattern believed to be self-defeating and one that might help explain some of the male-female disparity in depression rates. When Stanford University psychologist Susan Nolen-Hoeksema reviewed the literature, she was struck by the fact that "women generally seem to stay with negative emotions, like depression or anxiety, more than men do. It's often talked of as a woman's strength to be able to acknowledge negative emotions, but I started looking at how it works against them."

Dr. Nolen-Hoeksema concluded that people who obses-

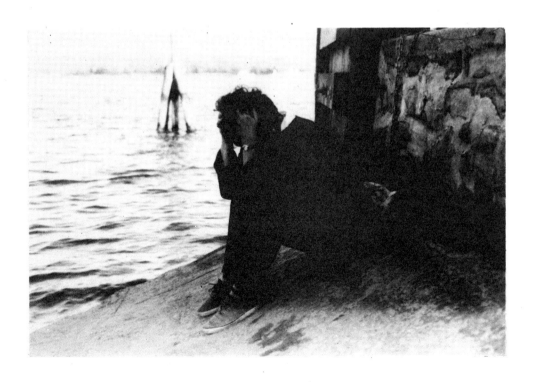

sively ponder a problem and its negative implications can find themselves sucked into a vicious circle of gloom. Those who distract themselves with sports or other enjoyable activities—as many men seem to do instinctively—emerge from unhappy moods faster and in a better state to tackle problems. Why do women tend to be brooders and men doers? "One of our guesses is that young boys aren't allowed to ruminate," says Nolen-Hoeksema. "They're taught to be active from an early age. Research on preschoolers seems to show that one thing parents will not tolerate is emotionality in boys. It's also possible that the things girls worry about actually are harder to deal with than the things boys worry about. Girls think a lot more about interpersonal relationships than boys do, and those are hard to control."

The logic behind cognitive therapy may sound simplistic, but it boasts many enthusiastic converts. Angela Wolf, the woman whose depression was triggered by her husband's infidelities, says cognitive therapy saved her life. " I was assaulted by automatic negative thoughts and my therapist would have me try to prove them to myself, the way you would to a jury. I'd think, 'If I leave this marriage, no man will ever be attracted to me.' Then I'd have to write down why I thought that statement was true, and also why I thought it wasn't. Inevitably, I'd wind up proving it *wasn't* true." Now divorced, Wolf says, "I'm infinitely happier today."

One particularly controversial issue among scientists who debate the merits of psychological vs. drug treatments is recurrence: At least 50% of those who suffer an attack will experience another. "Our whole concept of the disorder is shifting from thinking of it as time-limited to recognizing that it's much more chronic than we thought," says Brown's Dr. Shea. "For many people, depression won't be a one-shot deal." She adds that a few months of treatment with drugs or therapy, until fairly recently considered standard, often aren't enough to keep a patient well: "People shouldn't think of depression as something that can necessarily be cured in 16 weeks."

Therapy proponents argue that patients have a better chance of staying depression-free over time if they learn psychological techniques to help ward off relapses. "Pharmacology [drug therapy] is marvelous," says Hollon, "but it mostly suppresses symptoms. It's like taking aspirin. If you want to take it every day, it will do a very good job of stopping your headache. But if you learn to meditate and you reduce your overall stress level, maybe you won't get headaches to begin with. In that sense, cognitive therapy may be analogous to learning to meditate."

In a recent study published in the *Archives of General Psychiatry*, Hollon and colleague Mark Evans, a University of Minnesota psychologist, found that about 75% of depressed people in each of two groups treated either with medication or cognitive therapy felt well enough to stop treatment after three months. But over the next two years, 50% of those treated with medication relapsed into depressions, while only 20% of those treated with therapy did.

A growing number of doctors, however, are dealing with the threat of recurrence by keeping patients on medication for much longer periods of time—in some instances, many years beyond the six to nine months typically allotted for treating an episode of depression. Some 90% of those who stay on antidepressants remain symptom-free, but it has yet to be seen if prolonged antidepressant use carries undiscovered risks. "I'm a little nervous about the amount of time people are kept on drugs these days," says Hollon. "There probably aren't any really nasty complications lurking out there, but we're mucking around with complex physiology. You always wonder about the risk of side effects."

Clearly, there are complex questions remaining about depression that can only be answered through years of research. One point, however, is clear: Today, no one need stoically endure the lethargy and sense of futility that descend with an episode of depression. "I don't think long-term suffering is very therapeutic," sums up Dr. Zisook of UC-San Diego. "It doesn't help someone become a better person. And it's not something that people need to go through when we have treatments for it."

For more information on mood disorders, contact the following organizations: D/ART (Depression Awareness, Recognition, and Treatment), 800-421-4211; the National Depressive and Manic-Depressive Association, 800-826-3632; and the Depression and Related Affective Disorders Association, 410-955-4647.

ADDICTION
A Whole New View

*Our addiction theories and policies are woefully outdated. New research shows that there are no demon drugs. Nor are addicts innately defective. Nature has supplied us **all** with the ability to become hooked—and we all engage in addictive behaviors to some degree.*

Joann Ellison Rodgers

Joann Ellison Rodgers, M.S., *is deputy director of public affairs and director of media relations for the Johns Hopkins Medical Institutions. She is also president of the Council for the Advancement of Science Writing and a lecturer in the Department of Epidemiology at the Johns Hopkins School of Hygiene and Public Health on science and the mass media. A past president of the National Association of Science Writers and winner of a Lasker Award for medical journalism, Rodgers has written six books and innumerable articles.*

Millions of Americans are apparently "hooked," not only on heroin, morphine, amphetamines, tranquilizers, and cocaine, but also nicotine, caffeine, sugar, steroids, work, theft, gambling, exercise, and even love and sex. The War on Drugs alone is older than the century. In the last four years, the United States spent $45 billion waging it, with no end in sight, despite every kind of addiction treatment from psychosurgery, psychoanalysis, psychedelics, and self-help to acupuncture, group confrontation, family therapy, hypnosis, meditation, education, and tough love.

There seems no end to our "dependencies," their bewildering intractability, the glib explanations for their causes and even more glib "solutions."

The news, however, is that brain, mind, and behavior specialists are rethinking the whole notion of addiction. With help from neuroscience, molecular biology, pharmacology, psychology, and genetics, they're challenging their own hard-core assumptions and popular "certainties" and finding surprisingly common characteristics among addictions.

They're using new imaging techniques to see how addiction looks and feels and where cravings "live" in the brain and mind. They're concluding that things are far from hopeless and they are rapidly replacing conjecture with facts.

For example, scientists have learned that every animal, from the ancient hagfish to reptiles, rodents, and humans, share the same basic pleasure and "reward" circuits in the brain, circuits that all turn on when in contact with addictive substances or during pleasurable acts such as eating or orgasm. One conclusion from this evidence is that addictive behaviors are normal, a natural part of our "wiring." If they weren't, or if they were rare, nature would not have let the capacity to be addicted evolve, survive, and stick around in every living creature.

"Everyone engages in addictive behaviors to some extent because such things as eating, drinking, and sex are essential to survival and highly reinforcing," says G. Alan Marlatt, Ph.D., director of the Addictive Behaviors Research Center at the University of Washington. "We get immediate gratificaton from them and find them very hard to give up indeed. That's a pretty good definition of addiction."

"The inescapable fact is that nature gave us the ability to become hooked because the brain has clearly evolved a reward system, just as it has a pain system," says physiologist and pharmacologist Steven Childers, Ph.D., of Bowman Gray School of Medicine in North Carolina. "The fact that some things may accidentally or inadvertently trigger that system is somewhat beside the point.

"Our brains didn't develop opiate receptors to tempt us with heroin addiction. The coca plant didn't develop cocaine to produce what we call crack addicts. This plant doesn't care two hoots about our brain. But heroin and cocaine addiction certainly tell us a great deal about how brains work. And how they work is that if you taste or experience something that you like, that feels good, you're reinforced to do that again. Basic drives, for food, sex, and pleasure, activate reward centers in the brain. They're part of human nature."

6. ENHANCING HUMAN ADJUSTMENT: LEARNING TO COPE EFFECTIVELY

NEW THINKING, OLD PROBLEM

What we now call "addictions," in this sense, Childers says, are cases of a good and useful phenomenon taken hostage, with terrible social and medical consequences. Moreover, that insight is leading to the identification of specific areas of the brain that link feelings and behavior to reward circuits. "In the case of addictive drugs, we know that areas of the brain involved in memory and learning and with the most ancient part of our brain, the emotional brain, are the most interesting. I'm very optimistic that we will be able to develop new strategies for preventing and treating addictions."

The new concept of addiction is in sharp contrast to the conventional, frustrating, and some would say cynical view that everything causes addiction.

Ask 10 Americans what addiction is and what causes it and you might get at least 10 answers. Some will insist addiction is a failure of morality or a spiritual weakness, a sin and a crime by people who won't take responsibility for their behavior. If addicts want to self-destruct, let them. It's their fault; they choose to abuse.

For the teetotaler and politicians, it's a self-control problem; for sociologists, poverty; for educators, ignorance. Ask some psychiatrists or psychologists and you're told that personality traits, temperament, and "character" are at the root of addictive "personalities." Social-learning and cognitive-behavior theorists will tell you it's a case of conditioned response and intended or unintended reinforcement of inappropriate behaviors. The biologically oriented will say it's all in the genes and heredity; anthropologists that it's culturally determined. And Dan Quayle will blame it on the breakdown of family values.

The most popular "theory," however, is that addictive behaviors are diseases. In this view, an addict, like a cancer patient or a diabetic, either has it or does not have it. Popularized by Alcoholics Anonymous, the disease theory holds that addictions are irreversible, constitutional, and altogether abnormal and that the only appropriate treatment is total avoidance of the alcohol or other substance, lifelong abstinence, and constant vigilance.

ABSOLVING THE DISEASED

The problem with all of these theories and models is that they lead to control measures doomed to failure by mixing up the process of addiction with its impact. Worse, from the scientific standpoint, they don't hold up to the tests of observation, time, and consistent utility. They don't explain much and they don't account for a lot. For example:

• Not all drugs of abuse create dependence. LSD and other hallucinogens, caffeine, and tranquilizers are examples. Rats, for example, which can be easily addicted to heroin and cocaine just like humans, "just can't appreciate a psychedelic experience," notes Childers. "The same is true of marijuana and caffeine; it's hard to get animals to take them. People take these drugs for different reasons, not to feel pleasure."

At the same time, rats and other animals can become physically dependent on alcohol, but won't seek out alcohol even when they are in convulsions of withdrawal. Says Jack Henningfield, Ph.D., an addiction researcher at the National Institute of Drug Abuse in Baltimore, "we can get rats physically dependent on alcohol and even get them to go through DTs by withdrawing them. But we can't get them to crave alcohol naturally." Apparently, they have to learn, to be taught to want it. "Only when we give them the rat equivalent of smoke-filled rooms, soft jazz, and other rewards will they seek out alcohol."

• Some substances with clearly addictive properties are almost universally used and socially acceptable. Giving up coffee and colas containing caffeine can yield rapid heart beats, sweating, irritability, and headaches—markers of withdrawal.

• People can experience withdrawal syndromes with drugs that don't addict them or make them physically or psychologically dependent. Postsurgical morphine is always withdrawn gradually in the hospital, but most people who get morphine still undergo so-called white flu—flu-like symptoms after they leave the hospital. They are actually undergoing withdrawal symptoms, but they have to become dependent on or addicted to the morphine. There is also no evidence that terminal cancer patients in severe pain get "high" on heavy doses of morphine, although they do become dependent.

• Some drugs of abuse produce tolerance and some don't. Heroin addicts need more and more of it to avoid withdrawal symptoms. Cocaine produces no tolerance, yet most would say cocaine is far more addictive because craving accelerates to sometimes lethal doses. If permitted, lab rats will continue to take cocaine until they die.

• Some people, notably celebrities, check in regularly at the Betty Ford Center to overcome addiction to painkillers, alcohol, and barbiturates. Yet one of the most famous studies on Vietnam veterans shows that very few of those who returned addicted to heroin stayed addicted. Lots of planning went on for intensive treatment for them. But on follow-up back home, their rate of continuing addiction dropped to levels no different than those of the general population, despite their exposure to lots of drugs, stress, high-risk environments, youth, and other risk factors that predicted a serious addiction epidemic. They had no trouble for the most part leaving their addictions behind in the jungles, while in the U.S., relapses are legendary and widespread.

For decades, we've sent heroin addicts to Lexington, Kentucky, for treatment in an isolated treatment facility; the idea was to remove them for long periods from their conducive environments. Almost all got "clean" and stayed that way, but when released, still sought out their old haunts and relapsed. Yet the majority of people living in drug-infested cultures never get addicted.

• The children of alcoholics have a much higher risk of alcohol abuse than children of nonalcoholics. Some studies show that alcoholics have an enzyme abnormality related to alcohol activity that doesn't seem to exist in people who've never had a drink. Yet some people who are classic alcoholics can and do learn to drink moderately and safely. Others quit even when they know they can drink moderately.

DEBUNKING THE DOMINO THEORY

I began to understand the bankruptcy of many addiction theories when a lot of my predictions about alcoholism and treatment for it were dead wrong," says William R. Miller, Ph.D. A professor of psychology and psychiatry and director of the Center on Alcoholism, Substance Abuse, and Addictions at the University of New Mexico, his controversial studies of "controlled drinking" in the early 1970s were among the first to clash with the "disease" theory of addictions.

"I developed a reasonably successful program that taught alcoholics how to drink moderately. Lots of them eventually totally quit and became abstainers. I would never have predicted that. The prevalent theories were that they would either eventually relapse and lose control of their drinking or that they would quit because moderation did not work. We knew from blood and urine tests that they were able to moderate but quit anyhow. The old domino theory that one drink equals a drunk proved, for some, to be baloney. We know with cigarette smoking and alcohol and other addictive behaviors that moderation, tapering, and 'warm turkey' can be very effective." Miller blames mostly the persistent strength of the addiction-as-disease concept on the peculiarly American experience with alcohol and Prohibition.

"During Prohibition, alcohol was marked as completely dangerous and the message was that no one could use it safely. At the end of Prohibition, we had a problem: a cognitive dissonance. Clearly many people could use it safely, so we needed a new model to make drinking permissible again. That led to the idea that only 'some' people can't handle it, those who have a disease called alcoholism."

Everyone likes this model, Miller says. People with alcohol problems like it because they get special status as victims of a disease and get treatment. Nonalcoholics like it because they can tell themselves they don't need to worry if they don't have the "disease." The treatment industry loves it because there's money to be made, and the liquor industry loves it because under this theory, it's not alcohol that's the problem but the alcoholic.

"What's really bizarre," says Miller, "is that the alcohol beverage industry spends a lot of money to help teach us about the disease model. It's the inverse of the temperance movement, which many now laugh at, but which saw alcohol more realistically as a dangerous drug. It is."

Today, Miller notes, heroin and cocaine are looked upon the way the temperance movement once looked on alcohol. "Ironically, too," he says, "we are treating nicotine and gluttony the way we once treated alcohol. It's easy to see how the disease model and all other single-cause theories of addiction can lead to blind alleys and bad treatments in which therapists adopt every fad and reach into a bulging bag of tricks for whatever is in hand or intuitively meets the immediate moment. But what we wind up with are three myths about alcoholism and other addictions: that nothing works, that one particular approach is superior to all others, and that everything works about equally well. That's nonsense."

No Easy Targets

The most likely truth about addiction is that it's not a single, basic mechanism, but several problems we label 'addiction,'" says Michael F. Cataldo, Ph.D., chief of behavioral psychology at Johns Hopkins Medical Institutes. "No one thing explains addiction," echoes Miller. "There are things about individuals, about the environment in which they live, and about the substances involved that must be factored in." Experts today prefer the term "addictive behaviors," rather than addiction, to underscore their belief that while everyone has the capacity for addiction, it's what people do that should drive treatment.

So while all addictions display common properties, the proportions of those factors vary widely. And certainly not all addictions have the same effect on the quality of our lives or capacity to be dangerous. Everyday bad habits, compulsions, dependencies, and cravings clearly have something in common with heroin and cocaine addiction, in terms of their mechanisms and triggers. But what about people who are Type A personalities; who eat chocolate every day; who, like Microsoft's Bill Gates, focus almost pathologically on work; who feel compelled to expose themselves in public, seek thrills like race-car driving and fire fighting, or obsess constantly over hand washing, hair twirling, or playing video games. They have—from the standpoint of what their behavior actually means to themselves and others—very little in common with heroin and crack addicts.

Or consider two of the more fascinating candidates for addiction—sex and love. Anthropologist Helen Fisher, Ph.D., of the American Museum of Natural History, suggests that the initial rush of arousal and romantic, erotic love, the "chemistry" that hooks a couple to each other, produces effects in the brain parallel to what happens when a brain is exposed to morphine or amphetamines.

In the case of love, the reactions involve chemicals such as endorphins, the brain's own opiates, and oxytocin and vasopressin, naturally occurring hormones linked to male and female bonding. After a while, though, this effect diminishes as the brain's receptor sites for these chemicals become overloaded and thus desensitized. Tolerance occurs; attachment wanes and sets up the mind for separation, so that the "addicted" man or woman is ready to pursue the high elsewhere. In this scenario, divorce or adultery becomes the equivalent of drug-seeking behavior, addicts craving for the high. According to Fisher, the fact that most people stay married is "a triumph of culture over nature," much the way, perhaps, nonaddiction is.

Experts generally agree on the most common characteristics of addictions that trouble society:

• The substance or activity that triggers them must initially cause feelings of pleasure and changes in emotion or mood.
• The body develops a physical tolerance to the substance or activity so that addicts must take ever-larger amounts to get the same effects.
• Removal of the drug or activity causes painful withdrawal symptoms.
• Quite apart from physical tolerance, addiction involves physical and psychological dependence associated with craving that is independent of the need to avoid the pain of withdrawal.
• Addiction always causes changes in the brain and mind. These include physiological changes, chemical changes, anatomical changes, and behavioral changes.
• Addiction requires a prior experience with a substance or behavior. The first contact with the substance or activity is an initiation that may or may not lead to addiction, but must occur in order to set in motion the effects in the brain that are likely to encourage a person to try that experience again.
• Addictions cause repeated behavioral problems, take a lot of a person's time and energy, are openly sanctioned by the community, and are marked by a gradual obsession with the drug or behavior.
• Addictions develop their own motivations. For addicts, their tolerance and dependence in and of themselves become reinforcing and rewarding, independent of their actual use of the drug or the "high" they may get. "One way of understanding this," says Cataldo, "is to analyze what is happening behaviorally in withdrawal. Given that withdrawal is so punishing, why do addicts let themselves go through it more than once? One answer is that the withdrawal, when combined with relapse and returning to the use of the substance, itself may be 'rewarding.'"

Inside the Addict's Brain

Supporting the new view of addiction are the many details that have recently been worked out describing events in any brain exposed to the most common addictive drugs: heroin, morphine, barbiturates, tranquilizers, and alcohol (all depressants that slow down processes in the brain and central nervous system); and cocaine, amphetamines, nicotine, and marijuana (all stimulants that generally excite them).

As the target organ of addiction, brain cells react to stimuli, including substances introduced from outside and hormones and chemicals we make ourselves. Those reactions lead to other chemical reactions and to changes in movement, thought, feelings, and memory. Drugs of abuse abet, or interfere with the chemical messengers, or neurotransmitters. The neurotransmitters that facilitate addiction are released by the 10 billion neurons that deal with information transfer.

Neurotransmitters circulate, collect, and act at specific sites on nearby cell surfaces called receptor proteins, each of which is shaped to fit and receive a particular neurotransmitter and bind it the way a lock "recognizes" a key. Only after a neurotransmitter binds can the signal it carries travel to the next cell. If the cell is flooded with too much neurotransmitter, an elegant "control" system is normally activated so that the cell reabsorbs the excess for later use. This process, called "reuptake," prevents too many chemical signals from circulating and filling too many receptors, which can lead to overactivity and serious mental and physical problems.

Neuroscientists now know that some abused substances block reabsorption, leaving too much neurotransmitter around. Others block the release of neurotransmitters. Although many neurotransmitters and chemicals that act like them have been identified, those most notably linked to addiction are norepinephrine, dopamine, serotonin, substance P, and gamma-aminobutyric acid (GABA).

In 1973, Solomon Snyder, M.D., director of neuroscience at Johns Hopkins, and his then-graduate student Candace Pert, put a solid foundation under the new theory of addiction by finding receptors for opium in the brain. They accomplished this by tracking molecules of the drug with radioactive tags to their binding sites. Derivatives of heroin, and morphine bind to those same sites. Methadone, a weak synthetic opiate, binds less tightly; one reason it satisfies an addict's craving is that it is addictive but does not produce a "high."

But Snyder and Pert also understood that their discovery had far greater implications. For if the brain had opiate receptors, it surely wasn't because nature intended man to fall victim to heroin addiction, but because the body itself must produce opiates. The discovery in 1975 of the brain's own opiates, called endorphins or enkephalins, demonstrated neurochemical sites of pleasure in the brain activated naturally by human activity.

Soon, scientists would learn that opiates keep opiate receptors constantly full, producing the physical tolerance so characteristic of heroin addiction. They discovered that the opiate-addicted brain also appears to close off some receptors so that desensitization occurs, encouraging larger and larger doses.

They found that cocaine affects nerve cells in the limbic system, the most ancient part of the brain and one closely tied to emotions. But rather than bind to a receptor, it interrupts the process of reuptake that terminates the action of dopamine. Cocaine is not only a blocker of dopamine uptake but of the reuptake of serotonin and norepinephrine as well.

All of this leads to vast overstimulation of nerve cells and creates intense feelings of excitement and joy. With cocaine, dopamine spills forth and floods our pleasure receptors. On the downside, cocaine eventually wipes out the brain's existing supply of these neurotransmitters temporarily, leading to a hellish withdrawal marked by severe depression, paranoia, intense irritability, and craving.

According to Steven Childers, psychedelic drugs of abuse such as LSD and "mushrooms" don't activate the ancient reward system regulated by dopamine, serotonin, and norepinephrine. Moreover, they appear to influence different parts of the brain involved in higher functions than emotions and pleasure. "For people who use these drugs, they are less an addiction than an intellectual drive to alter mood and produce higher levels of consciousness," he says. "And when we look at how they act in the brain, we can begin to understand why."

The two most common types of tranquilizers, barbiturates and benzodiazepines (Valium and its cousins), also act differently in the brain. They don't have their own receptors, but act on a "foster" receptor, GABA, which is predominantly an inhibitory, or slow-down, neurotransmitter. These drugs "deinhibit" and, in sort of a double-negative effect, increase inhibition, sedating the user. "What these drugs do is hyperactivate inhibition," notes Childers. "Increase GABA enough and you shut down the brain. That's what sedatives do." Alcohol also appears to act on GABA receptors, amphetamines interrupt dopamine balance, and nicotine stimulates the release of endorphins, at least at high doses.

HAIR OF THE DOG

The withdrawal and relapse cycle suggests that like any behavior, the addict "gets something out of" the pain of withdrawal—attention, perhaps, or help. But, in any case, enough so that he not only is willing to do it again, but also may seek out the cycle the way he once sought out the drug.

In gambling addictions and certain eating disorders, particularly, says Toni Farrenkopf, Ph.D., a Seattle psychologist, the "rush" for the addict often comes from pursuit of the activity after "getting clean and clear" for a while, along with eluding police, spouses, parents, bill collectors, and employers.

"We know this is the case with animals we can train to do something, even if they never get a positive reward out of it," Cataldo says. The "reward" is escape from or absence of an electric shock or punishment, even if it's only occasional escape or unpredictable escape. The cocaine addict may be addicted to the pursuit of cocaine and stealing to get money to buy the drug; using coke may be secondary to the reward of not getting caught and the "high" of pursuing the drug life-style.

If addictions have characteristics in common, so do addicts, the experts say.

They have particular vulnerabilities or susceptibilities, opportunity to have contact with the substance or activity that will addict them, and a risk of relapse no matter how successfully they are treated. They tend to be risk takers and thrill seekers and expect to have a positive reaction to their substance of abuse before they use it.

Addicts have distinct preferences for one substance over another and for how they use the substance of abuse. They have problems with self-regulation and impulse control, tend to use drugs as a substitute for coping strategies in dealing with both stress and their everyday lives in general, and don't seek "escape" so much as a way to manage their lives. Finally, addicts tend to have higher-than-normal capacity for such drugs. Alcoholics, for example, often can drink friends "under the table" and appear somewhat normal, even drive (not safely) on doses of alcohol that would put most people to sleep or kill them.

The biological, psychological, and social processes by which addictions occur also have common pathways, but with complicated loops and detours. All addictions appear now to have roots in genetic susceptibilities and biological traits. But like all human animal behaviors, including eating, sleeping, and learning, addictive behavior takes a lot of handling. The end product is a bit like Mozart's talent: If he'd never come in contact with a piano or with music, it's unlikely he would have expressed his musical gifts.

Floyd E. Bloom, M.D., chairman of neuropharmacology at the Scripps Clinical and Research Foundation in La Jolla, California, once gave a talk called "The Bane of Pain Is Mainly in the Brain." His point was that both pain and pain relief occur in the brain, triggered by the release, control, uptake, and quantity of assorted brain chemicals and other natural substances. The same might be said for addiction. Regardless of the source of addiction, the effects are "mainly in the brain," physically, chemically, and psychologically affecting emotions and energy levels.

The new view of addiction ties together biology, chemistry, behavior, and emotions in the brain. Among others, Edythe London, Ph.D., chief of neuroimaging and the drug-action section of NIDA, has conducted experiments demonstrating that such links are in fact formed and offering some clues as to how that happens.

In her work, the first of its kind funded by the Office of National Drug Control Policy, she is using positron emission tomographic (PET) scans to figure out how drugs and behaviors produce the rewards that create addicts and keep them addicted even when the euphoria ends, the tolerance builds, and the withdrawals occur. She is homing in on areas of the brain where craving lives both neurochemically and psychologically.

PET scans measure the brain's uptake of glucose, the principal source of energy used by the brain to function, and locate areas of the brain affected by various experiences. By tagging glucose molecules with radioactive and other "tracers," scientists like London can watch the brain react to stimuli such as drugs, noise, stress, and work.

In early studies, she and he colleagues gave addictive drugs under carefully controlled conditions to addicts and gauged their mood and feelings while monitoring the rate of glucose use. "The surprising thing we found is that *all* drugs of abuse—even those that differ radically in structure such as morphine and cocaine—do the same thing. They reduce use of glucose in the brain, so providing a way to observe which areas of the brain are involved in specific psycho-

A TRIAL OF PRAYER

With a $30,000 grant from the National Institutes of Health's Office of Alternative Medicine, Scott Walker, M.D., is embarking on a study of prayer against substance abuse. It's not that alcoholics do the praying. Outsiders totally unknown to them will pray on their behalf.

Walker says his interest in the potential healing effects of intercessory prayer was triggered by his own strong spiritual beliefs.

There are more than 130 trials of "spiritual healing." Daniel J. Benor, M.D., reports in his 1993 book *Healing Research,* that 56 of the trials show "statistically significant results."

"Even if a therapist is atheistic, the majority of Americans have some spiritual or religious belief. If your patients believe, you need to address this faith factor if there is any chance it can help them," Walker says.

In the one-year study he is conducting, Walker will work with 40 adults about to enter a treatment program with a clinically verified substance abuse problem. At random, half the group will receive outside prayer, the other half will not.

All subjects will have urine drug screens and careful analysis of such factors as their treatment expectations, religious behavior, membership in support groups, and to what degree they are contemplating sobriety, are relapsed, and so on.

Walker is recruiting the pray-ers from the Albuquerque Faith Initiative. The group will include pray-ers of many religions.

They will get a specific suggestion about content: Thy Will Be Done. But they can improvise and must keep time sheets about content, duration, and location of sessions.

Walker will not reveal to any of the pray-ers or churches which or whose prayers did anything, if in fact that happens.

"We must absolutely minimize the possibility of any group saying it has a direct line to God."—J.E.R.

logical effects. The amount of glucose used in certain parts of the brain's cortex, moreover, was closely related to how good people felt, regardless of where any drug binds.

London says this common pathway of reduced brain metabolism should not really have surprised her. "If you think about it, it makes sense," she says, "because glucose is an index of brain activity and brain activity in any given area is a function of not only what drugs are binding right there, but of nerve connections feeding into that area. The final picture of drug action usually looks quite different than the pattern of where a drug binds. That's because the brain is a highly interconnected organ. Clearly, if a drug acts on dopamine-neurotransmitter systems in part of the limbic brain initially, it's easy to see that there would be wider distribution through the brain's networks and that the impact of the drug could be very diffuse and varied."

So far, London and others have seen this reduction in glucose use with morphine, cocaine, nicotine, buprenorphine (a treatment for opiate addicts), amphetamine, benzodiazepine, barbiturates, and alcohol. "All drugs of abuse do this."

From these studies, London moved on to experiments designed to show that an addict's brain is permanently different from what it was before and after the initial exposure. "I wanted to know where craving lived in the brain," she says.

Her first idea was wrong. "I thought that drug addicts had the same kind of situation as people with obsessive-compulsive disorder (OCD) in terms of where the brain was affected," she says, "because all OCD victims, like drug abusers, had a lack of impulse control. Studies had shown that they had disorders of the orbital frontal cortex, the part of the brain near the temple, and that's where I went looking."

She conducted experiments in which she gave a lot of drug-related cues—but not drugs—to cocaine addicts. These cues included videotapes showing crack houses, mounds of white powder, $10 bills, and people "high." "We thought that would make them crave the drug and we'd be able to see glucose use diminish in the orbital frontal cortex."

The bad news was that the orbital frontal cortex showed nothing. The good news was that they got a "pretty dramatic effect" in two other areas of the brain, the amygdala and the hippocampus.

The hippocampus is a bundle of fibers linked to learning and short-term memory and carries signals in and around the limbic system, forming electrochemical junctions for the emotional seat of the brain. The amygdala, located in the lower arc of the limbic system, is the seat of "fight or flight" reactions, and impairment or injury can lead to profound behavior changes. There is also evidence that the amygdala has a role in recalling pleasant or painful consequences of experiences and damage to this may flatten or remove some of this recall.

London hasn't entirely abandoned her notion that the orbital frontal cortex also is involved in addicts' recall of their drug experience and the onset of craving. Recent research suggests this part of the brain may be the anatomical location of "source memory," the place that helps people remember when and where and how a memory was formed, or whether it is a "real" memory at all.

London says she is convinced that addiction takes place in stages and requires not only initiation to a substance or to an activity that brings great pleasure, physically and/or psychologically, but also creation of nondrug "incentives" to keep using the drug and craving it. The incentives include the creation of memories—via the creation of neural pathways—of the pleasure and good mood and the excitement of getting the drug, preparing it, or sharing it with others.

"What we're talking about is like conditioning," says London. "Over time, events that happen concurrently with the euphoria begin to contribute to the drug experience and are involved in a sensitization process. They too probably produce a biochemical effect in the brain and become very important in the addiction process."

IF THAT HAPPENS, IT GOES A LONG WAY to explaining why relapse rates are so high, even for addicts who are "detoxified" and off drugs for long periods. Even when people clean up their act and stay clean for some time, they are still very vulnerable and this may have something to do not only with receptor sites and neurotransmitters, but also with biochemical processes that produce long-term, stored memories of the drug experience. Says London: "In my view, biochemical and psychological memories act in the same way. What we're talking about is learning at the molecular level—and the reason that addicts, long after they are free of a drug, can experience intense craving when presented with stimuli—even photographs or sounds—that remind them of the drug experience."

If there is a hitch in this new picture of addiction it is that it is far from simple. It is also politically incorrect, unlikely to make the "Just Say No" and "law and order" crowd very happy. But it is putting solid foundations under prevention and treatment programs and promising entirely new strategies to combat drug abuse. The implications of this new view of addiction are in fact profound for treatment, prevention, and public policy.

L.H.R. Drew, an Australian addiction expert, notes that "if the idea prevails that drug use—and more particularly drug addiction—is a special type of behavior which is highly contagious, irreversible, inevitably leads to disease, and is due to the special seductive properties of certain drugs, then our approach to reducing drug problems is not going to change. If, however, the ideas prevail that drug use is more similar than different to other behaviors and that there is little that is special about drug addiction compared with other addictions that are universally experienced, then the drug hysteria may abate and a rational approach to policies to reduce drug problems may be possible. It must be known that people get into trouble with drugs in the same way that they do with many other things...particularly behaviors giving short-term rewards."

In the new view of addiction, says Childers, people vary in their ability to manage problems and pleasures, "but we must recognize that we all share the same circuits of pleasure, rewards, and pain. Anyone who takes cocaine will enjoy it; anyone who has sex will enjoy it. There is nothing abnormal about getting high on cocaine. Everyone will. There is a natural basis of addiction and we need to get away from the concept that only bad or weak or diseased people have probems with addiction. Telling someone to 'just say no' is like telling someone to just say no to eating and drinking and sex. We must begin to see how very human and very hard this is. But it is far from hopeless."

STRESS
IT'S WORSE THAN YOU THINK

Psychological stress doesn't just put your head in a vise. New studies document exactly how it tears away at every body system—including your brain. But get this: The experience of stress in the past magnifies your reactivity to stress in the future. So take a nice deep breath and find a stress-stopping routine this instant.

John Carpi

JOHN CARPI writes on health, medicine, and the environment for a variety of publications. His articles have appeared in magazines as diverse as *Scientific American, Parenting,* and *Earth,* as well as in dozens of daily newspapers in the United States and abroad. He was the founding editor and later Editor-in-Chief of a *New York Times* medical news service. He teaches writing at New York University's graduate program in Science and Environmental Reporting. Between deadlines, Carpi is usually covering meetings around the world. The week he turned in his article on stress, he left town—on his honeymoon.

Technologic advances have expanded the business day. Leisure time has shrunk. Bathing-suited business men walk beaches on Sundays with cellular phones stuck to their ears, planning the next morning's meetings. Laptop computers find their way on vacations. The family icons of the 1990s are working couples picking up their children on their way home to dinners prepared by caterers or fast food chefs. Grieving time has shrunk. The divorce rate hovers near its highest in history. The concept of job security has gone the way of the dirigible. Yet there is no time to pick up the pieces. "Just snap out of it," yells the therapist as he slaps his patient in a newspaper cartoon. The caption: Time-saving single-visit psychotherapy.

Stress has become so endemic it is worn like a badge of courage. The business of stress reduction, from workshops to relaxation tapes to light and sound headsets, is booming. If ours is a culture without deep intimacy, then our relationship with stress is the exception.

Yet not even this familiarity can cushion the findings of the latest research: The effects of stress are even more profound than imagined. It penetrates to the core of our being. Stress is not something that just grips us and, with time or effort, then lets go. It changes us in the process. It alters our bodies—and our brains.

We may respond to stress as we do an allergy. That is, we can become sensitized, or acutely sensitive, to stress. Once that happens, even the merest intimation of stress can trigger a cascade of chemical reactions in brain and body that assault us from within. Stress is the psychological equivalent of ragweed. Once the body becomes sensitized to pollen or ragweed, it takes only the slightest bloom in spring or fall to set off the biochemical alarm that results in runny noses, watery eyes, and the general misery of hay fever. But while only some of us are genetically programmed to be plagued with hay fever, all of us have the capacity to become sensitized to stress.

Stress sensitization is uncharitably subversive. While the chemical signaling systems of body and brain are running amok in a person sensitized to stress, that person's perception of stress remains unchanged. It's as if the brain, aware that the burner on the stove is cool, still signals the body to jerk its hand away. "What happens is that sensitization leads the brain to re-circuit itself in response to stress," says psychologist Michael Meaney, Ph.D., of McGill University. "We know that what we are encountering may be a normal, everyday episode of stress, but the brain is signaling the body to respond inappropriately." We may not think we are getting worked up over running late for an appointment, but our brain is treating it as though our life were on the line.

Because some stress is absolutely necessary in living creatures, everyone has a built-in gauge that controls our reaction to it. It's a kind of biological thermostat that keeps the body from launching an all-out response literally over spilled milk. Sensitization, however, lowers the thermostat's set point, says psychologist Jonathan C. Smith, Ph.D., founder and director of the Stress Institute at Roosevelt University in Chicago. As a result, the body response typically reserved for life-threatening events is turned on by life's mundane aggravations. In this hothouse of hyperreactivity, biochemicals unleashed by stress may boil over at the most trivial of events, like our missing a train or being shunted to voice mail.

6. ENHANCING HUMAN ADJUSTMENT: LEARNING TO COPE EFFECTIVELY

"Years of research has told us that people do become sensitized to stress and that this sensitization actually alters physical patterns in the brain," says Seymour Levine, Ph.D., of the University of Delaware. "That means that once sensitized, the body just does not respond to stress the same way in the future. We may produce too many excitatory chemicals or too few calming ones; either way we are responding inappropriately."

The revelation that stress itself alters our ability to cope with stress has produced yet another remarkable finding: Sensitization to stress may occur before we are old enough to prevent it ourselves. New studies suggest that animals from rodents to monkeys to humans may experience still undetermined developmental periods during which exposure to stress is more damaging than in later years. "For example, we have known that losing a parent when you are young is harder to get over than if your parent dies when you are an adult," says Jean King, Ph.D., of the University of Massachusetts Medical School. "What we now believe is that a stress of that magnitude occurring when you are young may permanently rewire the brain's circuitry, throwing the system askew and leaving it less able to handle normal, everyday stress."

It is the stew of chemicals released by such provocations that ultimately explains the noose stress ties between mind and body. "This new paradigm of stress demonstrates that there is a link between psychological events and physical eruptions, between mind and body," King says. "The psychological events that are most deleterious probably occur during infancy and childhood—an unstable home environment, living with an alcoholic parent, or any other number of extended crises." The new paradigm also firmly ties everyday psychological stress to such suspect complaints as ulcers, headaches, and fatigue.

The new blueprint of how we respond to stress also may explain why people have different tolerances for stress. In the past stress tolerance may have been chalked up to mental fortitude: "He's a rock," or "She's really bearing up under pressure." Now it's clear that our ability to withstand stress has less to do with whether we are strong-willed than with how much and what kind of stress we encountered in the past.

Whether we end up stressed-out executives or laid-back surfers, we all start out with the same biological machinery for responding to stress. Stress activates primitive

Stress does not just grip us and let go. It changes us. It alters our bodies — and our brains.

regions of the brain, the same areas that control eating, aggression, and immune response. It switches on nerve circuits that ignite the body's fight-or-flight response as if there were a life-threatening danger.

From this evidence researchers have concluded that the stress response is "wired" into the brain, that we inherit the same ancient reactions that jump-started hunter-gatherers to escape a charging sabertooth tiger without having to give their actions time-consuming thought. Only this same life-or-death reaction is now called into play largely by non–life-threatening situations. Studies have found the same fight-or-flight circuits all working overtime in response to such varied stressors as extreme exercise, the death of a loved one, an approaching deadline.

One conclusion from the evidence is that we may be victims of evolution, saddled with a stress response system that's better suited to a life filled with occasional life-threatening events than one filled with everyday irritations like failing a test or blowing a sales call. Unfortunately, when stresses become routine, the constant biochemical pounding takes its toll on the body; the system starts to wear out at an accelerated rate.

By responding to the stress of everyday life with the same surge of biochemicals released during major threats, the body is slowly killing itself. The biochemical onslaught chips away at the immune system, opening the way to cancer, infection, and disease. Hormones unleashed by stress eat at the digestive tract and lungs, promoting ulcers and asthma. Or they may weaken the heart, leading to strokes and heart disease. "Chronic stress is like slow poison," King observes. "It is a fact of modern life that even people who are not sensitized to stress are adversely affected by everything that can go wrong in the day."

If stress has a central command post, it is the hypothalamus, a primitive area of the brain located near where the spine runs into the skull. By way of a dazzling array of hormonals signals, the hypothalamus is closely connected with the nearby pituitary gland and the distant adrenal glands, perched atop the kidneys. The so-called hypothalamic-pituitary axis (HPA) has a virtual monopoly on basic body functions. It regulates blood pressure, heart rate, body temperature, sleep patterns, hunger and thirst, and reproductive functions, among many other activities.

About the size of a grape, the hypothalamus does its work by releasing two types of signaling hormones; those that stimulate glands to release other hormones and those that inhibit the glands from performing their job. Among the best known of these hormones are follicle-stimulating and luteinizing hormones, which, dispatched on a strict schedule from the pituitary, begin the monthly process that prepares women for pregnancy or menstruation.

Like a cherry attached by its stem, the pituitary gland hangs off the hypothalamus, waiting to receive instructions on which of its many hormones to release and in what quantity. In hormonal terms it is the little gland that could. The pituitary releases substances that regulate growth, sex, skin color, bone length, and muscle strength. It also releases adrenocorticotropin, a hormone that activates the third part of the body's stress system, the adrenal glands.

When stress sets off the usual ferocious communication between the hypothalamus and the pituitary, the buck stops at the adrenal glands. They manufacture and release the true stress hormones—dopamine, epinephrine (also known as adrenaline), norepinephrine (noradrenaline), and especially cortisol. So responsive to the adrenal hormones are basic body functions like blood flow and breathing that even minute changes in levels of these substances can significantly affect health.

Slight overproduction of dopamine can constrict blood vessels and raise blood pressure; a shift in epinephrine could precipitate diabetes, or asthma, by constricting tiny airways in the lungs. If the adrenal gland slacks off on cortisol production the result may be obesity, heart disease, or osteoporosis; too much of the hormone can cause women to take on masculine traits like hair growth and muscle development and lead to one of the greatest fears of all for aging men—baldness. High levels of cortisol also may kill off brain cells crucial for memory.

The adrenal gland is also home of the granddaddy of all stress reactions, the fight-or-flight response. Sensing impending danger the hypothalamus presses out cortisol-releasing factor, a hormone that prompts the pituitary gland to release adrenocorticotropin (ACTH). Carried in the bloodstream to the adrenal glands, ACTH triggers production of cortisol and epinephrine. The end result of this hormonal relay is a sudden surge in blood sugar, heart rate, and blood pressure—everything the body needs to flee or confront the imminent danger.

The problem is, what we call the stress system is actually responsible for coordinating much more than just our response to stress. "Initiating a response to stress is just one of many things the system controls," says Jean King. "These hormones are carefully regulated substances that direct everything from the immune system to the cardiovascular system to our behavioral system."

For example, cortisol directly impacts storage of short-term memory in the hippocampus. The stress hormones dopamine and epinephrine are also neurotransmitters widely active in enabling communication among brain cells. Directly and indirectly, they act on numerous neural networks in the brain and throw off levels of other neurotransmitters. Stress, it's now known, alters serotonin pathways. And through effects on serotonin, stress is now linked with depression on one hand, aggression on the other.

The developing picture of the biochemistry of stress in some ways takes the heat off psychology. "We used to say that physical manifestations of stress were psychological defense mechanisms employed as a way to shield the person from revisiting a particularly troubling event in their past," says Roosevelt's Smith. "What is far more likely is that the same chemicals being released in response to stress are triggering physical reactions throughout the body."

A torrent of new studies catalogue how even a little stress can have wide-ranging effects on the body. Researchers have recently found that:

• Epinephrine, released by the adrenal glands in response to stress, instigates potentially damaging changes in blood cells. Epinephrine triggers blood platelets, the cells responsible for repairing blood vessels, to secrete large quantities of a substance called ATP. In large amounts, ATP can trigger a heart attack or stroke by causing blood vessels to rapidly narrow, thus cutting off blood flow, says Thomas Pickering, M.D., a cardiologist at the New York Hospital-Cornell Medical Center.

• Other substances released in the stress response impair the body's ability to fight infections. In one study, researchers tracked the neurohormones of parachute jumpers. They found an 84 percent surge in nerve growth factor (NGF) among young Italian soldiers attempting their first jump, compared with nonjumpers. Up to six hours after they hit ground, the jumpers' NGF levels were 107 percent higher than in nonjumping soldiers. Released by the pituitary gland as part of the stress response, NGF is attracted like a magnet to disease-fighting cells, where it hinders their ability to ward off infections. An immune system thus suppressed can raise susceptibility to colds—or raise the risk of cancer.

• Cortisol activation can similarly damage the immune system. Sheldon Cohen, Ph.D., professor of psychology at Carnegie Mellon University, gave 400 people a questionnaire designed to quantify the amount of stress they were under. He then exposed them to nose drops containing cold viruses. About 90 percent of the stressed subjects (versus 74 percent of those not under stress) caught a cold. He found they had elevated levels of corticotrophin-releasing factor (CRF). "We know that CRF interferes with the immune system," Cohen says. "That is likely the physical explanation why people under stress are more likely to catch a cold."

• Stress hormones are also implicated in rheumatoid arthritis. The hormone prolactin, released by the pituitary gland in response to stress, triggers cells that cause swelling in joints. In a study of 100 people with rheumatoid arthritis, Kathleen S. Matt, Ph.D., and colleagues at Arizona State University found that levels of prolactin were twice as high among those reporting high degrees of interpersonal stress than among those not stressed. Other studies have shown that prolactin migrates to joints, where it initiates a cascade of events leading to swelling, pain, tenderness. "This is clearly what people mean when they say stress is worsening their arthritis," Matt says. "Here we have the hormone released during stress implicated in the very thing that causes arthritis pain, swollen joints."

• After being released by the pituitary gland, the stress hormone ACTH can impede production of the body's natural pain relievers, endorphins, leading to a general feeling of discomfort and heightened pain after injury. High levels of ACTH also trigger excess serotonin, now linked to bursts of violent behavior.

By charting the pathways stress hormones take throughout the body, biological cartographers are doing more than mapping the links between stress and disease. Having caught cascades of biochemicals in flagrante delicto, researchers are diagraming the exact lines of communication between mind and body. Ultimately, they will force us to erase the dividing line between what is biological and what is psychological.

Important as they are, elucidating the neurohormones released during stress and relating them to body systems is not even the whole story. If that were all there was to how stress works, you would expect any physical reaction to occur immediately, since these hormones typically remain elevated for only a short time. And you would expect everyone to show some physical reaction. Certainly, not all people suffer a heart attack or asthma attack when they get upset. Some seem able to take stress in their stride, while others routinely are hobbled.

In studies only recently completed, Lawrence Brass, M.D., associate professor of neurology at Yale Medical School, found that severe stress is one of the most potent risk factors for stroke—more so than high blood pressure—even 50 years after the initial trauma. Brass studied 556 veterans of World War II and found that the rate of stroke among those who had been prisoners of war was eight times higher than among those veterans who had not been captured.

Stress is like an allergy; once we're sensitized, just a touch triggers a blitz from within.

6. ENHANCING HUMAN ADJUSTMENT: LEARNING TO COPE EFFECTIVELY

"If you counter stress after it hits, that's too late. You must be proactive, not reactive."

● ● ●

The findings at first confused Brass. After all, the stress hormones that cause heart disease and stroke are elevated only for a few hours after a stressful event. "I began to realize we would have to take our understanding of stress farther when I began to see that in some people stress can cause disease years after the initial event," he says. He concluded that the immediate effect of the war trauma on the stress response system had to have been permanent. "The stress of being a POW was so severe it changed the way these folks responded to stress in the future—it sensitized them."

Their neurohormonal system was kicked off-kilter. Instead of churning out the normal amount of hormones in the face of stress, their systems were now so dysregulated that at the slightest provocation, they either pumped out too much of some chemicals needed or not enough of others. "Years of this kind of hormonal assault may have weakened their cardiovascular systems and led to the strokes," Brass says.

Brass was unable to document actual changes in the neurohormonal system. But another study, of child abuse victims, reported last June at the meeting of the American Psychiatric Association, provides some of the earliest proof that stress can physically alter people. With magnetic resonance imaging, researchers took pictures of the brains of 38 women, 20 with a documented history of sexual abuse, 18 without. Among those women sexually abused as children, the researchers discovered, the hippocampus is actually smaller than normal. A tiny seahorse-shaped structure in the middle of the brain, the hippocampus is partially responsible for storing short-term memory. It is activated by some of the same neurohormones released during stress. "What we are seeing," says Murray Stein, Ph.D., of the University of California at San Diego, "is evidence that psychological stress can change the brain's makeup."

If stress sensitization begins with a major trauma and results in wholesale neurochemical and neuroanatomical changes, there should be other examples of its ravages. Perhaps, but they won't be easy to find, says UMass's King. "Most kids who suffer a trauma are not brought to the doctor," she says. "They get through the problem, go on with their lives, and wind up in our offices years later, suffering from depression or heart disease. And unless we were able measure amounts of hormones released before the initial exposure to stress, we wouldn't know if the levels were elevated." So researchers are looking at laboratory animals.

Even the lowly rat appears to become sensitized to stress. One study at UMass found that rats repeatedly stressed by exposure to life-threatening cold and being deprived of maternal contact immediately after birth became hyperresponsive to stress. "Rats stressed from birth had a blunted release of ACTH in response to later stress," reports King. Then she reexposed them to cold after the age of 14 days, when their hypothalamic-pituitary axis matures. "Without enough ACTH, the rats were less able to mount a fight-or-flight response. The trauma of the early stress seems to have altered their response system."

"Hormonal changes from stress sensitization are quite clear in animals," notes Delaware's Levine. His own studies of monkeys document permanent changes in cortisol output in response to stress among monkeys subjected to early psychological trauma. "What's interesting are the fine variations in the changes depending on the type and time of the trauma," Levine says.

For instance, monkeys separated from their mothers for a mere 15 minutes a day during the first few months of life develop a stress response system that is slightly muted, compared with monkeys reared normally. But if the monkeys are separated from their mothers for a full three hours a day during the first few months, their later response to stress is hyperreactive. These sensitized monkeys literally run around the cage or cower in a corner in the presence of other nonthreatening animals.

"At first this may appear contradictory, but actually it is logical," Levine explains. "Being separated from their mothers for a few minutes a day is stressful, but not traumatic. It is not life-threatening, and so the animals did not have to develop a different set of mechanisms to get through that time. The muting of their stress response can be seen as a kind of defense against this daily intrusion," as if the monkeys are telling themselves "why get all worked up over this when I know it soon will be over."

"On the other hand, being separated from their mother for three hours a day is very traumatic," observes Levine. "Anything can happen during that time, so the monkeys must develop a heightened sense of awareness to protect themselves. This need may permanently alter their response so it is hyperresponsive all the time."

Is the same true for us? "We do know that sensitization happens, but we don't know what kind of stress it takes or when the stress must take place in order to produce the changes. There are a lot of variables in humans that are very difficult to control for, like the emotional environment in the home, genetic susceptibilities, and more. Some factors may cancel out the effects of an early trauma. We don't know."

The most likely truth about stress sensitization is that it is not a simple alteration in the amount of any single stress hormone. "It takes finely-tuned amounts of many neurohormones for the hypothalamic-pituitary axis to remain in balance," says Georgia Witkin, Ph.D., director of the Stress Program at Mt. Sinai Medical Center in New York. "No one thing is going to explain stress because there is not just one chemical reaction to stress. And it also does not mean that everyone who loses a parent or is the victim of a violent crime will suffer from stress the rest of his life. There are things about individuals—genetic susceptibilities, pre-existing medical conditions, the environment they were brought up in, any alteration that may have taken place in their HPA axis—that must all be factored in.

"But the first pieces of the puzzle are being put into place. Looking at stress as a chemical reaction and realizing that this reaction, if strong enough, can change how we react in the future, offers the possibility of explaining many things we have witnessed regarding stress. For instance, the reactions we see in rats that are exposed to early trauma may give us a biological perspective on the phenomenon of learned helplessness. Perhaps what we call learned helplessness is biologically-programmed helplessness. If these animals become physically unable to respond to stress because trauma has altered their biology, we can't really call that learned behavior."

If this new picture of stress is not yet quite in full focus, that's because it requires the melding of disciplines ranging from genetics to psychology to medicine, and demands a new theory of mind/body interactions. But it holds the promise of entirely new strategies to combat stress.

Roosevelt's Smith envisions the day when "we may be able to develop drugs that can retune the entire neurochemical system. I think it's going to take years more research to better understand how an early trauma actually alters the neurochemical system. What is the mechanism by which psychological stress changes the way the brain communicates with the body? Does the same stress cause the same changes all the time? When are the developmental periods during which stress may be most harmful? As we continue to unveil the complex interactions between the mind and body, we may be able to isolate these reactions. That raises the possibility we can develop drugs to change them."

For now, says UMass's Jean King, "we have to remember that the reason some people deal poorly with current events is because of a past trauma. We must remember that there are physical reactions in our bodies when we are under stress and the extent to which we endure these reactions may be dictated by our past. Telling someone to 'just take it easy' is of no help. We are still a long way from knowing just what to say, but we are getting there."

A Smorgasbord of Stress-Stoppers

The future may hold specific ways of desensitizing brain and body so that they do not automatically hyperrespond to minor provocations. But for now, recognition of stress sensitization requires one all-important change in the way most of us approach de-stressing.

"If you wait until you're feeling stressed before you employ some technique for managing stress," contends psychologist Robert Epstein, Ph.D., "it's already too late. You need to have a bag of tricks that you can deploy proactively. If you turn to them throughout the day, that changes your threshold of stress tolerance."

Epstein, director emeritus of the Cambridge Center for Behavioral Studies and a researcher at San Diego State University, insists that "it's more important than ever to learn as many antistress techniques as possible, as young as possible."

"What we can now get out of the notion of sensitization is that people being treated for stress need individualized therapies," adds Saki F. Santorelli, Ed.D., associate director of the Stress Reduction Clinic at the University of Massachusetts Medical Center. "If we are saying that everyone responds to stress differently because of past experiences, then as therapists we need to be flexible and allow each person to focus on the part of therapy that works best for them. The only way to find that out is by trying different stress-reduction techniques."

There is no one-size-fits-all way to reduce stress. For example, "study upon study has shown that simple relaxation does not work in many people," says Rachel Yehuda, Ph.D., of Mt. Sinai Medical Center in New York. "Telling someone who has been sensitized to stress to just relax is like telling an insomniac to just fall asleep."

"What you don't want to do is resort to quick fixes that have no staying power," says Santorelli. "Smoking cigarettes, drinking alcohol, bringing on food; these are sure-fire stress failures. They may give the impression that they are relieving tension, but they will not work over time and sooner or later you will be right back where you started." He also advises those who feel stressed to avoid coffee and high-fat foods. "Caffeine is a stimulant and foods high in fat make the body work overtime to digest them, so both will probably add to your level of stress."

Mindfulness Meditation

At Santorelli's clinic, patients are taught mindfulness meditation, which comes out of the Buddhist tradition. Practitioners set aside 20 to 40 minutes a day when they focus on calming and becoming aware of their bodies with the aim of catching them—and interrupting them—in the act of hyperresponding to stress. "But the meditation really becomes a way of life. Once you begin practicing you realize that whenever you start feeling stressed during the day you are able to retrieve the feelings of relaxation you get during deep meditation. It becomes a way to take a few breaths and settle down just when you feel like you are beginning to explode."

Other forms of meditation use other devices to bring on moments of quiet contemplation, but all are designed to get you to focus on your body. "The most important thing is becoming aware of your body so you can sense when you are getting stressed. Meditation is an excellent way to do that" says Santorelli. "But it's not for everyone."

Biofeedback

If meditation is not for you, maybe biofeedback is. There are three main forms of it: electromyography (EMG), galvanic skin response (GSR), and electroencephalography (EEG). By attaching electrodes to a body system that readily reacts to stress—muscles, skin, and brain waves, respectively—you can monitor your actual stress level and learn to control, even reduce it. Modern biofeedback devices give off some signal—a blinking light, a bell—that announces a high level of tension. You concentrate on slowing the blinking light or bell.

Studies have found that each form of biofeedback works best for specific stress-related problems. EMG biofeedback, for example, reduces tension headaches; it allows people to focus and relax the muscles in the forehead that cause head pain. GSR seems to work best for stress-induced migraines, which tend to coincide with a rise in body temperature. EEG biofeedback leads to the deepest relaxation states.

What Calms You

But you don't have to meditate or go to a biofeedback clinic to avoid stress. "I meditate regularly, but when I am feeling unusually stressed I practice yoga or go exercise or tend to my garden, or I hang out with family or even just read and write," Santorelli says. "You have to become aware of what calms you best."

For Jean King, Ph.D., of the UMass Medical School, listening to music, going for a walk, or exercising always seems to put her mind at ease. "I love the water, so if I'm having a rough day I just go and look at it. I don't even have to go in, all I have to do is be near it."

Boston University biologist Eric Widmaier, Ph.D., confides that he used to combat stress by running and exercising. "But I've changed to a more thoughtful approach." He is an advocate of "internal conversations" in which he asks himself, "am I doing the right thing?" But the most important technique, he says, is "to learn to say no. People are constantly pushing at us by asking for favors."

Relaxation Response

One of the best-studied stress-relievers is the relaxation response, first described by Harvard's Herbert Benson, M.D., more than 20 years ago. Its great advantage is that it requires no special posture or place. Say you're stuck in traffic when you're expected at a meeting. Or you're having trouble falling asleep because your mind keeps replaying some awkward situation.

- Sit or recline comfortably. Close your eyes if you can, and relax your muscles.
- Breathe deeply. To make sure that you are breathing deeply, place one hand on your abdomen, the other on your chest. Breath in slowly through your nose, and as you do you should feel your abdomen (not your chest) rise.
- Slowly exhale. As you do, focus on your breathing. Some people do better if they silently repeat the word *one* as they exhale; it helps clear the mind.
- If thoughts intrude, do not dwell on them; allow them to pass on and return to focusing on your breathing.

Although you can turn to this exercise any time you feel stressed, doing it regularly for 10 to 20 minutes at least once a day can put you in a generally calm mode that can see you through otherwise stressful situations.

Cleansing Breath

Epstein, who has searched the world literature for techniques people have claimed valuable for coping, focuses on those that are simple and powerful. He calls them "gems," devices that work through differing means, can be learned in minutes, can be done anytime, anywhere, and have a pronounced physiologic effect. At the top of his list is the quickest of all—a cleansing breath.

Take a huge breath in. Hold it for three to four seconds. Then let it out v-e-r-y s-l-o-w-l-y. As you blow out, blow out all the tension in your body.

Relaxing Postures

"The research literature demonstrates that sitting in certain positions, all by itself, has a pronounced effect," says Epstein. Sit anywhere. Relax your shoulders so that they are comfortably rounded. Allow your arms to drop by your sides. Rest your hands, palm side up, on top of your thighs. With your knees comfortably bent, extend your legs and allow your feet, supported on the heels, to fall gently outward. Let your jaw drop. Close your eyes and breathe deeply for a minute or two.

Passive Stretches

It's possible to relax muscles without effort; gravity can do it all. Start with your neck and let your head fall forward to the right. Breathe in and out normally. With every breath out, allow your head to fall more. Do the same for shoulders, arms, back.

Imagery

Find a comfortable posture and close your eyes. Imagine the most relaxed place you've ever been. We all have a place like this and can call it to mind anywhere, any time. For everyone it is different. It may be a lake. It may be a mountain. It may be a cottage at the beach. Are you there?

Five—Count 'Em, Five—Tricks

Since you can never have too many tricks in your little bag, here are some "proven stress-busters" from Paul Rosch, M.D., president of the American Institute of Stress:

- Curl your toes against the soles of your feet as hard as you can for 15 seconds, then relax them. Progressively tense and relax the muscles in your legs, stomach, back, shoulders, neck.
- Visualize lying on a beach, listening to waves coming in and feeling the warm sun and gentle breezes on your back. Or, if you prefer, imagine an erotic fantasy or picture yourself in whatever situation makes you happiest.
- Set aside 20 to 30 minutes a day to do anything you want—even nothing.
- Take a brisk walk.
- Keep a Walkman handy and loaded with relaxing, enjoyable music.

"Beating stress is a matter of removing yourself from the situation and taking a few breaths," says Rosch. "If I find myself getting stressed I ask myself 'is this going to matter to me in five years?' Usually the answer is no. If so, why get worked up over it?"

The Power of Understanding

Simply knowing about stress sensitization seems to help some. "We tell patients about stress sensitization and I see a change in them," Yehuda says. "We explain that they have inappropriate reactions to stress because something has gone wrong with control mechanisms in the brain. It is like a light goes on and they can see:'Oh, so that may be the problem.' They do the same meditation and therapy but they are aware of the basis of their problem. There is something for them to focus on. There is a reason for them to say 'I'm not crazy. This is something real.'"

So You Think This Is the "Age of Stress"?

Quick, which would you rather be: late to work or lunch for a lion? The stress response we have today is out of synch with current needs. But it once was a Jurassic perk.

Eric P. Widmaier, Ph.D.

Nowadays, we are bombarded with what might be called the mythology of stress, which suggests that our psychological and physiological well-being is constantly threatened by degrees of stress unparalleled in history. Nothing could be farther from the truth.

What are some of these real or perceived stressors with which we continually do battle? Coping with rush-hour traffic, job and financial difficulties, troubled relationships, and family problems are just a few of hundreds of stressful stimuli that can be identified.

Anxiety over personal problems (will I be able to pay the rent this month?), or more global concerns (will there be another war?) is another type of stress that we all encounter much too often.

Nonetheless, anxiety and these other stressors are not immediate threats to survival, even if they do raise our blood pressure a bit now and then. Of greater concern is that the internal defense mechanisms of the body respond to these types of psychological stimuli in the same way as they would respond to life-threatening ones.

Why is this unfortunate? Because over the long haul, excess release of potent stress-fighting factors like the adrenal-gland hormones cortisol and epinephrine (also known as adrenaline) can suppress the immune system, cause ulcers, produce muscle atrophy, elevate blood sugar, place excessive demands on the heart, and eventually lead to the death of certain brain cells.

A person in the midst of a divorce does not require the hormonal, neuronal, and metabolic responses of someone who falls through thin ice on a wintery pond—yet in both cases the same internal changes are occurring.

Why do emotionally stressful events elicit the same chemical changes in our bodies as do events that are actual threats to survival? The answer may lie in a comparison of stress as we know it today and stress as it must have been when vertebrate animals were first evolving.

Are we really any more "stressed out" than our prehistoric ancestors? Presumably not, since the defense mechanisms that developed in mammals like ourselves did so very early in the evolution of life. We even see similar biological responses to stress in non-mammalian vertebrates like birds and reptiles.

These defenses consist of hormonal and neuronal signals that increase breathing, accelerate heart rate, increase blood pressure, increase the liver's ability to pump sugar into the bloodstream, and open up blood vessels in the large muscles to maximize the delivery of nutrients and oxygen.

The net effect is an animal that has lots of fuel in its blood, a more forceful heart to pump the blood around, plenty of oxygen, and efficient muscles. For an antelope in the wild that has spotted a nearby lion, these changes are exactly what the antelope needs to avoid becoming a meal.

Not surprisingly, then, animals evolved internal mechanisms to combat the stresses of infection, starvation, dehydration and pain, to name a few. Cortisol breaks down bone, muscle, fat, and other body tissues to provide material for the liver to convert into sugar. This sugar, essentially formed by the body's own self-digestion, can supply the needs of the heart and brain during a crisis. The natural pain-killer endorphin developed to combat severe pain.

Picture the antelope being attacked by the lion, but escaping to live another day. Its endorphin would allow the animal to cope with the pain of its wound, if only temporarily, and continue with the herd. Other hormones enable the kidney to retain more water than normal during periods of drought and dehydration.

All of these varied measures are short-term responses to very different types of stress. But they act in a concerted way to give an organism a fighting chance to get back on its feet.

Imagining the types of stress our paleolithic forebears must have encountered makes our daily aggravations seem much less overwhelming. Prior to the advent of agriculture, the typical cave-dweller would rarely have had the luxury of a steady and nutritious diet. On the contrary, malnutrition, vitamin and mineral deficiencies, even starvation would have been extremely common in the winter months, and sporadic dehydration from lack of clean or available water may have been common in the summer.

Hypothermia was a constant threat in the winter, especially in northern climes during the many ice ages. Injuries and infections that resulted from untreated minor wounds or parasite invasion would not only have been physiologically stressful but often lethal. Anthropological data suggest that our ancestors suffered many of the same maladies that continue to plague us today (arthritis, back problems, tooth decay, osteoporosis, to name a few).

However, as stressful as those conditions are for modern man, they would have been far more stressful at a time when no medical treatment of any kind was available.

What about the other type of stress that is not life-threatening, but is *perceived* to be of potential danger? When the antelope spotted the lion, there are not yet physical damage to the antelope's body. Nonetheless, the hormonal systems responded as if the damage was already done, in *anticipation* of impending doom. If the crisis were luckily averted, a complex system of

6. ENHANCING HUMAN ADJUSTMENT: LEARNING TO COPE EFFECTIVELY

hormonal feedback loops would apply a brake on the stress response to prevent unabated secretion of cortisol and other stress hormones.

Our prehistoric ancestors did not need to negotiate city traffic and deal with short-tempered bosses, but they had their share of psychological stress that produced no actual physical bodily insult.

Not knowing when (or *if*) your next meal will come would have been (and for much of the world's population continues to be) a chronic source of anxiety. Each empty-handed trip back to the cave would have increased the tribe's fears for the next day.

For that matter, obtaining a meal might have meant coping with the terror of chasing down a herd of animals much faster and larger than oneself, using a puny flint arrowhead tied to a stick.

Prehistoric man also differed in one profound way from modern man. Although an awareness of the cycles of nature and physical principles like gravity would likely have been present in even our most primitive ancestors, an *understanding* of the forces of nature would have completely eluded them.

Having no understanding of science meant having no sense of control over one's environment. Ancient man appears to have worried endlessly about celestial "beings" (sun gods, moon gods, etc.), and we know that until relatively recent times it was common for people to assign human traits to these deities.

This would have implied that it was within the realm of possibility for, say, the sun god to feel angry or neglected one day, thus deciding not to rise and plunging the world into darkness and chaos. Imagine going to sleep each night fretting that you may have failed to properly perform a certain worshipful ritual and that as a consequence your entire tribe or family might be forever doomed to darkness and misery.

From both a physical and psychological vantage point, our ancestors lived a much more stressful existence that we do today. The mechanisms that evolved to combat the deleterious effects of those stressors are still intact and usually serve us well.

However, we clearly make things worse for ourselves. Take compulsive exercisers. These people can actually become addicted to strenuous exercise, because this behavior imposes a severe stress on metabolism and results in the steady release of endorphin. Responsible for "runner's high," this pain-killer is similar to morphine in its addictive capabilities.

Extreme exercise also releases cortisol, which though useful in maintaining circulatory and respiratory function, can lead to immunosuppression, bone loss, hypertension, and death of brain cells. In yet another scenario, meeting a deadline at work is a source of pressure, but is not life-threatening, and yet it contributes to ill health by invoking an unnecessary release of stress hormones.

Are we stressed in today's society? Of course we are. But the important thing to remember is that all animals, including ourselves, are confronted with innumerable types of stress and always have been. We should ignore the incessant mantra of ours being the Age of Stress and put things in a more historical and evolutionary perspective.

Given the choice, who wouldn't prefer the aggravation of two working parents getting their kids off to day care or school on time to the dread of being eaten in one's sleep by a lion?

The New Frontiers of Happiness... Happily Ever Laughter

Laughter may help make you happier and healthier. But not everybody benefits from humor equally. Here's how to harness laughter's powers.

Peter Doskoch

While the 1980s were the decade in which the humor-is-healthy viewpoint finally gained scientific respectability, the 1990s may be the one in which humor's therapeutic limits become defined, its weaknesses understood. That may sound like a glum take on a cheerful subject, but it's not. For the better we understand when laughter is useful, the more effectively we can deploy it—something we can all be happy about.

Laughter is such an intrinsic part of our lives that we sometimes forget how very odd it is. Despite the development of newfangled imaging machines like MRI and PET scans, neuroscientists still have little idea what's happening in our brain when we laugh. Certainly the brain stem plays a role. People who've suffered strokes in this primitive brain region have been known to have prolonged bouts of pathological laughter. And some anencephalic infants—babies born missing their higher brain circuitry—will, when tickled, make faces that appear to be smiles or laughs, again implicating the primitive brain.

But laughing in response to something funny also calls on more sophisticated brain functions. One of the few brain studies conducted so far in humor research looked at the electrical activity that occurs as we chuckle, giggle, or guffaw. About four-tenths of a second after we hear the punch line of a joke—but before we laugh—a negatively charged wave of electricity sweeps through the cortex, reports Peter Derks, Ph.D., professor of psychology at the College of William and Mary.

What Derks finds most significant about this electrical wave is that it carpets our entire cerebral cortex, rather than just one region. So all or most of our higher brain may play a role in laughter, Derks suggests, perhaps with the left hemisphere working on the joke's verbal content while the analytic right hemisphere attempts to figure out the incongruity that lies at the heart of much humor.

In the Mood

That laughter is a full-cortex experience is only fitting considering the wide-ranging effects it has on us psychologically and physiologically. Perhaps the most obvious effect of laughter is on our mood. After all, with even the most intellectual brands of humor, laughter is ultimately an expression of emotion—joy, surprise, nervousness, amusement. More than a decade of research has begun unraveling the details of the laughter-mood connection:

- Stressed-out folks with a strong sense of humor become less depressed and anxious than those whose sense of humor is less well developed, according to a study by psychologists Herbert Lefcourt, Ph.D., of the University of Waterloo, and Rod Martin, Ph.D., now at the University of Western Ontario.

- Researchers at West Chester University in Pennsylvania found that students who used humor as a coping mechanism were more likely to be in a positive mood.

- In a study of depressed and suicidal senior citizens, the patients who recovered were the ones who demonstrated a sense of humor, reports psychiatrist Joseph Richman, M.D., professor emeritus at Albert Einstein Medical Center in Bronx, New York.

All of this makes sense in light of laughter's numerous physiological effects. "After you laugh, you go into a relaxed state," explains John Morreall, Ph.D., president of HUMORWORKS Seminars in Tampa, Florida. "Your blood pressure and heart rate drop below normal, so you feel profoundly relaxed. Laughter also indirectly stimulates endorphins, the brain's natural painkillers."

In addition to its biological effects, laughter may also improve our mood through social means. Telling a joke, particularly one that illuminates a shared experience or problem, increases our sense of "belonging and social cohesion," says Richman. He believes that by psychologically connecting us to others, laughter counteracts "feelings of alienation, a major factor in depression and suicide."

Some of laughter's other psychological effects are less obvious. For one thing, says Morreall, it helps us think more creatively. "Humor loosens up the mental gears. It encourages out-of-the-ordinary ways of looking at things."

Humor guru William Fry, M.D., professor emeritus of psychiatry at Stanford University, takes this idea one step further. "Creativity and humor are identical," he contends. "They both involve bringing together two items which do not have an obvious connection, and creating a relationship."

Finally, humor helps us contend with the unthinkable—our mortality. Lefcourt recently found that people's willingness to sign the organ donor consent on their driver's license rises with their tendency to laugh. "Very few people are ready to think, even for a moment, about death," he says. "But those who have a sense of humor are more able to cope with the idea."

A Healthy Sense of Humor

The idea that laughter promotes good health first received widespread attention through Norman Cousins's 1979 best-seller, *Anatomy of an Illness*. But centuries earlier astute observers had ascribed physical benefits to humor. Thomas Sydenham, a seventeenth-century British physician, once observed: "The arrival of a good clown into a village does more for its health than 20 asses laden with drugs."

Today, scientific belief in laughter's effects on health rest largely on the shoulders of Lee Berk, M.D., and Stanley Tan, M.D., both of the Loma Linda School of Medicine, in Loma Linda, California. Laughter, they find, sharpens most of the instruments in our immune system's tool kit. It activates T lymphocytes and natural killer cells, both of which help destroy invading microorganisms. Laughter also increases production of immunity-boosting gamma interferon and speeds up the production of new immune cells. And it reduces levels of the stress hormone cortisol, which can weaken the immune response.

Meanwhile, studies by Lefcourt and others have found that levels of immunoglobulin A, an antibody secreted in saliva to protect against respiratory invaders, drops during stress—but it drops far less in people who score high on a humor scale.

While these findings suggest how laughter might benefit our health, nobody has yet proven that these immune effects translate into faster healing, because humor's impact on actual recovery has never been scientifically confirmed.

A study now underway at Columbia-Presbyterian Medical Center in New York should shed some more light on this issue. Researchers in the pediatric wards are literally sending in the clowns to see if humor hastens healing in kids with cancer and other serious illnesses. A 35-member Clown Care Unit, composed of members **of the Big Apple Circus, makes thrice-weekly visits to Columbia's Babies and Children's Hospital while researchers monitor the kids' vital signs and rate of recovery.** Preliminary data should be available early next year.

Laughter: The Proper Dose

Now that we know what laughter can do, it's important to recognize when it's most effective. Here are some things to keep in mind to live life happily ever laughter.

Humor may help some people more than others.

There's one problem with nearly all the research that links humor and mood; it's what scientists call "correlational." The fact that two things happen at the same time doesn't mean one caused the other. So if folks with a strong sense of humor are less affected by stress, "it doesn't mean laughing is what's helping them cope," says Martin. Rather, it could be that if they're coping well, they can laugh a lot.

In Martin's view, by adulthood our sense of humor has essentially reached its final form. And for those of us whose internal humor settings are on the low side, he believes laughter may not help as much. For example, in one study, participants' levels of immunoglobulin A increased when they viewed humorous videos. But they rose most in people whose tendency to laugh was greatest to begin with. So the serious and sober among us may benefit less from laughter.

Others dispute this idea, asserting that humor is an equal-opportunity life-enhancer. "Anybody who has normal mental development can engage in and benefit from humor," insists Morreall. "All they have to do is put themselves in this more playful state of mind. We have to give ourselves permission to do something we did very easily when we were three years old."

Martin, though, remains unconvinced. "My sense is that research hasn't been as successful as people had hoped. It seems to be pretty hard to teach someone to change their sense of humor." Nonetheless, if you're a natural humor powerhouse, laughter's force may be especially at your command.

Control and choice may enhance laughter's benefits.

Numerous studies show that psychological and physical health improve when people feel a sense of control in their lives, whether over their jobs, future, relationships, or even their medical treatment. Laughter's benefits may have a similar origin, suggests Morreall.

"When we're stressed, we often feel like we have no control of the situation," he says. "We feel helpless. But when we laugh, at least in our minds, we assume some control. We feel able to handle it."

One implication of this is that the more control people have over the type of humor to which they're exposed, the more they may benefit from it. At least one study bears this out. When patients recovering from surgery at a Florida hospital were allowed to choose the humorous movies they saw, they required less painkillers than a control group that saw no movies. But a third set of patients, force-fed comedies that may not have been to their liking, did worst of all.

Perhaps that should come as no surprise. Humor is intensely personal. Jim Carrey's comedy has little in common with Woody Allen's. "To harness laughter's benefits, it's essential that each person is matched to his or her favorite brand of humor," says Lefcourt. Often, that's remarkably difficult, even for folks close to you. I'm sometimes very surprised at what people I know find funny," he says.

In the long run, conscientiousness may outperform laughter as a health aid.

Even if laughter proves to aid recovery, it may not be an asset in the long run, contends Howard Friedman, Ph.D., professor of psychology at the University of California at Riverside. Friedman and colleagues have been following the fates of the "Termites," a group of 1,528 eleven-year-olds that the legendary psychologist Louis Terman, Ph.D., began studying in 1921. Terman asked teachers and parents to assess various personality traits of his preteen subjects. Friedman's team found that individuals judged as being cheerful and having a good sense of humor as children have been dying sooner than their less jovial classmates.

The reason, he thinks, is that cheerful people may pay less attention to threats to their physical and psychological well-being. "In the short term, I think it is helpful to be optimistic about a particular illness," says Friedman. But the same good-natured attitude that helps us laugh off the threat of illness ("I'm going to be just fine.") may work against us when we're presented with the opportunity to eat unhealthy foods or light up a cigarette ("I'm going to be just fine.").

In fact, the only personality trait that consistently increased longevity among the Termites, Friedman says, was conscientiousness, possibly because folks with this trait are more likely to avoid hazardous behaviors. So laugh all you like —but temper it with a bit of caution.

The average six-year-old laughs 300 times a day, the average adult, just 17.

Prescription for Happiness

While laughter may not be a panacea, there's still much to be gained from it. And, truth be told, there's room **for plenty of additional chortles in our lives:** Fry found that by the time the average kid reaches kindergarten, he or she is laughing some 300 times each day. Compare that to the typical adult, whom Martin recently found laughs a paltry 17 times a day. (Men and women laugh equally often, Martin adds, but at different things.)

Fortunately, if you're attracted by the idea of using laughter to improve your spirit and health, chances are you've already got a good sense of humor. Meaning, of course, that you're just the type of person who might benefit from what Fry calls "prophylactic humor"—laughter as preventative medicine.

For people who want to inoculate themselves with laughter, Fry recommends this two-step process.

First, figure out your humor profile. Listen to yourself for a few days and see what makes you laugh out loud. Be honest with yourself; don't affect a taste for sophisticated French farces if your heartiest guffaws come from watching Moe, Larry, and Curly.

Next, use your comic profile to start building your own humor library: books, magazines, videos, what have you. If possible, set aside a portion of your bedroom or den as a "humor corner" to house your collection. Then, when life gets you down, don't hesitate to visit. Even a few minutes of laughter, says Fry, will provide some value.

"We're teaching people a skill that they can use when, say, deadline pressures are getting close," explains nurse/clown Patty Wooten, R.N., author of *Compassionate Laughter* (Commune-a-Key) and president of the American Association for Therapeutic Humor.

"The deadline will remain, but by taking time out to laugh, you adjust your mood, your physiology, your immune system. And then you go back to work and face what you have to do."

On the Power of Positive Thinking: The Benefits of Being Optimistic

Michael F. Scheier and Charles S. Carver

Michael F. Scheier is Professor of Psychology at Carnegie Mellon University. **Charles S. Carver** is Professor of Psychology at the University of Miami. Address correspondence to Michael F. Scheier, Department of Psychology, Carnegie Mellon University, Pittsburgh, PA 15213; e-mail: ms0a@andrew.cmu.edu.

If believing in something can make it so, then there really would be power in positive thinking. From the little train in the children's tale who said, "I think I can," to popular writers such as Norman Cousins and Norman Vincent Peale, to wise grandmothers everywhere—many people have espoused the benefits of positive thinking. But are these benefits real? Do people who think positively really fare better when facing challenge or adversity? Do they recover from illness more readily? If so, how and why do these things happen?

We and a number of other psychologists who are interested in issues surrounding stress, coping, and health have for several years focused our research attention on questions such as these. The primary purpose of this brief review is to provide a taste of the research conducted on this topic. We first document that positive thinking can be beneficial. We then consider why an optimistic orientation to life might confer benefits. After considering how individual differences in optimism might arise, we take up the question of whether optimism is always good and pessimism always bad. We close by discussing the similarities between our own approach and other related approaches.

CHARACTERIZING POSITIVE THINKING

Psychologists have approached the notion of positive thinking from a variety of perspectives. Common to most views, though, is the idea that positive thinking in some way involves holding positive expectancies for one's future. Such expectancies are thought to have built-in implications for behavior. That is, the actions that people take are thought to be greatly influenced by their expectations about the likely consequences of those actions. People who see desired outcomes as attainable continue to strive for those outcomes, even when progress is slow or difficult. When outcomes seem sufficiently unattainable, people withdraw their effort and disengage themselves from their goals. Thus, people's expectancies provide a basis for engaging in one of two very different classes of behavior: continued striving versus giving up.

People can hold expectancies at many levels of generality. Some theoretical views focus on expectancies that pertain to particular situations, or even to particular actions.[1] Such an approach allows for considerable variation in the positivity of one's thinking from one context to the next. Thus, a person who is quite optimistic about recovering successfully from a car accident may be far less optimistic about landing the big promotion that is up for grabs at work.

Our own research on positive and negative thinking began with a focus on situation-specific expectancies, but over the years we began to consider expectancies that are more general and diffuse. We believe that generalized expectancies constitute an important dimension of personality, that they are relatively stable across time and context. We refer to this dimension as optimism and construe it in terms of the belief that good, as opposed to bad, things will generally occur in one's life. We focus on this dimension for the rest of this article.

MEASURING OPTIMISM

We measure individual differences in optimism with the Life Orientation Test, or LOT.[2] The LOT consists of a series of items that assess the person's expectations regarding the favorability of future outcomes (e.g., "I hardly ever expect things to go my way," "In uncertain times, I usually expect the best"). LOT scores correlate positively with measures of internal control and self-esteem, correlate negatively with measures of depression and hopelessness, and are relatively unrelated to measures of social desirability.[2]

If dispositional optimism is in fact a personality characteristic, it should be relatively stable across time. We have reported a test–retest correlation of .79 across a 4-week period.[2] More recently, Karen Matthews has found a correlation of .69 between LOT scores assessed 3 years apart in a sample of 460 healthy, middle-aged women. Indeed, LOT scores seem to remain relatively stable even in the face of catastrophes. For example, Schulz, Tompkins, and

Rau[3] tracked LOT scores in a group of stroke patients and their primary caregivers across a 6-month period. Although the LOT scores of both the patients and the support persons dropped over time (significantly so for the latter), the absolute magnitude of the drop was exceedingly small (less than 1 point on a 32-point scale). Thus, optimism as measured by the LOT seems to be a relatively enduring characteristic that changes little with the vagaries of life.

Factor analyses of the LOT routinely yield two separate factors,[2,4] comprised of positively worded (optimistic) items and negatively worded (pessimistic) items, respectively. Identification of two factors raises the question of whether it is better to view optimism and pessimism as opposite poles of a single dimension or as constituting two separate but correlated dimensions.[4] Though this is an interesting question, we have thus far taken the former view.

PSYCHOLOGICAL WELL-BEING

A growing number of studies have examined the effects of dispositional optimism on psychological well-being.[5] These studies have produced a remarkably consistent pattern of findings: Optimists routinely maintain higher levels of subjective well-being during times of stress than do people who are less optimistic. Let us briefly describe two illustrative cases.

One study[6] examined the development of postpartum depression in a group of women having their first children. Women in this study completed the LOT and a standard measure of depression in the third trimester of pregnancy. They completed the same depression measure again 3 weeks postpartum. Initial optimism was inversely associated with depression 3 weeks postpartum, even when the initial level of depression was controlled statistically. In other words, optimism predicted changes in depression over time. Optimistic women were less likely to become depressed following childbirth.

Conceptually similar findings have recently been reported in a study of undergraduate students' adjustment to their first semester of college.[7] A variety of factors were assessed when the students first arrived on campus, including dispositional optimism. Several measures of psychological well-being were obtained 3 months later. Optimism had a substantial effect on future psychological well-being: Higher levels of optimism upon entering college were associated with lower distress levels 3 months later. Notably, the effects of optimism in this study were distinct from those of the other personality factors measured, including self-esteem, locus of control, and desire for control. Thus, an optimistic orientation to life seemed to provide a benefit over and above that provided by these other personality characteristics.

PHYSICAL WELL-BEING

If the effects of optimism were limited to making people feel better, perhaps such findings would not be very surprising. The effects of optimism seem to go beyond this, however. There is at least some evidence that optimism also confers benefits on physical well-being.

Consider, for example, a study conducted on a group of men undergoing coronary artery bypass graft surgery.[8] Each patient was interviewed on the day prior to surgery, 6 to 8 days postsurgery, and again 6 months later. Optimism was assessed on the day prior to surgery by the LOT. A variety of medical and recovery variables were measured at several times, beginning before surgery and continuing through surgery and several months thereafter.

The data showed a number of effects for dispositional optimism. One notable finding concerns reactions to the surgery itself. Optimism was negatively related to physiological changes reflected in the patient's electrocardiogram and to the release of certain kinds of enzymes into the bloodstream. Both of these changes are widely taken as markers for myocardial infarction. The data thus suggest that optimists were less likely than pessimists to suffer heart attack during surgery.

Optimism was also a significant predictor of the rate of recovery during the immediate postoperative period. Optimists were faster to achieve selected behavioral milestones of recovery (e.g., sitting up in bed, walking around the room), and they were rated by medical staff as showing better physical recovery.

The advantages of an optimistic orientation were also apparent at the 6-month follow-up. Optimistic patients were more likely than pessimistic patients to have resumed vigorous physical exercise and to have returned to work full-time. Moreover, optimists returned to their activities more quickly than did pessimists. In sum, optimists were able to normalize their lifestyles more fully and more quickly than were pessimists. It is important to note that all of the findings just described were independent of the person's medical status at the outset of the study. Thus, it was not the case that optimists did better simply because they were less sick at the time of surgery.

HOW DOES OPTIMISM HELP?

If an understanding can be gained of why optimists do better than pessimists, then perhaps psychologists can begin to devise ways to help pessimists do better. One promising line of inquiry concerns differences between optimists and pessimists in how they cope with stress. Research from a variety of sources is beginning to suggest that optimists cope in more adaptive ways than do pessimists.[5] Optimists are more likely than pessimists to take direct action to solve their problems, are more planful in dealing with the adversity they confront, and are more focused in their coping efforts. Optimists are more likely to accept the reality of the stressful situations they encounter, and they also seem intent on growing personally from negative experiences and trying to make the best of bad situations. In contrast to these positive coping reactions, pessimists are more likely than optimists to react to stressful events by trying to deny that they exist or by trying to avoid dealing with problems. Pessimists are also more likely to quit trying when difficulties arise.

We now know that these coping differences are at least partly responsible for the differences in distress that optimists and pessimists experience in times of stress. When Aspinwall and Taylor[7] studied adjustment to college life, they collected information about the coping tactics the students were using to help themselves adjust to college, as well as measuring their optimism and eventual adjustment. Optimists were more likely than pessimists to rely on active coping techniques and less likely to engage in avoidance. These two general coping orientations were both related to later adjustment, in opposite directions. Avoidance coping was associated with poorer adjustment, whereas active coping was associated with better adjustment. Further analysis revealed that these two coping tendencies mediated the link between optimism and adjustment. Thus, optimists did better than pessimists at least partly because optimists used more effective ways of coping with problems.

A similar conclusion is suggested by a study of breast cancer patients that we and our colleagues recently completed. The women in this study reported on their distress and coping reactions before surgery, 10 days after surgery, and at 3-month, 6-month, and 12-month follow-ups. Throughout this period, optimism was associated with a coping pattern that involved accepting the reality of the situation, along with efforts to make the best of it. Optimism was inversely associated with attempts to act as though the problem was not real and with the tendency to give up on the life goals that were being threatened by the diagnosis of cancer. Further analyses suggested that these differences in coping served as paths by which the optimistic women remained less vulnerable to distress than the pessimistic women throughout the year.

ANTECEDENTS OF OPTIMISM

Where does optimism come from? Why do some people have it and others not? At present, not much is known about the origins of individual differences on this dimension. The determinants must necessarily fall in two broad categories, however: nature and nurture.

On the nature side, the available evidence suggests that individual differences in optimism-pessimism may be partly inherited. A translated version of the LOT was given to a sample of more than 500 same-sex pairs of middle-aged Swedish twins, and the heritability of optimism and pessimism was estimated to be about 25% using several different estimation procedures.[9] Thus, at least part of the variation in optimism and pessimism in the general population seems due to genetic influence.

On the environmental side, less is known. It is certainly reasonable to argue that optimism and pessimism are partly learned from prior experiences with success and failure. To the extent that one has been successful in the past, one should expect success in the future. Analogously, prior failure might breed the expectation of future failure. Children might also acquire a sense of optimism (or pessimism) from their parents, for example, through modeling. That is, parents who meet difficulties with positive expectations and who use adaptive coping strategies are explicitly or implicitly modeling those qualities for their children. Pessimistic parents also provide models for their children, although the qualities modeled are very different. Thus, children might become optimistic or pessimistic by thinking and acting in ways their parents do.

Parents might also influence children more directly by instructing them in problem solving. Parents who teach adaptive coping skills will produce children who are better problem solvers than children of parents who do not. To the extent that acquiring adaptive coping skills leads to coping success, the basis for an optimistic orientation is provided. We have recently begun a program of research designed to examine how coping strategies are transmitted from parent to child, with particular emphasis on the manner in which parental characteristics affect the kinds of coping strategies that are taught.

IS OPTIMISM ALWAYS GOOD? IS PESSIMISM ALWAYS BAD?

Implicit in our discussion thus far is the view that optimism is good for people. Is this always true? There are at least two ways in which an optimistic orientation might lead to poorer outcomes. First, it may be possible to be too optimistic, or to be optimistic in unproductive ways. For example, unbridled optimism may cause people to sit and wait for good things to happen, thereby decreasing the chance of success. We have seen no evidence of such a tendency among people defined as optimistic on the basis of the LOT, however. Instead, optimistic people seem to view positive outcomes as partially contingent on their continued effort.

Second, optimism might also prove detrimental in situations that are not amenable to constructive action. Optimists are prone to face problems with efforts to resolve them, but perhaps this head-on approach is maladaptive in situations that are uncontrollable or that involve major loss or a violation of one's world view. Data on this question are lacking, yet it is worth noting that the coping arsenal of optimists is not limited to the problem-focused domain. Optimists also use a host of emotion-focused coping responses, including tendencies to accept the reality of the situation, to put the situation in the best possible light, and to grow personally from their hardships. Given these coping options, optimists may prove to have a coping advantage even in the most distressing situations.

What about the reverse question? Can pessimism ever work in one's favor? Cantor and Norem[10] recently coined the term *defensive pessimism* to reflect a coping style in which people expect outcomes that are more negative than their prior reward histories in a given domain would suggest. Defensive pessimism may be useful because it helps to buffer the person against future failure, should failure occur. In addition, defensive pessimism may help the person perform better because the worry over anticipated failure prompts remedial action in preparation for the event.

Defensive pessimism does seem to work. That is, the performance of defensive pessimists tends to be better than the performance of real pessimists, whose negative expectations are anchored in prior failure. On the other hand, defensive pessimism never works better than optimism. Moreover, this style apparently has some hidden costs: People who use defensive pessimism in the short run report more psychological symptoms and a lower quality of life in the long run than do optimists.[10] Such findings call into serious question the adaptive value of defensive pessimism.

RELATIONSHIP TO OTHER APPROACHES

The concept of optimism, as discussed here, does not stand apart from the rest of personality psychology. There are easily noted family resemblances to several other personality constructs and approaches that have arisen in response to the same questions that prompted our line of theorizing. Two well-known examples are attributional style[11] and self-efficacy.[1] It may be useful to briefly note some similarities and differences between our conceptualization and these other approaches.

Attributional Style

Work on attributional style derives from the cognitive model[11] that was proposed to account for the phenomenon of learned helplessness[12] in humans. In this model, people's causal explanations for past events influence their expectations for controlling future events. The explanations thus influence subsequent feelings and behavior. As the attributional theory developed, it evolved toward a consideration of individual differences and began to focus on the possibility that an individual may have a stable tendency toward using one or another type of attribution. A tendency to attribute negative outcomes to causes that are stable, global, and internal has come to be known as pessimistic. A tendency to attribute negative events to causes that are unstable, specific, and external has come to be known as optimistic.

There is a clear conceptual link between this theory and the approach that we have taken. Both theories rely on the assumption that the consequences of optimism versus pessimism derive from differences in people's expectancies (at least in part). This assumption has been focal in our theory, and it is also important—albeit less focal—in the attributional approach. Moreover, despite differences in the types of measures used to assess optimism and attributional style, research findings relating attributional style to psychological and physical well-being have tended to parallel findings obtained for dispositional optimism.[13] Thus, the data converge on the conclusion that optimism is beneficial for mental and physical functioning.

Self-Efficacy

Self-efficacy expectancies are people's expectations of being either able or unable to execute desired behaviors successfully. Although there are obvious similarities between self-efficacy and optimism-pessimism, there are also two salient differences. One difference involves the extent to which the sense of personal agency is seen as the critical variable underlying behavior. Our approach to dispositional optimism intentionally deemphasizes the role of personal efficacy. Statements on self-efficacy make personal agency paramount.[1]

The second difference concerns the breadth of the expectancy on which the theory focuses. Efficacy theory holds that people's behavior is best predicted by focalized, domain-specific (or even act-specific) expectancies. Dispositional optimism, in contrast, is thought to be a very generalized tendency that has an influence in a wide variety of settings. Interestingly, relevant research[8] suggests that both types of expectancies (specific and general) are useful in predicting behavior.

CONCLUDING COMMENT

Our purpose in writing this article (perhaps in line with its subject matter) was to put a positive foot forward in presenting work on the benefits of optimism. In so doing, we may have created a false sense that the important questions about positive thinking have all been answered. Such is not the case. Understanding of the nature and effects of optimism is still in its infancy, and there is much more to learn. For example, although the effects of optimism seem attributable in part to differences in the ways optimists and pessimists cope with stress, this cannot be the complete answer. It is impossible to account fully for differences between optimists and pessimists on the basis of this factor alone.

Similarly, more work is needed to tease apart the effects of optimism from the effects of related variables. As noted earlier, a number of personality dimensions bear a conceptual resemblance to optimism-pessimism. Some of these dimensions, such as personal coherence, hardiness, and learned resourcefulness, have appeared in the literature only recently. Other dimensions, such as neuroticism, self-esteem, and self-mastery, have a longer scientific past. Given the existence of these related constructs, it is reasonable to ask whether their effects are distinguishable. This question cannot be resolved easily on the basis of one or two studies alone. An answer must await the gradual accumulation of evidence from many studies using different methodologies and assessing different outcomes.

There does seem to be a power to positive thinking. It surely is not as simple and direct a process as believing in something making it so. But believing that the future holds good things in store clearly has an effect on the way people relate to many aspects of life.

Acknowledgments—Preparation of this article was facilitated by National Science Foundation Grants BNS-9010425 and BNS-9011653, by National Institutes of Health Grant 1R01HL44432-01A1, and by American Cancer Society Grant PBR-56.

Notes

1. A. Bandura, *Social Foundations of Thought and Action: A Social Cognitive Theory* (Prentice-Hall, Englewood Cliffs, NJ, 1986).
2. M.F. Scheier and C.S. Carver, Optimism, coping, and health: Assessment and implications of generalized outcome expectancies, *Health Psychology, 4*, 219–247 (1985).
3. R. Schulz, C.A. Tompkins, and M.T. Rau, A longitudinal study of the psychosocial impact of stroke on primary support persons, *Psychology and Aging, 3*, 131–141 (1988).
4. G.N. Marshall, C.B. Wortman, J.W. Kusulas, L.K. Hervig, and R.R. Vickers, Jr., Distinguishing optimism from pessimism: Relations to fundamental dimensions of mood and personality, *Journal of Personality and Social Psychology, 62*, 1067–1074 (1992).
5. See M.F. Scheier and C.S. Carver, Effects of optimism on psychological and physical well-being: Theoretical overview and empirical update, *Cognitive Therapy and Research, 16*, 201–228 (1992).
6. C.S. Carver and J.G. Gaines, Optimism, pessimism, and postpartum depression, *Cognitive Therapy and Research, 11*, 449–462 (1987).
7. L.G. Aspinwall and S.E. Taylor, Modeling cognitive adaptation: A longitudinal investigation of the impact of individual differences and coping on college adjustment and performance, *Journal of Personality and Social Psychology* (in press).
8. M.F. Scheier, K.A. Matthews, J.F. Owens, G.J. Magovern, Sr., R. Lefebvre, R.C. Abbott, and C.S. Carver, Dispositional optimism and recovery from coronary artery bypass surgery: The beneficial effects of optimism on physical and psychological well-being, *Journal of Personality and Social Psychology, 57*, 1024–1040 (1989).
9. R. Plomin, M.F. Scheier, C.S. Bergeman, N.L. Pedersen, J.R. Nesselroade, and G.E. McClearn, Optimism, pessimism and mental health: A twin/adoption analysis, *Personality and Individual Differences* (in press).
10. N. Cantor and J.K. Norem, Defensive pessimism and stress and coping, *Social Cognition, 7*, 92–112 (1989).
11. L.Y. Abramson, M.E.P. Seligman, and J.D. Teasdale, Learned helplessness in humans: Critique and reformulation, *Journal of Abnormal Psychology, 87*, 49–74 (1978).
12. M.E.P. Seligman, *Helplessness: On Depression, Development, and Death* (Freeman, San Francisco, 1975).
13. For a review, see C. Peterson and L.M. Bossio, *Health and Optimism: New Research on the Relationship Between Positive Thinking and Physical Well-Being* (Free Press, New York, 1991).

Recommended Reading

Scheier, M.F., and Carver, C.S. (1992). Effects of optimism on psychological and physical well-being: Theoretical overview and empirical update. *Cognitive Therapy and Research, 16*, 201–228.

Seligman, M.E.P. (1991). *Learned Optimism* (Knopf, New York).

Taylor, S.E. (1989). *Positive Illusions: Creative Self-Deception and the Healthy Mind* (Basic Books, New York).

Glossary

This glossary of psychology terms is included to provide you with a convenient and ready reference as you encounter general terms in your study of personal growth and behavior that are unfamiliar or require a review. It is not intended to be comprehensive, but, taken together with the many definitions included in the articles themselves, it should prove to be quite useful.

Abnormal Irregular, deviating from the norm or average. Abnormal implies the presence of a mental disorder that leads to behavior that society labels as deviant. There is a continuum between normal and abnormal. These are relative terms in that they imply a social judgment. See Normal.

Accommodation Process in cognitive development; involves altering or reorganizing the mental picture to make room for a new experience or idea.

Acetylcholine A neurotransmitter involved in memory.

Achievement Drive The need to attain self-esteem, success, or status. Society's expectations strongly influence the achievement motive.

ACTH (Adrenocorticotropic Hormone) The part of the brain called the hypothalamus activates the release of the hormone ACTH from the pituitary gland when a stressful condition exists. ACTH in turn activates the release of adrenal corticoids from the cortex of the adrenal gland.

Action Therapy A general classification of therapy (as opposed to insight therapy) in which the therapist focuses on symptoms rather than on underlying emotional states. Treatment aims at teaching new behavioral patterns rather than at self-understanding. See Insight Therapy.

Actor-Observer Attribution The tendency to attribute the behavior of other people to internal causes and the behavior of yourself to external causes.

Adaptation The process of responding to changes in the environment by altering one's responses to keep one's behavior appropriate to environmental demands.

Addiction Physical dependence on a drug. When a drug causes biochemical changes that are uncomfortable when the drug is discontinued, when one must take ever larger doses to maintain the intensity of the drug's effects, and when desire to continue the drug is strong, one is said to be addicted.

Adjustment How we react to stress; some change that we make in response to the demands placed upon us.

Adrenal Glands Endocrine glands involved in stress and energy regulation.

Affective Disorder Affect means feeling or emotion. An affective disorder is mental illness marked by a disturbance of mood (e.g., manic depression.)

Afferent Neuron (Sensory) A neuron that carries messages from the sense organs toward the central nervous system.

Aggression Any act that causes pain or suffering to another. Some psychologists believe that aggressive behavior is instinctual to all species, including man, while others believe that it is learned through the processes of observation and imitation.

Alienation Indifference to or loss of personal relationships. An individual may feel estranged from family members, or, on a broader scale, from society.

All-or-None Law The principle that states that a neuron only fires when a stimulus is above a certain minimum strength (threshold), and that when it fires, it does so at full strength.

Altered State of Consciousness (ASC) A mental state qualitatively different from a person's normal, alert, waking consciousness.

Altruism Behavior motivated by a desire to benefit another person. Altruistic behavior is aided by empathy and is usually motivated internally, not by observable threats or rewards.

Amphetamine A psychoactive drug that is a stimulant. Although used in treating mild depressions or, in children, hyperactivity, its medical uses are doubtful, and amphetamines are often abused. See Psychoactive Drug.

Anal Stage Psychosexual stage, during which, according to Freud, the child experiences the first restrictions on his impulses.

Antisocial Personality Disorder Personality disorder in which individuals who engaged in antisocial behavior experience no guilt or anxiety about their actions; sometimes called sociopathy or psychopathy.

Anxiety An important term that has different meanings for different theories (psychoanalysis, behavior theory); a feeling state of apprehension, dread, or uneasiness. The state may be aroused by an objectively dangerous situation or by a situation that is not objectively dangerous. It may be mild or severe.

Anxiety Disorder Fairly long-lasting disruptions of the person's ability to deal with stress; often accompanied by feelings of fear and apprehension.

Applied Psychology The area of psychology that is most immediately concerned with helping to solve practical problems; includes clinical and counseling psychology, and industrial, environmental, and legal psychology.

Aptitude Tests Tests which are designed to predict what can be accomplished by a person in the future with the proper training.

Arousal A measure of responsiveness or activity; a state of excitement or wakefulness ranging from deepest coma to intense excitement.

Aspiration Level The level of achievement a person strives for. Studies suggest that people can use internal or external standards of performance.

Assertiveness Training Training which helps individuals stand up for their rights while not denying rights of other people.

Assimilation Process in cognitive development; occurs when something new is taken into the child's mental picture of the world.

Association Has separate meanings for different branches of psychology. Theory in cognitive psychology suggests that we organize information so that we can find our memories systematically, that one idea will bring another to mind. In psychoanalysis, the patient is asked to free associate (speak aloud all consecutive thoughts until random associations tend of themselves to form a meaningful whole). See Cognitive Psychology; Psychoanalysis.

Association Neurons Neurons that connect with other neurons.

Associationism A theory of learning suggesting that once two stimuli are presented together, one of them will remind a person of the other. Ideas are learned by association with sensory experiences and are not innate. Among the principles of associationism are contiguity (stimuli that occur close together are more likely to be associated than stimuli far apart), and repetition (the more frequently stimuli occur together, the more strongly they become associated).

Attachment Process in which the individual shows behaviors that promote the proximity or contact with a specific object or person.

Attention The tendency to focus activity in a particular direction and to select certain stimuli for further analysis while ignoring or possibly storing for further analysis all other inputs.

Attitude An overall tendency to respond positively or negatively to particular people or objects in a way that is learned through experience and that is made up of feelings (affects), thoughts (evaluations), and actions (conation).

Attribution The process of determining the causes of behavior in a given individual.

Autism A personality disorder in which a child does not respond socially to people.

Autonomic Nervous System The part of the nervous system (the other part is the central nervous system) that is for emergency functions and release of large amounts of energy (sympathetic division) and regulating functions such as digestion and sleep (parasympathetic division). See Biofeedback.

Aversion Therapy A counterconditioning therapy in which unwanted responses are paired with unpleasant consequences.

Avoidance Conditioning Situation in which a subject learns to avoid an aversive stimulus by responding appropriately before it begins.

Barbiturates Sedative-hypnotic, psychoactive drugs widely used to induce sleep and to reduce tension. Overuse can lead to addiction. See Addiction.

Behavior Any observable activity of an organism, including mental processes.

Behavior Therapy The use of conditioning processes to treat mental disorders. Various techniques may be used, including positive reinforcement in which rewards (verbal or tangible) are given to the patient for appropriate behavior, modeling in which patients unlearn fears by watching models exhibit fearlessness, and systematic desensitization in which the patient is taught to relax and visualize anxiety-producing items at the same time. See Insight Therapy; Systematic Desensitization.

Behaviorism A school of psychology stressing an objective approach to psychological questions, proposing that psychology be limited to observable behavior and that the subjectiveness of consciousness places it beyond the limits of scientific psychology.

Biofeedback The voluntary control of physiological processes by receiving information about those processes as they occur, through instruments that pick up these changes and display them to the subject in the form of a signal. Blood pressure, skin temperature, etc. can be controlled.

Biological (Primary) Motives Motives that have a physiological basis; include hunger, thirst, body temperature regulation, avoidance of pain, and sex.

Biological Response System System of the body that is particularly important in behavioral responding; includes the senses, endocrines, muscles, and the nervous system.

Biological Therapy Treatment of behavior problems through biological techniques; major biological therapies include drug therapy, psychosurgery, and electronconvulsive therapy.

Bipolar Disorder Affective disorder that is characterized by extreme mood swings from sad depression to joyful mania; sometimes called manic-depression.

Body Language Communication through position and movement of the body.

Brain Mapping A procedure for identifying the function of various areas of the brain; the surgeon gives tiny electrical stimulation to a specific area and notes patient's reaction.

Brain Stimulation The introduction of chemical or electrical stimuli directly into the brain.

Brain Waves Electrical responses produced by brain activity that can be recorded directly from any portion of the brain or from the scalp with special electrodes. Brain waves are measured by an electroencephalograph (EEG). Alpha waves occur during relaxed wakefulness and beta waves during active behavior. Theta waves are associated with drowsiness and vivid visual imagery, delta waves with deep sleep.

Cannon-Bard Theory of Emotion Theory of emotion that states that the emotional feeling and the physiological arousal occur at the same time.

Causal Attribution Process of determining whether a person's behavior is due to internal or external motives.

Cautious Shift Research suggests that the decisions of a group will be more conservative than that of the average individual member when dealing with areas for which there are widely held values favoring caution (e.g., physical danger or family responsibility). *See* Risky Shift.

Central Nervous System The part of the human nervous system that interprets and stores messages from the sense organs, decides what behavior to exhibit, and sends appropriate messages to the muscles and glands; includes the brain and spinal cord.

Central Tendency In statistics, measures of central tendency give a number that represents the entire group or sample.

Cerebellum The part of the brain responsible for muscle and movement control and coordination of eye-body movement.

Cerebral Cortex The part of the brain consisting of the outer layer of cerebral cells. The cortex can be divided into specific regions: sensory, motor, and associative.

Chaining Behavior theory suggests that behavior patterns are built up of component parts by stringing together a number of simpler responses.

Character Disorder (or Personality Disorder) A classification of psychological disorders (as distinguished from neurosis or psychosis). The disorder has become part of the individual's personality and does not cause him or her discomfort, making that disorder more difficult to treat psychotherapeutically.

Chromosome *See* Gene.

Chunking The tendency to code memories so that there are fewer bits to store.

Classical Conditioning *See* Pavlovian Conditioning.

Client-Centered Therapy A nondirective form of psychotherapy developed by Carl Rogers in which the counselor attempts to create an atmosphere in which the client can freely explore herself or himself and her or his problems. The client-centered therapist reflects what the client says back to him, usually without interpreting it.

Clinical Psychology The branch of psychology concerned with testing, diagnosing, interviewing, conducting research and treating (often by psychotherapy) mental disorders and personality problems.

Codependency The relationship of one person to a second person who is often a substance abuser. The codependent assists or enables the abuser to continue the drug dependency or problem behavior. The codependent becomes as addicted to the enabling life-style as the abuser is to the problem behavior or substance.

Cognitive Appraisal Intellectual evaluation of situations or stimuli. Experiments suggest that emotional arousal is produced not simply by a stimulus but by how one evaluates and interprets the arousal. The appropriate physical response follows this cognitive appraisal.

Cognitive Behavior Therapy A form of behavior therapy that identifies self-defeating attitudes and thoughts in a subject, and then helps the subject to replace these with positive, supportive thoughts.

Cognitive Dissonance People are very uncomfortable if they perceive that their beliefs, feelings, or acts are not consistent with one another, and they will try to reduce the discomfort of this dissonance.

Cognitive Psychology The study of how individuals gain knowledge of their environments. Cognitive psychologists believe that the organism actively participates in constructing the meaningful stimuli that it selectively organizes and to which it selectively responds.

Comparative Psychology The study of similarities and differences in the behavior of different species.

Compulsive Personality Personality disorder in which an individual is preoccupied with details and rules.

Concept Learning The acquisition of the ability to identify and use the qualities that objects or situations have in common. A class concept refers to any quality that breaks objects or situations into separate groupings.

Concrete-Operational Stage A stage in intellectual development, according to Piaget. The child at approximately seven years begins to apply logic. His or her thinking is less egocentric, reversible, and the child develops conservation abilities and the ability to classify.

Conditioned Reinforcer Reinforcement that is effective because it has been associated with other reinforcers. Conditioned reinforcers are involved in higher order conditioning.

Conditioned Response (CR) The response or behavior that occurs when the conditioned stimulus is presented (after the conditioned stimulus has been associated with the unconditioned stimulus).

Conditioned Stimulus (CS) An originally neutral stimulus that is associated with an unconditioned stimulus and takes on its capability of eliciting a particular reaction.

Conditioned Taste Aversion (CTA) Learning an aversion to particular tastes by associating them with stomach distress; usually considered a unique form of classical conditioning because of the extremely long interstimulus intervals involved.

Conduction The ability of a neuron to carry a message (an electrical stimulus) along its length.

Conflict Situation that occurs when we experience incompatible demands or desires.

Conformity The tendency of an individual to act like others regardless of personal belief.

Conscience A person's sense of the moral rightness or wrongness of behavior.

Consciousness Awareness of experienced sensations, thoughts, and feelings at any given point in time.

Consensus In causal attribution, the extent to which other people react the same way the subject does in a particular situation.

Consistency In causal attribution, the extent to which the subject always behaves in the same way in a particular situation.

Consolidation The biological neural process of making memories permanent; possibly short-term memory is electrically coded and long-term memory is chemically coded.

Continuum of Preparedness Seligman's proposal that animals are biologically prepared to learn certain responses more readily than others.

Control Group A group used for comparison with an experimental group. All conditions must be identical for each group with the exception of the one variable (independent) that is manipulated. *See* Experimental Group.

Convergence Binocular depth cue in which we detect distance by interpreting the kinesthetic sensations produced by the muscles of the eyeballs.

Convergent Thinking The kind of thinking that is used to solve problems having only one correct answer. *See* Divergent Thinking.

Conversion Disorder Somatoform disorder in which a person displays obvious disturbance in the nervous system, however, a medical examination reveals no physical basis for the problem; often includes paralysis, loss of sensation, or blindness.

Corpus Callosum Nerve fibers that connect the two halves of the brain in humans. If cut, the halves continue to function although some functions are affected.

Correlation A measurement in which two or more sets of variables are compared and the extent to which they are related is calculated.

Correlation Coefficient The measure, in number form, of how two variables vary together. They extend from -1 (perfect negative correlation) to a $+1$ (perfect positive correlation).

Counterconditioning A behavior therapy in which an unwanted response is replaced by conditioning a new response that is incompatible with it.

Creativity The ability to discover or produce new solutions to problems, new inventions, or new works of art. Creativity is an ability independent of IQ and is opened-ended in that solutions are not predefined in their scope or appropriateness. *See* Problem Solving.

Critical Period A specific stage in an organism's development during which the acquisition of a particular type of behavior depends on exposure to a particular type of stimulation.

Cross-Sectional Study A research technique that focuses on a factor in a group of subjects as they are at one time, as in a study of fantasy play in subjects of three different age groups. *See* Longitudinal Study.

Culture-Bound The idea that a test's usefulness is limited to the culture in which it was written and utilized.

Curiosity Motive Motive that causes the individual to seek out a certain amount of novelty.

Cutaneous Sensitivity The skin senses: touch, pain, pressure and temperature. Skin receptors respond in different ways and with varying degrees of sensitivity.

Decay Theory of forgetting in which sensory impressions leave memory traces that fade away with time.

Defense Mechanism A way of reducing anxiety that does not directly cope with the threat. There are many types, denial, repression, etc., all of which are used in normal functioning. Only when use is habitual or they impede effective solutions are they considered pathological.

Delusion A false belief that persists despite evidence showing it to be irrational. Delusions are often symptoms of mental illness.

Dependent Variable Those conditions that an experimenter observes and measures. Called "dependent" because they depend on the experimental manipulations.

Depersonalization Disorder Dissociative disorder in which individuals escape from their own personalities by believing that they don't exist or that their environment is not real.

Depression A temporary emotional state that normal individuals experience or a persistent state that may be considered a psychological disorder. Characterized by sadness and low self-esteem. See Self-Esteem.

Descriptive Statistics Techniques that help summarize large amounts of data information.

Developmental Norms The average time at which developmental changes occur in the normal individual.

Developmental Psychology The study of changes in behavior and thinking as the organism grows from the prenatal stage to death.

Deviation, Standard and Average Average deviation is determined by measuring the deviation of each score in a distribution from the mean and calculating the average of the deviations. The standard deviation is used to determine how representative the mean of a distribution is. See Mean.

Diagnostic and Statistical Manual of Mental Disorders (DSM) DSM-III was published in 1980 by the American Psychiatric Association.

Diffusion of Responsibility As the number of witnesses to a help-requiring situation—and thus the degree of anonymity—increases, the amount of helping decreases and the amount of time before help is offered increases.

Discrimination The ability to tell whether stimuli are different when presented together or that one situation is different from a past one.

Displacement The process by which an emotion originally attached to a particular person, object, or situation is transferred to something else.

Dissociative Disorders Disorders in which individuals forget who they are.

Distal Stimuli Physical events in the environment that affect perception. See Proximal Stimuli.

Distinctiveness In causal attribution, the extent to which the subject reacts the same way in other situations.

Divergent Thinking The kind of thinking that characterizes creativity (as contrasted with convergent thinking) and involves the development of novel resolutions of a task or the generation of totally new ideas. See Convergent Thinking.

DNA See Gene.

Double Bind A situation in which a person is subjected to two conflicting, contradictory demands at the same time.

Down's Syndrome Form of mental retardation caused by having three number 21 chromosomes (trisomy 21).

Dreams The thoughts, images, and emotions that occur during sleep. Dreams occur periodically during the sleep cycle and are usually marked by rapid movements of the eyes (REM sleep). The content of dreams tends to reflect emotions (sexual feelings, according to Freud) and experiences of the previous day. Nightmares are qualitatively different from other dreams, often occurring during deep or Stage 4 sleep.

Drive A need or urge that motivates behavior. Some drives may be explained as responses to bodily needs, such as hunger or sex. Others derive from social pressures and complex forms of learning, for example, competition, curiosity, achievement, See Motivation.

Drive Reduction Theory Theory of motivation that states that the individual is pushed by inner forces toward reducing the drive and restoring homeostasis.

Drug Dependence A state of mental or physical dependence on a drug, or both. Psychoactive drugs are capable of creating psychological dependence (anxiety when the drug is unavailable), although the relationship of some, such as marijuana and LSD, to physical dependence or addiction is still under study. See Psychoactive Drug; Addiction.

Drug Tolerance A state produced by certain psychoactive drugs in which increasing amounts of the substance are required to produce the desired effect. Some drugs produce tolerance but not withdrawal symptoms, and these drugs are not regarded as physically addicting.

Effectance Motive The striving for effectiveness in dealing with the environment. The effectance motive differs from the need for achievement in that effectance depends on internal feelings of satisfaction while the need for achievement is geared more to meeting others' standards.

Efferent Neuron (Motor) A neuron that carries messages from the central nervous system to the muscles and glands.

Ego A construct to account for the organization in a person's life and for making the person's behavior correspond to physical and social realities. According to Freud, the ego is the "reality principle" that is responsible for holding the id or "pleasure principle" in check. See Id.

Egocentrism Seeing things from only one's own point of view; also, the quality of a child's thought that prevents her or him from understanding that different people perceive the world differently. Egocentrism is characteristic of a stage that all children go through.

Electra Complex The libidinal feelings of a child toward a parent of the opposite sex. See also Oedipus Complex

Electroshock Therapy A form of therapy used to relieve severe depression. The patient receives electric current across the forehead, loses consciousness, and undergoes a short convulsion. When the patient regains consciousness, his or her mood is lifted.

Emotion A complex feeling-state that involves physiological arousal; a subjective feeling which might involve a cognitive appraisal of the situation and overt behavior in response to a stimulus.

Empathy The ability to appreciate how someone else feels by putting yourself in her or his position and experiencing her or his feelings. Empathy is acquired normally by children during intellectual growth.

Empiricism The view that behavior is learned through experience.

Encounter Groups Groups of individuals who meet to change their personal lives by confronting each other, discussing personal problems, and talking more honestly and openly than in everyday life.

Endocrine Glands Ductless glands that secrete chemicals called hormones into the blood stream.

Equilibration According to Piaget, the child constructs an understanding of the world through equilibration. Equilibration consists of the interaction of two complementary processes, assimilation (taking in input within the existing structures of the mind, e.g., putting it into mental categories that already exist) with accommodation (the changing of mental categories to fit new input that cannot be taken into existing categories) and is the process by which knowing occurs. One's developmental stage affects how one equilibrates.

Ethnocentrism The belief that one's own ethnic or racial group is superior to others.

Experiment Procedures executed under a controlled situation in order to test a hypothesis and discover relationships between independent and dependent variables.

Experimental Control The predetermined conditions, procedures, and checks built into the design of an experiment to ensure scientific control; as opposed to "control" in common usage, which implies manipulation.

Experimental Group In a scientific experiment, the group of subjects that is usually treated specially, as opposed to the control group, in order to isolate just the variable under investigation. See Control Group.

Experimental Psychology The branch of psychology concerned with the laboratory study of basic psychological laws and principles as demonstrated in the behavior of animals.

Experimenter Bias How the expectations of the person running an experiment can influence what comes out of the experiment. Experimenter bias can affect the way the experimenter sees the subjects' behavior, causing distortions of fact, and can also affect the way the experimenter reads data, also leading to distortions.

Extinction The elimination of behavior by, in classical conditioning, the withholding of the unconditional stimulus, and in operant conditioning, the withholding of the reinforcement.

Extrasensory Perception (ESP) The range of perceptions that are "paranormal," (such as the ability to predict events, reproduce drawings sealed in envelopes, etc.).

Fixed Interval (FI) Schedule Schedule of reinforcement in which the subject receives reinforcement for the first correct response given after a specified time interval.

Fixed Ratio (FR) Schedule Schedule of reinforcement in which the subject is reinforced after a certain number of responses.

Fixed-Action Pattern Movement that is characteristic of a species and does not have to be learned.

Forgetting The process by which material that once was available is no longer available. Theory exists that forgetting occurs because memories interfere with one another, either retroactively (new memories block old) or proactively (old memories block new); that forgetting occurs when the cues necessary to recall the information are not supplied, or when memories are too unpleasant to remain in consciousness. See Repression.

Formal Operational Stage According to Piaget, the stage at which the child develops adult powers of reasoning, abstraction, and symbolizing. The child can grasp scientific, religious, and political concepts and deduce their consequences as well as reason hypothetically ("what if . . .").

Frustration A feeling of discomfort or insecurity aroused by a blocking of gratification or by unresolved problems. Several theories hold that frustration arouses aggression. See Aggression.

Functionalism An early school of psychology stressing the ways behavior helps one adapt to the environment and the role that learning plays in this adaptive process.

Gene The unit of heredity that determines particular characteristics; a part of a molecule of DNA. DNA (dioxyribonucleic acid) is found mainly in the nucleus of living cells where it occurs in threadlike structures called chromosomes. Within the chromosomes, each DNA molecule is organized into specific units that carry the genetic information necessary for the development of a particular trait. These units are the genes. A gene can reproduce itself exactly, and this is how traits are carried between generations. The genotype is the entire structure of genes that are inherited by an organism from its parents. The environment interacts with this genotype to determine how the genetic potential will develop.

General Adaptation Syndrome (GAS) The way the body responds to stress, as described by Hans Selye. In the first stage, an alarm reaction, a person responds by efforts at self-control and shows signs of nervous depression (defense mechanisms, fear, anger, etc.) followed by a release of ACTH. In stage 2, the subject shows increased resistance to the specific source of stress and less resistance to other sources. Defense mechanisms may become neurotic. With stage 3 comes exhaustion, stupor, even death.

Generalization The process by which learning in one situation is transferred to another, similar situation. It is a key term in behavioral modification and classical conditioning. *See* Pavlovian Conditioning.

Generalized Anxiety Disorder Disorder in which the individual lives in a state of constant severe tension; continuous fear and apprehension experienced by an individual.

Genetics The study of the transfer of the inheritance of characteristics from one generation to another.

Genotype The underlying genetic structure that an individual has inherited and will send on to descendants. The actual appearance of a trait (phenotype) is due to the interaction of the genotype and the environment.

Gestalt Psychology A movement in psychology begun in the 1920s, stressing the wholeness of a person's experience and proposing that perceiving is an active, dynamic process that takes into account the entire pattern of ("gestalt") of the perpetual field. *See* Behaviorism; Associationism.

Glia Cells in the central nervous system that regulate the chemical environment of the nerve cells. RNA is stored in glial cells.

Grammar The set of rules for combining units of a language.

Group Therapy A form of psychotherapy aimed at treating mental disorders in which interaction among group members is the main therapeutic mode. Group therapy takes many forms but essentially requires a sense of community, support, increased personal responsibility, and a professionally trained leader.

Growth The normal quantitative changes that occur in the physical and psychological aspects of a healthy child with the passage of time.

Gustation The sense of taste. Theory suggests that the transmission of sense information from tongue to brain occurs through patterns of cell activity and not just the firing of single nerve fibers. Also, it is believed that specific spatial patterns or places on the tongue correspond to taste qualities.

Habit Formation The tendency to make a response to a stimulus less variable, especially if it produced successful adaptation.

Hallucination A sensory impression reported by a person when no external stimulus exists to justify the report. Hallucinations are serious symptoms and may be produced by psychoses. *See* Psychosis.

Hallucinogen A substance that produces hallucinations, such as LSD, mescaline, etc.

Hierarchy of Needs Maslow's list of motives in humans, arranged from the biological to the uniquely human.

Higher Order Conditioning Learning to make associations with stimuli that have been previously learned (CSs).

Hippocampus Part of the cortex of the brain governing memory storage, smell, and visceral functions.

Homeostasis A set of processes maintaining the constancy of the body's internal state, a series of dynamic compensations of the nervous system. Many processes such as appetite, body temperature, water balance, and heart rate are controlled by homeostasis.

Hormones Chemical secretions of the endocrine glands that regulate various body processes (e.g., growth, sexual traits, reproductive processes, etc.).

Humanism Branch of psychology dealing with those qualities distinguishing humans from other animals.

Hypnosis A trancelike state marked by heightened suggestibility and a narrowing of attention that can be induced in a number of ways. Debate exists over whether hypnosis is a true altered state of consciousness and to what extent strong motivating instructions can duplicate so-called hypnosis.

Hypothalamus A part of the brain that acts as a channel that carries information from the cortex and the thalamus to the spinal cord and ultimately to the motor nerves or to the autonomic nervous system, where it is transmitted to specific target organs. These target organs release into the bloodstream specific hormones that alter bodily functions. *See* Autonomic Nervous System.

Hypothesis A hypothesis can be called an educated guess, similar to a hunch. When a hunch is stated in a way that allows for further testing, it becomes a hypothesis.

Iconic Memory A visual memory. Experiments suggest that in order to be remembered and included in long-term memory, information must pass through a brief sensory stage. Theory further suggests that verbal information is subject to forgetting but that memorized sensory images are relatively permanent.

Id According to Freud, a component of the psyche present at birth that is the storehouse of psychosexual energy called *libido*, and also of primitive urges to fight, dominate, destroy.

Identification The taking on of attributes that one sees in another person. Children tend to identify with their parents or other important adults and thereby take on certain traits that are important to their development.

Illusion A mistaken perception of an actual stimulus.

Imitation The copying of another's behavior; learned through the process of observation. *See* Modeling.

Impression Formation The process of developing an evaluation of another person from your perceptions; first, or initial, impressions are often very important.

Imprinting The rapid, permanent acquisition by an organism of a strong attachment to an object (usually the parent). Imprinting occurs shortly after birth.

Independent Variable The condition in an experiment that is controlled and manipulated by the experimenter; it is a stimulus that will cause a response.

Inferential Statistics Techniques that help researchers make generalizations about a finding based on a limited number of subjects.

Inhibition Restraint of an impulse, desire, activity, or drive. People are taught to inhibit full expression of many drives (for example, aggression or sexuality) and to apply checks either consciously or unconsciously. In Freudian terminology, an inhibition is an unconsciously motivated blocking of sexual energy. In Pavlovian conditioning, inhibition is the theoretical process that operates during extinction, acting to block a conditioned response. *See* Pavlovian Conditioning.

Insight A sudden perception of useful or proper relations among objects necessary to solve the problem.

Insight Therapy A general classification of therapy in which the therapist focuses on the patient's underlying feelings and motivations and devotes most effort to increasing the patient's self-awareness or insight into his or her behavior. The other major class of therapy is action therapy. *See* Action Therapy.

Instinct An inborn pattern of behavior, relatively independent of environmental influence. An instinct may need to be triggered by a particular stimulus in the environment, but then it proceeds in a fixed pattern. The combination of taxis (orienting movement in response to a particular stimulus) and fixed-action pattern (inherited coordination) is the basis for instinctual activity. *See* Fixed-Action Pattern.

Instrumental Learning *See* Operant Conditioning.

Intelligence A capacity for knowledge about the world. This is an enormous and controversial field of study, and there is no agreement on a precise definition. However, intelligence has come to refer to higher-level abstract processes and may be said to comprise the ability to deal effectively with abstract concepts, the ability to learn, and the ability to adapt and deal with new situations. Piaget defines intelligence as the construction of an understanding. Both biological inheritance and environmental factors contribute to general intelligence. Children proceed through a sequence of identifiable stages in the development of conceptual thinking (Piaget). The degree to which factors such as race, sex, and social class affect intelligence is not known.

Intelligence Quotient (IQ) A measurement of intelligence originally based on tests devised by Binet and now widely applied. Genetic inheritance and environment affect IQ, although their relative contributions are not known. IQ can be defined in different ways; classically it is defined as a relation between chronological and mental ages.

Interference Theory of forgetting in which information that was learned before (proactive interference) or after (retroactive interference) the material of interest causes the learner to be unable to remember the material.

Interstimulus Interval The time between the start of the conditioned stimulus and the start of the unconditioned stimulus in Pavlovian conditioning. *See* Pavlovian Conditioning.

Intrauterine Environment The environment in the uterus during pregnancy can affect the physical development of the organism and its behavior after birth. Factors such as the mother's nutrition, emotional, and physical state significantly influence offspring. The mother's diseases, medications, hormones, and stress level all affect the pre- and postnatal development of her young.

Intrinsic Motivation Motivation inside of the individual; we do something because we receive satisfaction from it.

Introspection Reporting one's internal, subjective mental contents for the purpose of further study and analysis.

James-Lange Theory of Emotion Theory of emotion that states that the physiological arousal and behavior come before the subjective experience of an emotion.

Labeling-of-Arousal Experiments suggest that an individual experiencing physical arousal that she or he cannot explain will interpret her or his feelings in terms of the situation she or he is in and will use environmental and contextual cues.

Language A set of abstract symbols used to communicate meaning. Language includes vocalized sounds or semantic units (words, usually) and rules for combining the units (grammar). There is some inborn basis for language acquisition, and there are identifiable stages in its development that are universal.

Language Acquisition Linguists debate how children acquire language. Some believe in environmental shaping, a gradual system of reward and punishment. Others emphasize the unfolding of capacities inborn in the brain that are relatively independent of the environment and its rewards.

Latency Period According to Freud, the psychosexual stage of development during which sexual interest has been repressed and thus is low or "latent" (dormant).

Law of Effect Thorndike's proposal that when a response produces satisfaction, it will be repeated; reinforcement.

Leadership The quality of exerting more influence than other group members. Research suggests that certain characteristics are generally considered essential to leadership: consideration, sensitivity, ability to initiate and structure, and emphasis on production. However, environmental factors may thrust authority on a person without regard to personal characteristics.

Learned Helplessness Theory suggests that living in an environment of uncontrolled stress reduces the ability to cope with future stress that *is* controllable.

Learned Social Motives Motives in the human that are learned, including achievement, affiliation, and autonomy.

Learning The establishment of connections between stimulus and response, resulting from observation, special training, or previous activity. Learning is relatively permanent.

Life Span Span of time from conception to death; in developmental psychology, a life span approach looks at development throughout an individual's life.

Linguistic Relativity Hypothesis Proposal by Whorf that the perception of reality differs according to the language of the observer.

Linguistics The study of language, its nature, structure, and components.

Locus of Control The perceived place from which come determining forces in one's life. A person who feels that he or she has some control over his or her fate and tends to feel more likely to succeed has an internal locus of control. A person with an external locus of control feels that it is outside himself or herself and therefore that his or her attempts to control his or her fate are less assured.

Longitudinal Study A research method that involves following subjects over a considerable period of time (as compared with a cross-sectional approach); as in a study of fantasy play in children observed several times at intervals of two years. *See* Cross-Sectional Study.

Love Affectionate behavior between people, often in combination with interpersonal attraction. The mother-infant love relationship strongly influences the later capacity for developing satisfying love relationships.

Manic-Depressive Reaction A form of mental illness marked by alternations of extreme phases of elation (manic phase) and depression.

Maternalism Refers to the mother's reaction to her young. It is believed that the female is biologically determined to exhibit behavior more favorable to the care and feeding of the young than the male, although in humans maternalism is probably determined as much by cultural factors as by biological predisposition.

Maturation The genetically-controlled process of physical and physiological growth.

Mean The measure of central tendency, or mathematical average, computed by adding all scores in a set and dividing by the number of scores.

Meaning The concept or idea conveyed to the mind, by any method. In reference to memory, meaningful terms are easier to learn than less meaningful, unconnected, or nonsense terms. Meaningfulness is not the same as the word's meaning.

Median In a set of scores, the median is that middle score that divides the set into equal halves.

Memory Involves the encoding, storing of information in the brain, and its retrieval. Several theories exist to explain memory. One proposes that we have both a short-term (STM) and a long-term memory (LTM) and that information must pass briefly through the STM to be stored in the LTM. Also suggested is that verbal information is subject to forgetting, while memorized sensory images are relatively permanent. Others see memory as a function of association—information processed systematically and the meaningfulness of the items. Debate exists over whether memory retrieval is actually a process of reappearance or reconstruction.

Mental Disorder A mental condition that deviates from what society considers to be normal.

Minnesota Multiphasic Personality Inventory (MMPI) An objective personality test that was originally devised to identify personality disorders.

Mode In a set of scores, the measurement at which the largest number of subjects fall.

Modeling The imitation or copying of another's behavior. As an important process in personality development, modeling may be based on parents. In therapy, the therapist may serve as a model for the patient.

Morality The standards of right and wrong of a society and their adoption by members of that society. Some researchers believe that morality develops in successive stages, with each stage representing a specific level of moral thinking (Kohlberg). Others see morality as the result of experiences in which the child learns through punishment and reward from models such as parents and teachers.

Motivation All factors that cause and regulate behavior that is directed toward achieving goals and satisfying needs. Motivation is what moves an organism to action.

Narcissism A strong tendency to glorify the self at the expense of other people or other more mentally healthy tendencies. The concept relates primarily to physical attractiveness but can also mean any strong self-glorification.

Narcotic A drug that relieves pain. Heroin, morphine, and opium are narcotics. Narcotics are often addicting.

Naturalistic Observation Research method in which behavior of people or animals in the normal environment is accurately recorded.

Nature vs. Nurture A controversy in psychology that centers on whether behaviors and traits are biologically determined (e.g., genes) or environmentally determined (e.g., learned).

Negative Reinforcement Any event that upon termination, strengthens the preceding behavior; taking from subject something bad will increase the probability that the preceding behavior will be repeated. Involves aversive stimulus.

Neuron A nerve cell. There are billions of neurons in the brain and spinal cord. Neurons interact at synapses or points of contact. Information passage between neurons is electrical and biochemical. It takes the activity of many neurons to produce a behavior.

Neurosis Any one of a wide range of psychological difficulties, accompanied by excessive anxiety (as contrasted with psychosis). Psychoanalytic theory states that neurosis is an expression of unresolved conflicts in the form of tension and impaired functioning. Most neurotics are in much closer contact with reality than most psychotics. Term has been largely eliminated from DSM-III.

Nonverbal Behaviors Gestures, facial expressions, and other body movements. They are important because they tend to convey emotion. Debate exists over whether they are inborn or learned.

Norm An empirically set pattern of belief or behavior. Social norm refers to widely accepted social or cultural behavior to which a person tends to or is expected to conform.

Normal Sane, or free from mental disorder. Normal behavior is the behavior typical of most people in a given group, and "normality" implies a social judgment.

Normal Curve When scores of a large number of random cases are plotted on a graph, they often fall into a bell-shaped curve; there are as many cases above the mean as below on the curve.

Object Permanence According to Piaget, the stage in cognitive development when a child begins to conceive of objects as having an existence even when out of sight or touch and to conceive of space as extending beyond his or her own perception.

Oedipus Complex The conflicts of a child in triangular relationship with his mother and father. According to Freud, a boy must resolve his unconscious sexual desire for his mother and the accompanying wish to kill his father and fear of his father's revenge in order that he proceed in his moral development. The analogous problem for girls is called the Electra complex.

Olfaction The sense of smell. No general agreement exists on how olfaction works, though theories exist to explain it. One suggests that the size and shape of molecules of what is smelled is a crucial cue. The brain processes involved in smell are located in a different and evolutionarily older part of the brain than the other senses.

Operant Conditioning The process of changing, maintaining, or eliminating voluntary behavior through the consequences of that behavior. Operant conditioning uses many of the techniques of Pavlovian conditioning but differs in that it deals with voluntary rather than reflex behaviors. The frequency with which a behavior is emitted can be increased if it is rewarded (reinforced) and decreased if it is not reinforced, or punished. Some psychologists believe that all behavior is learned through conditioning while others believe that intellectual and motivational processes play a crucial role. *See* Pavlovian Conditioning.

Operational Definitions If an event is not directly observable, then the variables must be defined by the operations by which they will be measured. These definitions are called operational definitions.

Organism Any living animal, human or subhuman.

Orienting Response A relatively automatic, "what's that?" response that puts the organism in a better position to attend to and deal with a new stimulus. When a stimulus attracts our attention, our body responds with movements of head and body toward the stimulus, changes in muscle tone, heart rate, blood flow, breathing, and changes in the brain's electrical activity.

Pavlovian Conditioning Also called classical conditioning, Pavlovian conditioning can be demonstrated as follows: In the first step, an *unconditioned stimulus* (UCS) such as food, loud sounds, or pain is paired with a neutral *conditioned stimulus* (CS) that causes no direct effect, such as a click, tone, or a dim light. The response elicited by the UCS is called the *unconditioned response* (UCR) and is a biological reflex of the nervous system (for example, eyeblinks or salivation). The combination of the neutral CS, the response-causing UCS, and the unlearned UCR is usually presented to the subject several times during conditioning. Eventually, the UCS is dropped from the sequence in the second step of the process, and the previously neutral CS comes to elicit a response. When conditioning is complete, presentation of the CS alone will result in a *conditioned response* (CR) similar but not always the same as the UCR.

Perception The field of psychology studying ways in which the experience of objects in the world is based upon stimulation of the sense organs. In psychology, the field of perception studies what determines sensory impressions, such as size, shape, distance, direction, etc. Physical events in the environment are called distal stimuli while the activity at the sense organ itself is called a proximal stimulus. The study of perceiving tries to determine how an organism knows what distal stimuli are like since proximal stimuli are its only source of information. Perception of objects remains more or less constant despite changes in distal stimuli and is therefore believed to depend on relationships within stimuli (size *and* distance, for example). Perceptual processes are able to adjust and adapt to changes in the perceptual field.

Performance The actual behavior of an individual that is observed. We often infer learning from observing performance.

Peripheral Nervous System The part of the human nervous system that receives messages from the sense organs and carries messages to the muscles and glands; everything outside of the brain and spinal cord.

Personal Space The area around the body that people feel is their own space. When interacting with others, we maintain a distance sufficient to protect our personal space or personal "bubble."

Persuasion The process of changing a person's attitudes, beliefs, or actions. A person's susceptibility to persuasion depends on the persuader's credibility, subtlety, and whether both sides of an argument are presented.

Phenotype The physical features or behavior patterns by which we recognize an organism. Phenotype is the result of interaction between genotype (total of inherited genes) and environment. *See* Genotype.

Phobia A neurosis consisting of an irrationally intense fear of specific persons, objects, or situations and a wish to avoid them. A phobic person feels intense and incapacitating anxiety. The person may be aware that the fear is irrational, but this knowledge does not help.

Pituitary Gland Is located in of the brain and controls secretion of several hormones: the antidiuretic hormone that maintains water balance, oxytocin that controls blood pressure and milk production, and ACTH that is produced in response to stress, etc. *See* ACTH.

Placebo A substance that in and of itself has no real effect but which may produce an effect in a subject because the subject expects or believes that it will.

Positive Reinforcement Any event that, upon presentation, strengthens the preceding behavior; giving a subject something good will increase the probability that the preceding behavior will be repeated.

Prejudice An attitude in which one holds a negative belief about members of a group to which he or she does not belong. Prejudice is often directed at minority ethnic or racial groups and may be reduced by contact with these perceived "others."

Premack Principle Principle that states that of any two responses, the one that is more likely to occur can be used to reinforce the response that is less likely to occur.

Prenatal Development Development from conception to birth. It includes the physical development of the fetus as well as certain of its intellectual and emotional processes.

Primary Reinforcement Reinforcement that is effective without having been associated with other reinforcers; sometimes called unconditioned reinforcement.

Probability (p) In inferential statistics, the likelihood that the difference between the experimental and control groups is due to the independent variable.

Problem Solving A self-directed activity in which an individual uses information to develop answers to problems, to generate new problems, and sometimes to transform the process by creating a unique, new system. Problem solving involves learning, insight and creativity.

Projective Test A type of test in which people respond to ambiguous, loosely structured stimuli. It is assumed that people will reveal themselves by putting themselves into the stimuli they see. The validity of these tests for diagnosis and personality assessment is still at issue.

Propaganda Information deliberately spread to aid a cause. Propaganda's main function is persuasion.

Prosocial Behavior Behavior that is directed toward helping others.

Proximal Stimulus Activity at the sense organ.

Psychoactive Drug A substance that affects mental activities, perceptions, consciousness, or mood. This type of drug has its effects through strictly physical effects and through expectations.

Psychoanalysis There are two meanings to this word: it is a theory of personality development based on Freud and a method of treatment also based on Freud. Psychoanalytic therapy uses techniques of free association, dream analysis, and analysis of the patient's relationship (the "transference") to the analyst. Psychoanalytic theory maintains that the personality develops through a series of psychosexual stages and that the personality consists of specific components energized by the life and death instincts.

Psychogenic Pain Disorder Somatoform disorder in which the person complains of severe, long-lasting pain for which there is no organic cause.

Psycholinguistics The study of the process of language acquisition as part of psychological development and of language as an aspect of behavior. Thinking may obviously depend on language, but their precise relationship still puzzles psycholinguists, and several different views exist.

Psychological Dependence Situation when a person craves a drug even though it is not biologically necessary for his or her body.

Psychophysiological Disorders Real medical problems (such as ulcers, migraine headaches, and high blood pressure) that are caused or aggravated by psychological stress.

Psychosexual Stages According to Freud, an individual's personality develops through several stages. Each stage is associated with a particular bodily source of gratification (pleasure). First comes the oral stage when most pleasures come from the mouth. Then comes the anal stage when the infant derives pleasure from holding and releasing while learning bowel control. The phallic stage brings pleasure from the genitals, and a crisis (Oedipal) occurs in which the child gradually suppresses sexual desire for the opposite-sex parent, identifies with the same-sex parent and begins to be interested in the outside world. This latency period lasts until puberty, after which the genital stage begins and mature sexual relationships develop. There is no strict timetable, but, according to Freudians, the stages do come in a definite order. Conflicts experienced and not adequately dealt with remain with the individual.

Psychosis The most severe of mental disorders, distinguished by a person being seriously out of touch with objective reality. Psychoses may result from physical factors (organic) or may have no known physical cause (functional). Psychoses take many forms, of which the most common are schizophrenia and psychotic depressive reactions, but all are marked by personality disorganization and a severely reduced ability to perceive reality. Both biological and environmental factors are believed to influence the development of psychosis, although the precise effect of each is not presently known. *See* Neurosis.

Psychosomatic Disorders A variety of body reactions that are closely related to psychological events. Stress, for example, brings on many physical changes and can result in illness or even death if prolonged and severe. Psychosomatic disorders can affect any part of the body.

Psychotherapy Treatment involving interpersonal contacts between a trained therapist and a patient in which the therapist tries to produce beneficial changes in the patient's emotional state, attitudes, and behavior.

Punishment Any event that decreases the probability of the preceding behavior being repeated. You can give something bad (positive punishment) to decrease the preceding behavior.

Rational-Emotive Therapy A cognitive behavior modification technique in which a person is taught to identify irrational, self-defeating beliefs and then to overcome them.

Rationalization Defense mechanism in which individuals make up logical excuses to justify their behavior rather than exposing their true motives.

Reaction Formation Defense mechanism in which a person masks an unconsciously distressing or unacceptable trait by assuming an opposite attitude or behavior pattern.

Reality Therapy A form of treatment of mental disorders pioneered by William Glasser in which the origins of the patient's problems are considered irrelevant and emphasis is on a close, judgmental bond between patient and therapist aimed to improve the patient's present and future life.

Reflex An automatic movement that occurs in direct response to a stimulus.

Rehearsal The repeating of an item to oneself and the means by which information is stored in the short-term memory (STM). Theory suggests that rehearsal is necessary for remembering and storage in the long-term memory (LTM).

Reinforcement The process of affecting the frequency with which a behavior is emitted. A reinforcer can reward and thus increase the behavior or punish and thus decrease its frequency. Reinforcers can also be primary, satisfying basic needs such as hunger or thirst, or secondary, satisfying learned and indirect values, such as money.

Reliability Consistency of measurement. A test is reliable if it repeatedly gives the same results. A person should get nearly the same score if the test is taken on two different occasions.

REM (Rapid-Eye Movement) Type of sleep in which the eyes are rapidly moving around; dreaming occurs in REM sleep.

Repression A defense mechanism in which a person forgets or pushes into the unconscious something that arouses anxiety. *See* Defense Mechanism; Anxiety.

Reticular Formation A system of nerve fibers leading from the spinal column to the cerebral cortex that functions to arouse, alert, and make an organism sensitive to changes in the environment. *See* Cerebral Cortex.

Retina The inside coating of the eye, containing two kinds of cells that react to light: the rods that are sensitive only to dim light and the cones that are sensitive to color and form in brighter light. There are three kinds of cones, each responsive to particular colors in the visible spectrum (range of colors).

Risky Shift Research suggests that decisions made by groups will involve considerably more risk than individuals in the group would be willing to take. This shift in group decision depends heavily on cultural values. *See* Cautious Shift.

Rod Part of the retina involved in seeing in dim light. *See* Retina.

RNA (Ribonucleic Acid) A chemical substance that occurs in chromosomes and that functions in genetic coding. During task-learning, RNA changes occur in the brain.

Role Playing Adopting the role of another person and experiencing the world in a way one is not accustomed to.

Role Taking The ability to imagine oneself in another's place or to understand the consequences of one's actions for another person.

Schachter-Singer Theory of Emotion Theory of emotion that states that we interpret our arousal according to our environment and label our emotions accordingly.

Schizoid Personality Personality disorder characterized by having great trouble developing social relationships.

Schizophrenia The most common and serious form of psychosis in which there exists an imbalance between emotional reactions and the thoughts associated with these feelings. It may be a disorder of the process of thinking. *See* Psychosis.

Scientific Method The process used by psychologists to determine principles of behavior that exist independently of individual experience and that are untouched by unconscious bias. It is based on a prearranged agreement that criteria, external to the individual and communicable to others, must be established for each set of observations referred to as fact.

Secondary Reinforcement Reinforcement that is only effective after it has been associated with a primary reinforcer.

Self-Actualization A term used by humanistic psychologists to describe what they see as a basic human motivation: the development of all aspects of an individual into productive harmony.

Self-Esteem A person's evaluation of oneself. If someone has confidence and satisfaction in oneself, self-esteem is considered high.

Self-Fulfilling Prophecy A preconceived expectation or belief about a situation that evokes behavior resulting in a situation consistent with the preconception.

Senses An organism's physical means of receiving and detecting physical changes in the environment. Sensing is analyzed in terms of reception of the physical stimulus by specialized nerve cells in the sense organs, transduction or converting the stimulus' energy into nerve impulses that the brain can interpret, and transmission of those nerve impulses from the sense organ to the part of the brain that can interpret the information they convey.

Sensitivity Training Aims at helping people to function more effectively in their jobs by increasing their awareness of their own and others' feelings and exchanging "feedback" about styles of interacting. Sensitivity groups are unlike therapy groups in that they are meant to enrich the participants' lives. Participants are not considered patients or ill. Also called T-groups.

Sensorimotor Stage According to Piaget, the stage of development beginning at birth during which perceptions are tied to objects that the child manipulates. Gradually the child learns that objects have permanence even if they are out of sight or touch.

Sensory Adaptation Tendency of the sense organs to adjust to continuous, unchanging stimulation by reducing their functioning; a stimulus that once caused sensation no longer does.

Sensory Deprivation The blocking out of all outside stimulation for a period of time. As studied experimentally, it can produce hallucinations, psychological disturbances, and temporary disorders of the nervous system of the subject.

Sex Role The attitudes, activities, and expectations considered specific to being male or female, determined by both biological and cultural factors.

Shaping A technique of behavior shaping in which behavior is acquired through the reinforcement of successive approximations of the desired behavior.

Sibling Rivalry A (somewhat psychoanalytic) concept which suggests that we compete with our brothers and sisters for our parents' attention and for other rewards.

Sleep A periodic state of consciousness marked by four brain-wave patterns. Dreams occur during REM sleep. Sleep is a basic need without which one may suffer physical or psychological distress. *See* Brain Waves; Dreams.

Social Comparison Theory proposed by Festinger that states that we have a tendency to compare our behavior to others to ensure that we are conforming.

Social Facilitation Phenomenon in which the presence of others increases dominant behavior patterns in an individual; Zajonc's theory of social facilitation states that the presence of others enhances the emission of the dominant response of the individual.

Social Influence The process by which people form and change the attitudes, opinions, and behavior of others.

Social Learning Learning acquired through observation and imitation of others.

Social Psychology The study of individuals as affected by others and of the interaction of individuals in groups.

Socialization A process by which a child learns the various patterns of behavior expected and accepted by society. Parents are the chief agents of a child's socialization. Many factors have a bearing on the socialization process, such as the child's sex, religion, social class, and parental attitudes.

Sociobiology The study of the genetic basis of social behavior.

Sociophobias Excessive irrational fears and embarrassment when interacting with other people.

Somatic Nervous System The part of the peripheral nervous system that carries messages from the sense organs and relays information that directs the voluntary movements of the skeletal muscles.

Somatoform Disorders Disorders characterized by physical symptoms for which there are no obvious physical causes.

Somesthetic Senses Skin senses; includes pressure, pain, cold, and warmth.

Species-Typical Behavior Behavior patterns common to members of a species. Ethologists state that each species inherits some patterns of behavior (e.g., birdsongs).

Stanford-Binet Intelligence Scale Tests that measure intelligence from two years of age through adult level. The tests determine one's intelligence quotient by establishing one's chronological and mental ages. *See* Intelligence Quotient.

State-Dependent Learning Situation in which what is learned in one state can only be remembered when the person is in that state.

Statistically Significant In inferential statistics, a finding that the independent variable did influence greatly the outcome of the experimental and control group.

Stereotype The assignment of characteristics to a person mainly on the basis of the group, class, or category to which he or she belongs. The tendency to categorize and generalize is a basic human way of organizing information. Stereotyping, however, can reinforce misinformation and prejudice. *See* Prejudice.

Stimulus A unit of the environment that causes a response in an individual; more specifically, a physical or chemical agent acting on an appropriate sense receptor.

Stimulus Discrimination Limiting responses to relevant stimuli.

Stimulus Generalization Responses to stimuli similar to the stimulus that had caused the response.

Stress Pressure that puts unusual demands on an organism. Stress may be caused by physical conditions but eventually will involve both. Stimuli that cause stress are called stressors, and an organism's response is the stress reaction. A three-stage general adaptation syndrome is hypothesized involving both emotional and physical changes. *See* General Adaptation Syndrome.

Sublimation Defense mechanism in which a person redirects his socially undesirable urges into socially acceptable behavior.

Subliminal Stimuli Stimuli that do not receive conscious attention because they are below sensory thresholds. They may influence behavior, but research is not conclusive on this matter.

Substance-Induced Organic Mental Disorders Organic mental disorders caused by exposure to harmful environmental substances.

Suggestibility The extent to which a person responds to persuasion. Hypnotic susceptibility refers to the degree of suggestibility observed after an attempt to induce hypnosis has been made. *See* Hypnosis; Persuasion.

Superego According to Freud, the superego corresponds roughly to conscience. The superego places restrictions on both ego and id and represents the internalized restrictions and ideals that the child learns from parents and culture. *See* Conscience; Ego; Id.

Sympathetic Nervous System The branch of the autonomic nervous system that is more active in emergencies; it causes a general arousal, increasing breathing, heart rate, and blood pressure.

Synapse A "gap" where individual nerve cells (neurons) come together and across which chemical information is passed.

Syndrome A group of symptoms that occur together and mark a particular abnormal pattern.

Systematic Desensitization A technique used in behavior therapy to eliminate a phobia. The symptoms of the phobia are seen as conditioned responses of fear, and the procedure attempts to decondition the fearful response until the patient gradually is able to face the feared situation. *See* Phobia.

TAT (Thematic Apperception Test) Personality and motivation test that requires the subject to devise stories about pictures.

Theory A very general statement that is more useful in generating hypotheses than in generating research. *See* Hypothesis.

Therapeutic Community The organization of a hospital setting so that patients have to take responsibility for helping one another in an attempt to prevent patients from getting worse by being in the hospital.

Token Economy A system for organizing a treatment setting according to behavioristic principles. Patients are encouraged to take greater responsibility for their adjustment by receiving tokens for acceptable behavior and fines for unacceptable behavior. The theory of token economy grew out of operant conditioning techniques. *See* Operant Conditioning.

Traits Distinctive and stable attributes that can be found in all people.

Tranquilizers Psychoactive drugs that reduce anxiety. *See* Psychoactive Drug.

Trial and Error Learning Trying various behaviors in a situation until the solution is hit upon; past experiences lead us to try different responses until we are successful.

Unconditioned Response (UR) An automatic reaction elicited by a stimulus.

Unconditioned Stimulus (US) Any stimulus that elicits an automatic or reflexive reaction in an individual; it does not have to be learned in the present situation.

Unconscious In Freudian terminology, a concept (not a place) of the mind. The unconscious encompasses certain inborn impulses that never rise into consciousness (awareness) as well as memories and wishes that have been repressed. The chief aim of psychoanalytic therapy is to free repressed material from the unconscious in order to make it susceptible to conscious thought and direction. Behaviorists describe the unconscious as an inability to verbalize. *See* Repression.

Undifferentiated Schizophrenia Type of schizophrenia that does not fit into any particular category, or fits into more than one category.

Validity The extent to which a test actually measures what it is designed to measure.

Variability In statistics, measures of variability communicate how spread out the scores are; the tendency to vary the response to a stimulus, particularly if the response fails to help in adaptation.

Variable Any property of a person, object, or event that can change or take on more than one mathematical value.

Wechsler Adult Intelligence Scale (WAIS) An individually administered test designed to measure adults' intelligence, devised by David Wechsler. The WAIS consists of eleven subtests, of which six measure verbal and five measure performance aspects of intelligence. *See* Wechsler Intelligence Scale for Children.

Wechsler Intelligence Scale for Children (WISC) Similar to the Wechsler Adult Intelligence Scale, except that it is designed for people under fifteen. Wechsler tests can determine strong and weak areas of overall intelligence. *See* Wechsler Adult Intelligence Scale (WAIS).

Withdrawal Social or emotional detachment; the removal of oneself from a painful or frustrating situation.

Yerkes-Dodson Law Prediction that the optimum motivation level decreases as the difficulty level of a task increases.

Source for the Glossary:
The majority of terms in this glossary are reprinted from *The Study of Psychology*, Joseph Rubinstein. © by The Dushkin Publishing Group, Inc., Guilford, CT 06437.

The remaining terms were developed by the Annual Editions staff.

Index

abortion, 181, 184
academic skills, day care and, 82–85
addiction theories, substance abuse and, 211–216
adrenaline, 218, 219
adrenocorticotropin (ACTH), 219, 220
Agape love style, 142
aggression, 153; self-esteem and, 17–19
aging: memory and, 110–112; sex and, 183
alcohol abuse, effect of prenatal, 76–81
alien abductions, repressed memories and, 95
altruism, 53
Alzheimer's disease, 46–47, 58, 59–60, 67, 110–112; decreases in memory during aging and, 110–112
amygdala, 64–67, 68, 70, 119, 216; fear and, 64–67
amyotrophic lateral sclerosis, 43
anger, 70, 119–120; heart disease and, 133–137
antidepressant drugs, 198–202
anxiety, 64, 68–69, 70, 223; guided imagery and, 29–30; panic attacks and, 188–193
apologies, importance of, 138–140
Arcus, Doreen, 127, 128, 131
Aristotle, 119
ATP, 219
avocados, 167

Bank, Stephen, 155, 156
bed nucleus of the stria terminalis (BNST), 130
behavior therapy, for panic attacks, 189–193
behaviorism, 8, 12–14
Belsky, Jay, 86, 87, 89, 90, 92
Benson, Herbert, 72
biofeedback, 221–222
bipolar disorder, 206
birth-order effects, 55–56
birthweight, low, and prenatal substance abuse, 77–78
blacks: sexual activity and teenage, 102–104; violent crime and, 164
"blood," folk concept of, and race, 167
Bowling Park Elementary School, 100–101
brain, 57–60, 130; addiction theories and, 211–216; gender differences in, 61–63; genetic vs. environmental influences on, 42–47; happiness and, 68–70; memory and aging of, 110–112; panic and, 153
Brass, Lawrence, 219–220
Brazil, race in, 168
bulimia, 193–194
Bush, George, 99
Bushmen, 166

C. elegans, 43
Campbell, Matthew, 152, 153
Carter, Jimmy, 121
Cataldo, Michael F., 213, 215
catastrophic thinking, panic attacks and, 188–189
catecholamines, 120
cell death, 43, 44, 58–59
cerebellum, 119
cerebral cortex, 66
Chagnon, Napoleon A., 54, 177

Chance, Paul, on rewards, 31–35
change, possibility of, 188–195
Childers, Steven, 211, 212, 214, 216
childlessness, 184–185
children: day care and, 82–85; effect of prenatal substance abuse of, 76–81; gender bias in education and, 97–99; media violence and, 170–176; sexual abuse of, 23–24, 93–96; sibling relationships and, 155–159
Chomsky, Noam A., 53–54
Civilization and Its Discontents (Freud), 179
Clark, David, 114, 189–191
cleansing breath, stress and, 222
clinical depression, 205
Clinton, Bill, 113, 121
cognitive psychology, 121
cognitive therapy, for panic attacks, 189–193
cognitivism, 8–9
cohabitation, 181, 184
Comer, James P., 101
computers, cybertherapy and, 203–204
Comstock, George, 171, 173
conditioning, 8, 175
conscience, apologies and, 139
"contextual" conditioning, 130
corpus callosum, 62
corticotropin releasing factor (CRF), 130
cortisol, 218, 219, 223, 224
Cosmides, Leda, 52, 53, 55, 178
CoZi school, 101
Crews, Frederick, 24
Crick, Francis, 9
crime, family and violent, 162–164
criminal justice, media violence and, 175–176
cybertherapy, 203–204
cyclical bi-directional model, media violence and, 173

Damasio, Antonio, 119
Darwinists, social, 51–56
Davidson, Richard, 70
Davis, Michael, 65, 66, 67
day care, positive effects of, 82–85
daydreams, 29–30
de Klerk, F. W., 139–140
delayed gratification, 118, 122
depression, 59, 68–69, 93, 189, 194–195, 205–210; suicide and, 113–115
Derks, Peter, 225
Descartes, René, 8, 119
developmental psychology, 8
dieting, change and, 193–194
discipline, positive, 32, 33–34
disgust, 119
divorce, 181, 184
DNA (deoxyribonucleic acid), 42, 48, 49, 50
domestic violence, 150–154
domino theory, alcoholism and, 212–213
dopamine, 60, 214, 216, 218
double-blind studies, 200–201
dreams, 7
drug abuse, effect of prenatal, 76–81
Dunn, Judy, 156, 157
Durkheim, Émile, 113–114
dysthymia, 205, 208

eating disorders, 122

education, 46–47, 100–101; gender biases in, 89–91
Einstein, Albert, 29
Ekman, Paul, 70
electroencephalography, 221, 222
electromyography (EMG), 221–222
Emerson, Ralph Waldo, 29, 30
empathy, 82, 121, 138
endorphins, 213, 214
environment, brain and, 44–47
ephinephrine, 218, 219
Epstein, Robert, 221, 222
Erikson, Erik, 38
Eron, Leonard, 174–175
Eros love style, 142
evil, 12
evolutionary psychology, 119, 177–180
excitotoxicity, 59
exercise: depression and, 205–206; stress and, 224
experiments: double-blind, 200–201; placebo effects and, 201–202
extrinsic rewards, 31, 32, 34

family: sexuality and, 181–185; violent crime and, 162–164
fantasy, 29–30
fathers, role of, in child development, 86–92
fear, amygdala and, 64–67
feminism, 96, 179, 182–183
fetal alcohol syndrome (FAS), 78
fictive kinships, 185
fight-or-flight response, 216, 220
First Adulthood, 105–106
Fisher, Helen, 213
Flaming Fifties, 107–108
Flourishing Forties, 106
folk taxonomies, 167
forgiveness, in intimate relationships, 148–149
Foster, Vincent, 113, 205
Freud, Sigmund, 71, 136, 177, 179; criticism of, 22–28
Friedman, Howard, 227
friendship, enduring power of, 123–125

GABA, 45
galvanic skin response (GSR), 221, 222
Ganaway, George, 94, 96
gangs, 164; self-esteem and, 18
Geffner, Robert, 151, 154
Gelles, Richard, 151, 154
gender bias, in education, 97–99
gender differences, in brain, 61–63
gender, social Darwinism and, 52–53
gene therapy, 46
genetics, 48–50; brain and, 57–58; depression and, 207; love and, 141–143; panic and, 189
George, Mark, 68, 69, 70
glutamate, 59
glutamic acid decarboxylase (GAD), 45, 46
Goleman, Daniel, 118–122
Goodwin, Frederick K., 114, 115
Gottman, John, 147, 148
gratification, delayed, 118, 122
Grunbaum, Adolph, 24–25
gun culture, 175
Gur, Ruben C., 61–62, 63

happiness, 68–70, 225–227
Harlow, Harry, 13, 14
Head Start, 46
health, prayer and, 71–73
heart disease, anger and, 133–137
heaven, 7–8
hell, 7–8
helplessness, learned, 220–221
Hemingway, Ernest, 113
Hernnstein, Richard, 170, 172
Hetherington, E. Mavis, 156, 157
Hill, Craig, 37–38
hippocampus, 70, 72, 130, 216
Holmes, Leonard, 203–204
Holtzworth-Monroe, Amy, 151–152
homosexuality, 50
Horwath, Ewald, 205, 207
hostility, heart disease and, 133–137
Huesmann, L. Rowell, 174–175
Hugh Grant Effect, 131
Human Behavior and Evolution Society (HBES), 51
humanistic psychology, 38
Huntington's disease, 49, 50, 57, 58, 59
hypo-descent, 167
hypothalamic-pituitary axis (HPA), 218, 220
hypothalamus, 72, 130, 218
hypothermia, 223

imagery, stress and, 222
incest, 93, 96
Independence, Missouri, 101
indigenous people, 177, 178
intelligence: emotions and, 118–122; genetics and, 43–44; race and, 168–169
intensity, anxiety and, 192
Internet, 179; cybertherapy on, 203–204
interracial families, 185
intimacy, 144–146
intimate relationships, preventing failures in, 147–149
intrinsic rewards, 32, 34
Israel, shyness in, 129–130

Jacobson, Neil S., 152
Japan, shy children in, 129
jealousy, 53
Johnson, Lyndon, 121
juvenile delinquency, self-esteem and, 18

Kagan, Jerome, 119, 127, 128
Kahn, Michael, 156, 159
Kennedy, John, 121
Kevorkian, Jack, 113, 115
King, Jean, 218, 220, 222
Kinsey, Alfred, 13, 181
Kramer, Peter, 208
Krantz, David, 134–135
Krasnegor, Norman, 62–63
Ku Klux Klan (KKK), 18–19
!Kung San, 177, 179

La Barre, Weston, 6, 7
language, social Darwinists and, 53–54
laughter, 225–226
learned helplessness, 220–221
learning: effect of prenatal substance abuse on, in children, 76–81; rewards of, 31–35
LeDoux, Joseph, 65, 66, 119
Lefcourt, Herbert, 225, 226
Letterman, David, 127
life cycle, stage theories of, 105–109
limbic system, 61–62, 68, 72, 119, 214, 216
Litwin, Dorothy, 203

Locke, John, 8, 115
Loftus, Elizabeth, 94–95
London, Edythe, 215–216
LOT (Life Orientation Test), 228, 229, 230
Lou Gehrig's disease, 43
love: genetic influences on, 141–143; limbic system and, 119
Ludus love style, 142

magnetic resonance imaging. See MRI
Manic love style, 142
Martin, Rod, 225, 226
Maslow, Abraham, interview with, 11–14
Masson, Jeffrey, 23
mate preference studies, 51, 52–53
McHugh, Paul, 93, 96, 118, 119, 122
media: sex and, 181; violence in, 170–176
meditation, 192, 193
memory, 216; aging and, 110–112; repressed, 23–24, 93–96
menopause, 106
men's movement, 183
metamotivation, 13
mind, soul and, 7
Minnesota Multiphasic Personality Inventory, 36
"mismatch theory," technology and, 177–180
Mitchell, Anne, 83–84
Morreall, John, 226
motivation, 32, 33
Mr. Mom, 185
MRI (magnetic resonance imaging), 70
multiple-personality disorder, sexual abuse and, 93–96
Munson, Ronald, 61, 62

natural weight, 193–194
near-death experiences, 6
negligible cause model, media violence and, 171–172
NEO Personality Inventory, 36
nerve growth factor (NFG), 219
Nesse, Randolph M., 51, 52
neuroprotective drugs, 59
neuroticism, personality and, 37
neurotransmitters, 9, 66, 120, 207, 214, 216
NMDA receptor, 59, 66
noncoding DNA, 50
norepinephrine, 207, 208, 214, 218
Norfolk, Virginia, 100–101
nuclear family, 184, 185

Oates, Joyce Carol, 113
obsessive-compulsive disorder (OCD), 216
only children, 159
optimism, 120–121, 228–232
out-of-body experiences, 6, 9
oxytocin, 213

panic attacks, 68, 188–193
Pannen, Donald, 124
paralysis, anxiety as, 192
parenting, shyness and, 128, 132
Parke, Ross, 86, 89, 90, 91, 92
Parkinson's disease, 46
Pavlov, Ivan, 8, 65
peak experience, 11, 13
penis envy, 93
performance-contingent rewards, 33, 34
perimenopause, 106
personality, stability of, 36–39
PET (positron emission topography), 68–70, 189, 215
Piaget, Jean, 8

Pilkonis, Philip, 127, 128
pineal gland, 8
pituitary gland, 218, 219
placebo effect, 72; antidepressant drugs and, 198–199, 201–202
Plath, Sylvia, 205
Plomin, Robert, 157, 158
police officers, domestic violence and, 153–154
pornography, 172
positive thinking, optimism and, 228–232
postmarital society, 181
post-menopausal zest, 106
post-traumatic stress disorder (PTSD), 64–65, 94, 189
poverty, violent crime and, 162–163
practice, rewards and, 31
Pragma love style, 142
prayer: health and, 71–73; substance abuse and, 215
prefrontal cortex, 70
prefrontal lobes, 68
pregnancy: substance abuse during, 76–81; teenage, and negative consequences of sexual activity, 102–104
prenatal substance abuse, effects of, 76–81
preoptic nucleus, 62
primary cause model, media violence and, 171–172
progressive relaxation, 191, 192, 193
prolactin, 219
protocol analysis, 8–9
Provisional Adulthood, 105
Prozac, 60, 198
Prusank, Diane, 123, 124
psyche, 7
PsychNet, of American Psychological Association, 204
psychoanalysis, criticism of, 22–28, 136
psychotherapy, 196–197
punishment: apologies and, 139; as alternative to rewards, 33–34
purgatory, 7

race: physical appearance and, 165–169; violent crime and, 163–164
Rachman, S. J., 188–189
race myth, 172
rational suicide, 113
Rawlins, William, 123, 124
Reagan, Ronald, 121
reason, soul and, 7
reciprocal altruism, 53
regret, apology and, 139
relaxation response, 222
religion: health and, 71–73; sex and, 183; soul and, 6–10
reparation, apology and, 138–140
repressed memories, 93–96
Retzinger, Suzanne, 147–148
reuptake, 214
reward center, in brain, and addiction theory, 211–216
reward(s): contingency, 33; costs of, 31–33; extrinsic, 31–32, 34; intrinsic, 32, 34; performance-contingent, 33; self-respect and, 31–35; success-contingent, 33; task-contingent, 33
Richelson, Elliot, 207, 209
Rip van Winkle study, 174–175
RNA (ribonucleic acid), 42
robust repression, 94
Romanoski, Alan, 206, 207
romantic love, 213

Rorschach test, 14
Rose, Mimi, 153, 154
Rule of Thumb, 150
Rush, A. John, 206, 207, 209

sadness, 68–70
Sage Seventies, 109
Salovey, Peter, 118, 122
same-sex families, 185
satanic rituals, 93, 96
Scheff, Thomas, 147–148
schizophrenia, 50, 60, 67
seasonal affective disorder (SAD), 206
Second Adulthood, 106
secular humanism, 6
self-actualization, 11, 13, 14
self-efficacy, optimism and, 231
self-esteem, perils of boosting, in education, 15–21
Seligman, Martin, 120–121
Serene Sixties, 108–109
serotonin, 66, 114, 115, 153, 207, 208, 214
sexual abuse, repressed memories and, 23–24, 93–96
sexual activity, teenagers and negative consequences of, 102–104
sexual harassment, 182
sexuality, family and, 181–185
sexually transmitted diseases (STDs), negative consequences of teenage sexual activity and, 103–104
shame, in intimate relationships, 148, 149
Shaver, Phillip, 141–143
Shaywitz, Sally and Bennett, 61, 62, 63
Shea, Tracie, 208, 210
Shrink-Link, 203, 204
shyness, 126–132
sibling relationships, 155–159
Simpson, O. J. and Nicole, domestic violence and, 150–154
Singer, Jerome, 29, 30

Singh, Devendra, 51
single-parent families, 184
Skinner, B. F., 32, 33
smoking, effect of, on prenatal development, 76–81
Snidman, Nancy, 127, 130
social Darwinism, 51–56
social skills, day care and, 82–85
sociobiology, 52
Socrates, 6, 7, 13
soul, modern psychological interpretations of, 6–10
source memory, 216
spousal abuse, 150–154
stage theories, of life cycles, 105–109
stepparents, 54–55
Storge love style, 142
streptavidin, 50
stress, 118, 119, 223–224; heart disease and, 133–137; preventing, 221–222; sensitization, 217–221
stretching, stress and, 222
stroke, 59
Styron, William, and depression, 205, 206
substance abuse: addiction theories and, 211–216; effects of, on prenatal development, 76–81
success-contingent rewards, 33
suicide, 113–115, 206
Sulloway, Frank J., 55–56, 157
Swann, William, 37–38
synapses, 66
synergy, 11, 14

Targ, Elisabeth, 71
task-contingent rewards, 33
technology: communication and, 131–132; evolutionary psychology and, 179–180
teenagers: negative consequences of sexual activity and, 102–104; shyness and, 128, 130

temperament, stability of, 36–39
temporal lobe, 68, 70
Terman, Louis, 227
"Termites," 227
Thorndike, E. L., 31
Tooby, John, 52, 53, 55, 178
transcription factors, 42, 43
21st Century model, 101
twin studies, 50; on genetic influence on love styles, 141–143
Type A behavior, 134, 205, 213

UFO abductions, repressed memories of, 95
Unabomber, 177, 178
unipolar depression, 205. See also depression

violence: domestic, 150–154; media and, 170–176; self-esteem and, 17–19
violent crime, family and, 162–164
virtual reality, sex and, 183–184
visualization, 93

Waardenburg's syndrome, 49
Walker, Lenore, 151, 152
Waller, Niels, 141–143
Watson, John, 8
white flu, 212
Whitehead, Alfred North, 13, 14
will: soul and, 7; work of, 119
Wilson, James I., 170, 172
Witelson, Sandra, 62, 64
withdrawal, addiction and, 213, 215
workplace, women in the, 185

Yanomamö people, 54, 177

Zigler, Edward, 101
Zimbardo, Philip, 126, 127, 129, 130, 132
Zisook, Sidney, 207, 210

Credits/Acknowledgments

Cover design by Charles Vitelli

1. Becoming a Person
Facing overview—Photo by Cheryl Greenleaf.

2. Determinants of Behavior
Facing overview—Dushkin Publishing Group illustration by Tom Goddard.

3. Problems Influencing Personal Growth
Facing overview—Stock Boston photo by Peter Vandermark.

4. Relating to Others
Facing overview—Photo by Louis P. Raucci.

5. Dynamics of Personal Adjustment
Facing overview—United Nations photo.

6. Enhancing Human Adjustment
Facing overview—United Nations photo by Margot Granitsas.
209—Photo by Louis P. Raucci.

*PHOTOCOPY THIS PAGE!!!**

ANNUAL EDITIONS ARTICLE REVIEW FORM

■ NAME: _____ DATE: _____

■ TITLE AND NUMBER OF ARTICLE: _____

■ BRIEFLY STATE THE MAIN IDEA OF THIS ARTICLE: _____
_____

■ LIST THREE IMPORTANT FACTS THAT THE AUTHOR USES TO SUPPORT THE MAIN IDEA:
_____
_____
_____
_____

■ WHAT INFORMATION OR IDEAS DISCUSSED IN THIS ARTICLE ARE ALSO DISCUSSED IN YOUR TEXTBOOK OR OTHER READINGS THAT YOU HAVE DONE? LIST THE TEXTBOOK CHAPTERS AND PAGE NUMBERS:
_____
_____
_____
_____
_____

■ LIST ANY EXAMPLES OF BIAS OR FAULTY REASONING THAT YOU FOUND IN THE ARTICLE:
_____
_____
_____
_____

■ LIST ANY NEW TERMS/CONCEPTS THAT WERE DISCUSSED IN THE ARTICLE, AND WRITE A SHORT DEFINITION:
_____
_____
_____
_____

*Your instructor may require you to use this ANNUAL EDITIONS Article Review Form in any number of ways: for articles that are assigned, for extra credit, as a tool to assist in developing assigned papers, or simply for your own reference. Even if it is not required, we encourage you to photocopy and use this page; you will find that reflecting on the articles will greatly enhance the information from your text.

We Want Your Advice

ANNUAL EDITIONS revisions depend on two major opinion sources: one is our Advisory Board, listed in the front of this volume, which works with us in scanning the thousands of articles published in the public press each year; the other is you—the person actually using the book. Please help us and the users of the next edition by completing the prepaid article rating form on this page and returning it to us. Thank you for your help!

ANNUAL EDITIONS: PERSONAL GROWTH AND BEHAVIOR 97/98
Article Rating Form

Here is an opportunity for you to have direct input into the next revision of this volume. We would like you to rate each of the 49 articles listed below, using the following scale:

1. Excellent: should definitely be retained
2. Above average: should probably be retained
3. Below average: should probably be deleted
4. Poor: should definitely be deleted

Your ratings will play a vital part in the next revision. So please mail this prepaid form to us just as soon as you complete it.
Thanks for your help!

Rating	Article	Rating	Article
	1. The 'Soul': Modern Psychological Interpretations		25. The Mystery of Suicide
	2. The Last Interview of Abraham Maslow		26. The EQ Factor
	3. Should Schools Try to Boost Self-Esteem?		27. The Enduring Power of Friendship
	4. The Shrink Is In		28. Are You Shy?
	5. How Useful Is Fantasy?		29. Hotheads and Heart Attacks
	6. Rewards of Learning		30. Go Ahead, Say You're Sorry
	7. The Stability of Personality: Observations and Evaluations		31. The Heart and the Helix
	8. Nature, Nurture, Brains, and Behavior		32. Back Off!
	9. Unraveling the Mystery of Life		33. Preventing Failure in Intimate Relationships
	10. The New Social Darwinists		34. Patterns of Abuse
	11. Revealing the Brain's Secrets		35. The Secret World of Siblings
	12. Man's World, Woman's World? Brain Studies Point to Differences		36. Disintegration of the Family Is the Real Root Cause of Violent Crime
	13. Kernel of Fear		37. Mixed Blood
	14. The Brain Manages Happiness and Sadness in Different Centers		38. Media, Violence, Youth, and Society
	15. Faith & Healing		39. The Evolution of Despair
	16. Clipped Wings		40. Psychotrends: Taking Stock of Tomorrow's Family and Sexuality
	17. How Kids Benefit from Child Care		41. What You Can Change and What You Cannot Change
	18. Fathers' Time		42. Frontiers of Psychotherapy
	19. Lies of the Mind		43. Prescriptions for Happiness?
	20. Why Schools Must Tell Girls: 'You're Smart, You Can Do It'		44. Upset? Try Cybertherapy
	21. It Takes a School		45. Defeating Depression
	22. Helping Teenagers Avoid Negative Consequences of Sexual Activity		46. Addiction: A Whole New View
	23. New Passages		47. Stress: It's Worse than You Think
	24. Is It Normal Aging—Or Alzheimer's?		48. The New Frontiers of Happiness . . . Happily Ever Laughter
			49. On the Power of Positive Thinking: The Benefits of Being Optimistic

(Continued on next page)

ABOUT YOU

Name _____ Date _____

Are you a teacher? ❏ Or a student? ❏

Your school name _____

Department _____

Address _____

City _____ State _____ Zip _____

School telephone # _____

YOUR COMMENTS ARE IMPORTANT TO US!

Please fill in the following information:

For which course did you use this book? _____

Did you use a text with this *ANNUAL EDITION*? ❏ yes ❏ no

What was the title of the text? _____

What are your general reactions to the *Annual Editions* concept?

Have you read any particular articles recently that you think should be included in the next edition?

Are there any articles you feel should be replaced in the next edition? Why?

Are there other areas of study that you feel would utilize an *ANNUAL EDITION*?

May we contact you for editorial input?

May we quote your comments?

ANNUAL EDITIONS: PERSONAL GROWTH AND BEHAVIOR 97/98

BUSINESS REPLY MAIL
First Class   Permit No. 84   Guilford, CT

Postage will be paid by addressee

**Dushkin Publishing Group/
Brown & Benchmark Publishers**
Sluice Dock
Guilford, Connecticut 06437

No Postage Necessary if Mailed in the United States